Endoscopic Diagnosis of Superficial Gastric Cancer for ESD

Tsuneo Oyama
Editor

Endoscopic Diagnosis of Superficial Gastric Cancer for ESD

Springer

Editor
Tsuneo Oyama
Saku Central Hospital
Saku, Nagano
Japan

ISBN 978-4-431-56630-4 ISBN 978-4-431-54469-2 (eBook)
DOI 10.1007/978-4-431-54469-2

Softcover reprint of the hardcover 1st edition 2016
Original Japanese edition published by Nankodo Co., Ltd, Tokyo, 2010

Printed on acid-free paper

This Springer imprint is published by Springer Nature
The registered company is Springer Japan KK

Contents

Part III Practices

Contributors

Keita Funakawa Department of Gastroenterology, Kagoshima City Hospital, Kagoshima-shi, Kagoshima, Japan

Kinichi Hotta Division of Endoscopy, Shizuoka Cancer Center, Sunto-gun, Shizuoka, Japan

Yoko Kitamura Department of Gastroenterology, Center for Digestive and Liver Diseases, Nara City Hospital, Nara-Shi, Nara, Japan

Kenji Kunieda Division of Oncology, Saku Central Hospital, Saku, Nagano, Japan

Tadashi Miike Department of Gastroenterology and Hematology (Internal Medicine), Faculty of Medicine of University of Miyazaki, Miyazaki, Japan

Shuko Morita Department of Gastroenterology, Kobe City Medical Center General Hospital, Kobe-city, Hyogo, Japan

Yuji Nishiyama Department of Internal Medicine, Watanabe Hospital, Kurashiki, Okayama, Japan

Koichi Okamoto Department of Gastroenterology and Oncology, University of Tokushima, Tokushima, Japan

Tsuneo Oyama Division of Endoscopy, Saku Central Hospital, Saku, Nagano, Japan

Ayako Seki Department of Gastroenterology, Nagano Municipal Hospital, Nagano-shi, Nagano, Japan

Kotaro Shibagaki Department of Endoscopy, Shimane University, Faculty of Medicine, Matsue, Shimane, Japan

Tomoaki Shinohara Department of Gastroenterology, Saku Central Hospital, Saku, Nagano, Japan

Akiko Takahashi Division of Endoscopy, Saku Central Hospital, Saku, Nagano, Japan

Masaki Tanaka Division of Endoscopy, Shizuoka Cancer Center, Sunto-gun, Shizuoka, Japan

Tokuma Tanuma Department of Gastroenterology, Teine Keijinkai Hospital, Sapporo, Hokkaido, Japan

Akihisa Tomori Department of Gastroenterology, Saku Central Hospital, Saku, Nagano, Japan

Tetsuro Yamazato Department of Gastroenterology, Tokyo Metropolitan Cancer Detection Center, Fuchu, Tokyo, Japan

Kou Yoshida Department of Internal Medicine, Obihiro Kosei General Hospital, Obihiro, Hokkaido, Japan

Shigetaka Yoshinga Endoscopy Division, National Cancer Center Hospital, Chuo-ku, Tokyo, Japan

Part I

Basic Understandings of Diagnostic Endoscopy of ESD for Gastric Cancer

Indications for Endoscopic Submucosal Dissection of Early Gastric Cancer

1

Kinichi Hotta

Endoscopic mucosal resection (EMR) of early gastric cancer (EGC) has developed in the early 1980s, such as strip biopsy method [1], endoscopic resection with local injection of hypersaline-epinephrine (ERHSE) method [2], endoscopic mucosal resection with a cap-fitted panendoscope (EMRC) method [3], endoscopic aspiration mucosectomy (EAM) method [4], and EMR with a ligating device (EMR-L) method [5]. These methods are classified into conventional EMR methods. These are simple and safe methods, but lesion size which can be resected in en bloc fashion is limited.

Endoscopic submucosal dissection (ESD), which is characterized by mucosal incision surrounding a lesion followed by submucosal dissection, has developed in the late 1990s. This new type of methods such as IT knife method [6], hook knife method [7], and flex knife method [8] resulted in extending indications for safe and large en bloc resection.

Indications for EMR/ESD of EGC were proposed by the Japanese gastric cancer treatment guidelines of the Japanese Gastric Cancer Association (JGCA) [9] based on published analysis of a large clinicopathological database combining surgical cases of EGCs obtained from two large Japanese cancer centers [10].

1.1 Absolute Indication for EMR/ESD (Endoscopic Resection as a Standard Treatment)

The principle behind indications for EMR/ESD is EGC which has negligible risk of lymph node metastasis and is suitable for en bloc resection. Therefore, the absolute indication for EMR/ESD is defined as an EGC which is a differentiated-type adenocarcinoma without ulcerative findings (UL(−)) and of which the depth of invasion is clinically diagnosed as T1a and the diameter is ≦2 cm. The necessary conditions for curative resection are lesions which can be resected en bloc, with tumor size ≦2 cm, adenocarcinoma of differentiated type, pT1a, horizontal/vertical margins negative, and without lymphatic or vascular involvements (Table 1.1).

Table 1.1 Endoscopic mucosal resection (EMR) indication

Principles of indication	Tumor with little possibility of lymph node metastasis, which can be removed en bloc according to its location and size
Criteria details	Macroscopic mucosal cancer (cM) of differentiated type (pap, tub1, tub2) less than 2 cm in diameter
	No ulceration or scar in cases of depressed type, irrespective of macroscopic type

1.2 Expanded Indications for ESD (Endoscopic Resection as an Investigative Treatment)

A previous report containing analyses of long-term prognosis of large number of patients with EGCs demonstrated that the 5-year cancer-specific survival rates of EGC limited to the mucosa or the submucosa were 99 % and 96 %, respectively [11]. Therefore, allowable risks of lymph node metastases for ESD of EGCs which are limited to the mucosa or the submucosa are less than 1 % and 4 %, respectively. The gastric cancer treatment guidelines of the JGCA [9] proposed three categories for expanded criteria for ESD: (1) intramucosal differentiated-type cancers (cT1a) >2 cm without ulcer findings, (2) intramucosal differentiated-type cancers (cT1a) ≦3 cm with ulcer findings, and (3) intramucosal undifferentiated-type cancers (cT1a) ≦2 cm without ulcer

K. Hotta (✉)
Division of Endoscopy, Shizuoka Cancer Center, 1007 Shimonagakubo, Nagaizumi-cho, Sunto-gun, Shizuoka 411-8777, Japan
e-mail: k.hotta@scchr.jp

T. Oyama (ed.), *Endoscopic Diagnosis of Superficial Gastric Cancer for ESD*, DOI 10.1007/978-4-431-54469-2_1

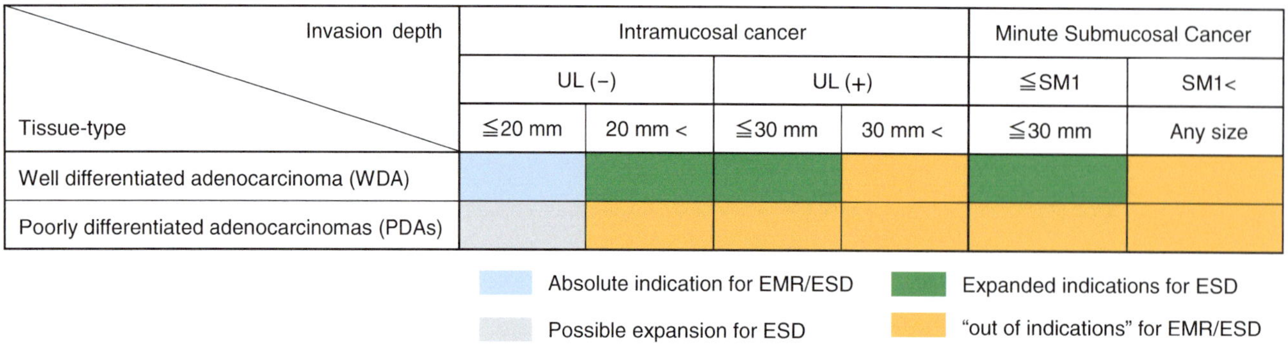

Fig. 1.1 Absolute indication for EMR/ESD and expanded indications for ESD

Table 1.2 Criteria for expansion of local treatment, derived from our results

Criteria	Intramucosal cancer	Intramucosal cancer	Minute submucosal penetration (SM1)	Undifferentiated intramucosal cancer
	Differentiated adenocarcinoma	Differentiated adenocarcinoma	Differentiated adenocarcinoma	
	No lymphovascular invasion	No lymphovascular invasion	No lymphovascular invasion	No lymphovascular invasion
	Irrespective of ulcer findings	Without ulcer findings		Without ulcer findings
	Tumor less than 3 cm in size	Irrespective of tumor size	Tumor less than 3 cm in size	Tumor less than 3 cm in size
Incidence	1/1230 (0 %)	0/929 (0 %)	0/145 (0 %)	0/141 (0 %)
95 % CI	0–0.3 %	0–0.4 %	0–2.5 %	0–2.6 %

Gitoda et al.: Gastric Cancer 3: 219–225, 2000

findings. The necessary conditions for curative resection are defined as below: (a) en bloc, tumor size >2 cm, differentiated type, pT1a, and without ulcer findings; (b) en bloc, tumor size ≦3 cm, differentiated type, pT1a, and with ulcer findings; (c) en bloc, tumor size ≦2 cm, undifferentiated type, pT1a, and without ulcer findings; and (d) en bloc, tumor size ≦3 cm, differentiated type, and pT1b (SM < 500 μm). Horizontal/vertical margins negative and no lymphatic or vascular involvements are common conditions in all categories (Fig. 1.1, Table 1.2).

Evidences concerning mixed histological types with differentiated- and undifferentiated-type gastric cancers are still insufficient. Therefore, conditions as below are considered as indications for additional surgical resection with lymph node dissection: (i) areas of undifferentiated-type carcinoma that exceed 2 cm in (a) above, (ii) any components of undifferentiated-type carcinoma in (b) above, and (iii) undifferentiated-type components in the submucosal invasion in (d) above.

1.3 Lesions Which Are "Out of Indications" for EMR/ESD (Endoscopic Resection in Special Situations)

Lesions which do not fulfill the absolute indication or the expanded indications are considered as "out-of-indication" lesions. Also, lesions which show lymphovascular invasions by histopathological evaluation are categorized as "out-of-indication" lesions.

"Out-of-indication" lesions, in general, are estimated to have risks of lymphatic invasion of at least 5–10 % and therefore are recommended for surgical resection by the gastric cancer treatment guidelines of the JGCA [9]. However, endoscopic resection may be considered as an alternative treatment in situations when surgical treatments are difficult because of old age or higher risk of complications.

1.4 Curative and Non-curative Resections

Curability status must be determined finally by pathological evaluations of endoscopically resected specimens. Pathologically speaking, complete curability must fulfill all of the abovementioned conditions of expanded indications as well as confirmation of cancer-free cut ends and absence of lymphatic and vascular invasions. Since divided resections make evaluation for cut ends, as well as depth of invasion, and lymphovascular involvements very difficult, en bloc resections are desirable. Even when pre-resection diagnosis based on biopsy is WDA, resection is non-curative if the final pathological diagnosis is undifferentiated adenocarcinomas. When ulcer scars are not detectible endoscopically but confirmed histologically, curability status must be considered as in ulcer-accompanied lesions.

1.5 Future Perspectives of ESD

There are a few reports about long-term prognosis about expanded criteria for ESD. Gotoda et al. reported that the 5-year overall survival of the expanded criteria group ($n = 625$) was 93.4 % and there was no significant difference with guideline criteria group ($n = 635$, 92.4 %) [12]. Multicenter prospective studies of expanded criteria for ESD were ongoing and final results were desired for more reliable evidences [13, 14]. The behavior of mixed-type EGCs is unclear. Takizawa et al. reported that a mixed type with a predominantly undifferentiated component should be managed the same way as a differentiated type. Further investigation is required to manage mixed-type EGCs [15].

References

1. Tada M, Shimada M, Murakami F, et al. Development of strip-off biopsy. Gastroenterol Endosc (in Japanese with English abstract). 1984;26:833–9.
2. Hirao M, Kobayashi T, Hase Y, et al. Endoscopic resection of early gastric carcinomas and other gastric lesions with malignant potential. Gastroenterol Endosc (in Japanese with English abstract). 1983;25:1942–53.
3. Inoue H, Takeshita K, Hori H, et al. Endoscopic mucosal resection with a cap-fitted panendoscope for esophagus, stomach and colon mucosal lesions. Gastrointest Endosc. 1993;39:58–62.
4. Torii A, Sakai M, Kajiyajma T, et al. Endoscopic aspiration mucosectomy as curative endoscopic surgery; analysis of 24 cases of early gastric cancer. Gastrointest Endosc. 1995;42:475–9.
5. Suzuki H, Masuda K, Fujisaki J, et al. Endoscopic treatment of gastrointestinal cancers–indication and limitation. Nihon Rinsho (in Japanese with English abstract). 1993;5:1215–9.
6. Hosokawa K, Yoshida S. Recent advances in endoscopic mucosal resection for early gastric cancer. Jpn J Cancer Chemother (in Japanese with English abstract). 1998;25:483.
7. Oyama T, Kikuchi Y. Aggressive endoscopic mucosal resection in the upper GI tract-Hook knife EMR method. Minim Invasive Ther Allied Technol. 2002;11:291–5.
8. Yahagi N, Fujishiro M, Kakushima N, et al. Merits and demerits of endoscopic submucosal dissection using a flex knife. Stomach and Intestine (in Japanese with English abstract). 2004;39:39–43.
9. Japanese Gastric Cancer Association. Japanese gastric cancer treatment guidelines 2010 (ver.3). Gastric Cancer. 2011;14:113–23.
10. Gotoda T, Yanagisawa A, Sasako M, et al. Incidence of lymph node metastasis from early gastric cancer: estimation with a large number of cases at two large centers. Gastric Cancer. 2000;3:219–25.
11. Sasako M, Kinoshita T, Maruyama K. Prognosis of early gastric cancer. Stomach and Intestine (in Japanese with English abstract). 1993;28:139–46.
12. Gotoda T, Iwasaki M, Kusano C, et al. Endoscopic resection of early gastric cancer treated by guideline and expanded National Cancer Centre criteria. Br J Surg. 2010;97:868–71.
13. Kurokawa Y, Hasuike N, Ono H, et al. A phase II trial of endoscopic submucosal dissection for mucosal gastric cancer: Japan Clinical Oncology Group Study JCOG0607. Jpn J Clin Oncol. 2009;39:464–6.
14. Takizawa K, Takashima A, Kimura A, et al. A phase II clinical trial of endoscopic submucosal dissection for early gastric cancer of undifferentiated type: Japan Clinical Oncology Group study JCOG1009/1010. Jpn J Clin Oncol. 2013;43:87–91.
15. Takizawa K, Ono H, Kakushima N, et al. Risk of lymph node metastases from intramucosal gastric cancer in relation to histological types: how to manage the mixed histological type for endoscopic submucosal dissection. Gastric Cancer. 2013;16:531–6.

Basic Technique of Endoscopic Diagnosis for Superficial Gastric Adenocarcinoma

2

Tsuneo Oyama

2.1 Basic Structure of Gastric Mucosa

There are three types of glands in the stomach. They are cardiac, fundic, and pyloric glands. Cardiac glands exist in the very narrow area just anal to the squamocolumnar junction (SCJ). Fundic and pyloric glands exist in the gastric body and the antrum, respectively. Since there are folds in the fundic gland areas (Fig. 2.1), the background gland type could be diagnosed by the endoscopic findings. Sometimes, gastric mucosa is replaced by intestinal metaplasia (IM) when a patient has *Helicobacter pylori* infection. The gastric mucosa becomes thinner with progression of atrophic gastritis making submucosal vessels visible (Fig. 2.2). IM is observed as white small elevations because of rich mucus contained within (Fig. 2.3).

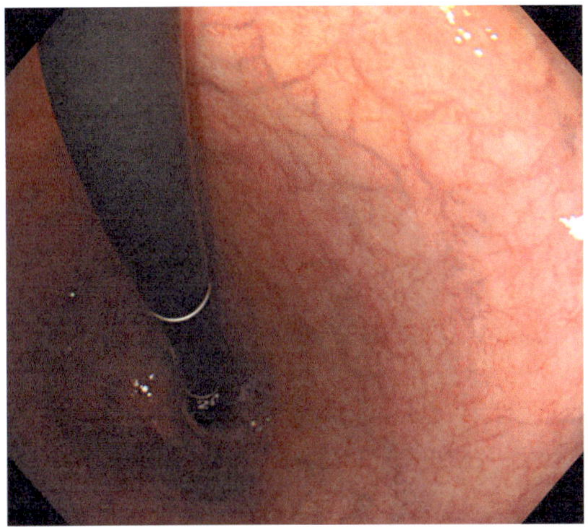

Fig. 2.2 Atrophic gastritis

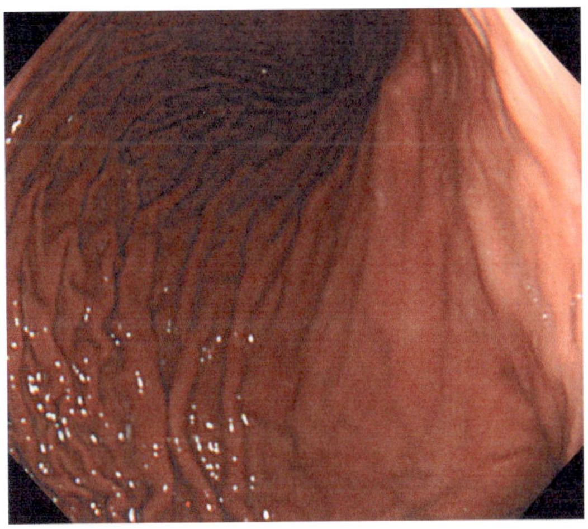

Fig. 2.1 Fundic gland area

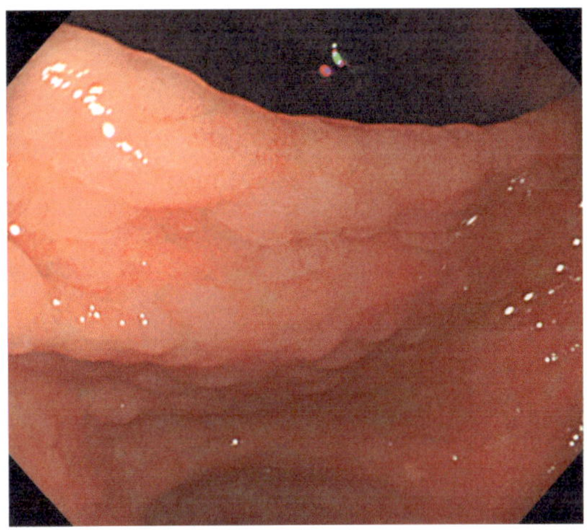

Fig. 2.3 Intestinal metaplasia

T. Oyama (✉)
Division of Endoscopy, Saku Central Hospital, 197 Usuda, Saku, Nagano 384-0301, Japan
e-mail: oyama@coral.ocn.ne.jp

T. Oyama (ed.), *Endoscopic Diagnosis of Superficial Gastric Cancer for ESD*, DOI 10.1007/978-4-431-54469-2_2

2.2 Basic Structure of Gastric Adenocarcinoma

According to the Japanese guidelines for gastric cancer, the histology of gastric cancer is classified into well- or poorly differentiated adenocarcinoma.

2.2.1 Basic Structure of Well-Differentiated Adenocarcinoma (WDA)

WDAs have glandular structures. Therefore, the color of WDAs often appears reddish because of many vessels noted within the parenchyma. The macroscopic type of WDA varies from 0-I to 0-III. Often, the background mucosa contains IM which appears pale compared to WDA. WDA replaces the full mucosal layer of the surrounding glands and appears at the surface of mucosa. Therefore, the lateral extension becomes well demarcated (Fig. 2.4 arrow).

2.2.2 Basic Structure of Poorly Differentiated Adenocarcinoma (PDA)

PDAs do not have glandular structures. The cancer cells are scattered, spreading laterally at the glandular neck level (Fig. 2.5) in the parenchyma resulting in unclear margins. The number of vessels is fewer than that of WDA because the cancer cells spread through the parenchyma without vascular neogenesis. Therefore, the color is basically pale. However, when PDAs result in ischemic erosions, the color may appear reddish. Sometimes PDAs spread as broadly depressed lesions, leaving some areas of nonneoplastic mucosa as slightly elevated islands within PDA.

Typical macroscopic type of PDA is a well-demarcated 0-IIc cancer in the fundic gland area. However, when PDA occurs in the background of atrophic gastritis, it may become a 0-IIb cancer with very unclear margin.

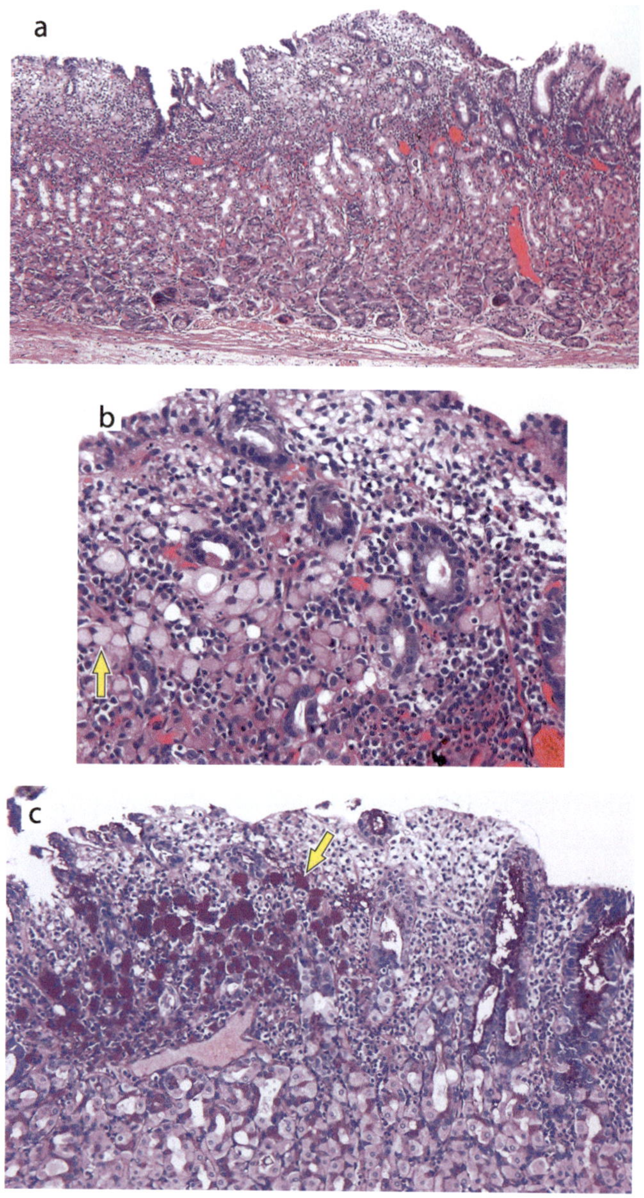

Fig. 2.5 PDA. (**a**) HE stain. (**b**) HE stain *arrow*: signet carcinoma. (**c**) ABPAS stain *arrow*: signet ring carcinoma

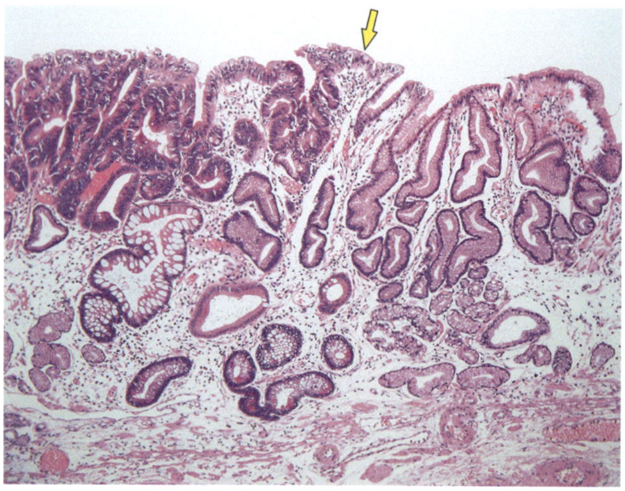

Fig. 2.4 Well-differentiated adenocarcinoma

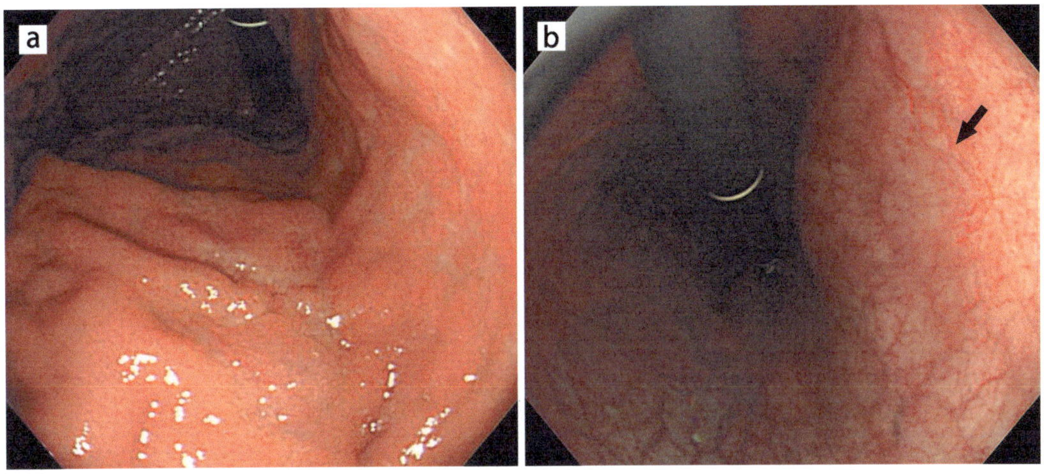

Fig. 2.6 (**a**) PDA (well-demarcated margin in fundic gland area). (**b**) PDA (unclear margin in atrophic area)

2.2.3 What Makes Cancer Borders Well Demarcated or Unclear?

PDAs spread laterally through the parenchyma of the nonneoplastic glands and mainly exist in the mid-mucosal layer. The surface is basically covered by nonneoplastic glands. Therefore, the lateral extension becomes obscure. On the other hand, WDAs make glands which spread laterally replacing surrounding nonneoplastic glands. The cancerous glands are exposed at the surface and the lateral extension becomes well demarcated.

The parenchyma of fundic glands is thinner than that of IM. Therefore, when a PDA exists in the fundic gland area, it is difficult to spread laterally through the parenchyma. Then, the PDA forms a mass within the mucosal layer, trying to expand laterally. Therefore, PDAs surrounded by fundic glands show well-demarcated 0-IIc lesions (Fig. 2.6a).

On the other hand, the parenchyma of IM is loose. Therefore, when PDAs exist within IM, the cancer cells can easily scatter laterally. Furthermore, the cancer cells remain in the mid-mucosal layer unexposed on the surface, covered by noncancerous glands. The macroscopic type of such lesions is 0-IIb with very unclear borders, making endoscopic diagnosis extremely difficult (Fig. 2.6b).

2.3 Are There *Helicobacter pylori*?

Endoscopic diagnosis of the infection of *Helicobacter pylori* (HP) is important because HP is an important risk factor of gastric cancer. Gastric folds disappear after HP infection because of atrophic gastritis. Therefore, when gastric folds are observed in the lesser curvature of gastric body, the likelihood of HP infection is low (Fig. 2.7a). And, regular arrangement of collecting venues (RAC) [1] is also an important finding because RAC disappears after HP infection (Fig. 2.7b) [1].

On the other hand, the endoscopic findings suggesting HP infection are thick mucus and atrophic gastritis. The endoscopic findings characteristic of atrophic gastritis are disappearing of folds and thinning mucosa with visible submucosal vessels (Fig. 2.8a). And, sometimes atrophy occurs in patches resulting in mixtures of reddish and whitish mucosal areas (Fig. 2.8b).

When you insert a scope into the stomach, the upper body is first observed. If gastric folds without thick mucus are observed in the lesser curvature of the gastric body, HP is likely negative (Fig. 2.9a). On the other hand, if gastric mucosa is covered with thick mucus and no folds are observed, HP is present (Fig. 2.9b). Endoscopic diagnosis

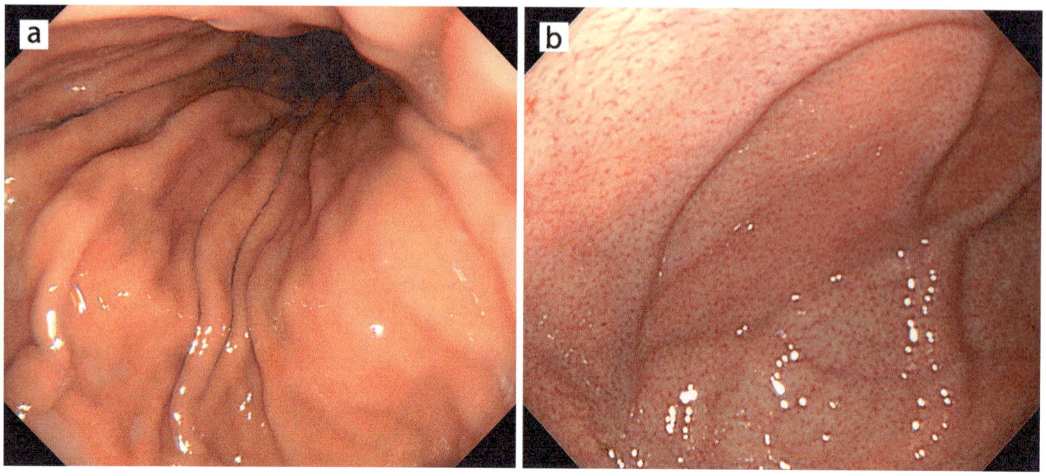

Fig. 2.7 Endoscopic view of normal stomach

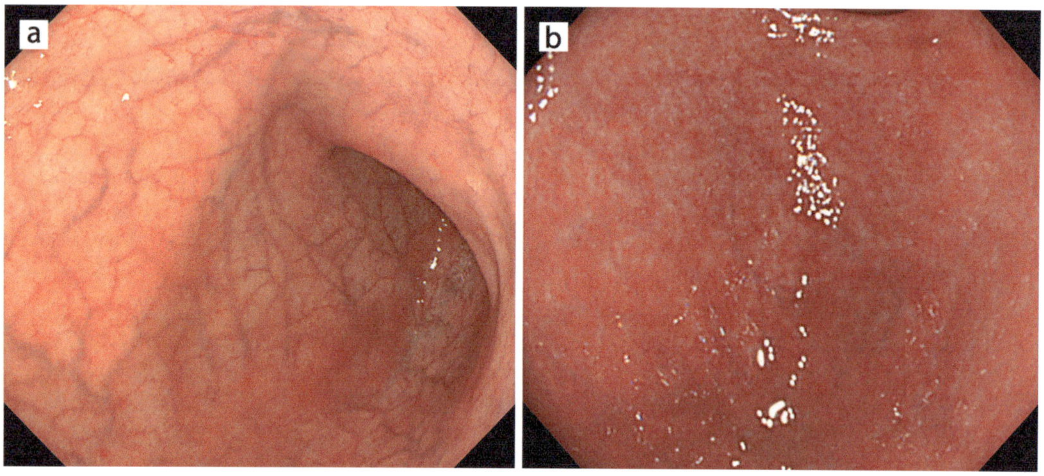

Fig. 2.8 Endoscopic view of *Helicobacter pylori*-infected stomach

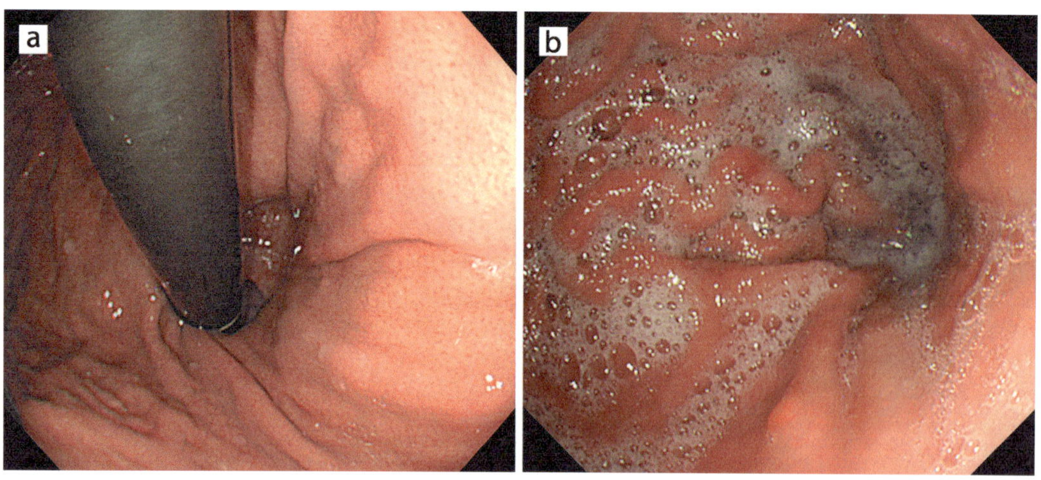

Fig. 2.9 (**a**) *H. pylori* negative: the mucosa was observed clearly without mucin, and RAC pattern was positive. (**b**) *H. pylori* positive: the lesion is covered by thick mucin

of HP infection could be possible just after you insert the scope into the stomach. If HP is present, the risk of gastric cancer is increased. So you must carefully observe for a possible EGC.

2.4 Points for Early Detection by White Light Image

2.4.1 The First Step Is Removal of Mucus

The surface of gastric mucosa is covered by thick mucus, when the patient has HP infection. Therefore, removal of mucus is the essential first step in detection of superficial cancers. Pronase (Kaken Pharmaceutical Co., Ltd., Tokyo) is a medicinal enzymatic preparation effective for removal of mucus. Not only gastric mucosa but also pharyngeal and esophageal walls could be cleaned by this medicinal enzymatic preparation. Pronase diluted by 100 ml of water should be taken orally 10–15 min before examination. If taken in upright position, only the lower portion of the stomach is cleaned. Ideally, the patient should be asked to lie down and roll around several times to apply the enzymatic solution to the entire gastric wall. This will make later removal of mucus easier with injections of water mixed with a small amount of dimethicone syrup.

2.4.2 Protrusions

Protuberant lesions are the easiest lesions to detect for beginners. WDAs and tubular adenomas (TAs) are the main lesions for differential diagnosis. And, hyperplastic polyp, fundic gland polyp, or IM should be ruled out. The key points to observe are color, shape, demarcation, and surface patterns.

2.4.2.1 Color

WDAs, HPs, or inflammation should be considered for red protuberant lesions. Adenomas, fundic gland polyps, IM, or submucosal tumors (SMTs) should be considered for white protuberant lesions. Key points to differentiate among these are surface pattern, demarcation, and background mucosa.

2.4.2.2 Shape

Regularity of shape must be carefully observed. A whitish protuberant lesion is observed at the posterior side of the antrum (Fig. 2.10a). The shape of this pale protrusion is regular and smooth, and its demarcation is unclear. And the lesion is diagnosed as IM (Fig. 2.10b). On the other hand, Fig. 2.13 shows a WDA. While this is also flat and protuberant, the demarcation around this lesion is irregular and sharp. It is important not only to evaluate the general overall shape but also the shape of the demarcation between the lesion and its background mucosa.

2.4.2.3 Demarcation of Rising Border

Generally speaking, superficial neoplasms such as gastric adenocarcinoma or tubular adenoma show a well-demarcated rise at their margins. And inflammatory changes and neoplasms of non-epithelial origins such as gastritis, malignant lymphoma, or SMTs show gradual rise without clear demarcations. Yamada's classification is often used to describe rising patterns.

2.4.2.4 Surface Patterns

Next to be observed are surface patterns. Is the surface flat and smooth or nodular? Are the sizes and shapes of nodules even or variable? Also note if there are depressions in the central areas. It is helpful to apply indigo carmine spray, which makes detailed observation of the surface patterns possible.

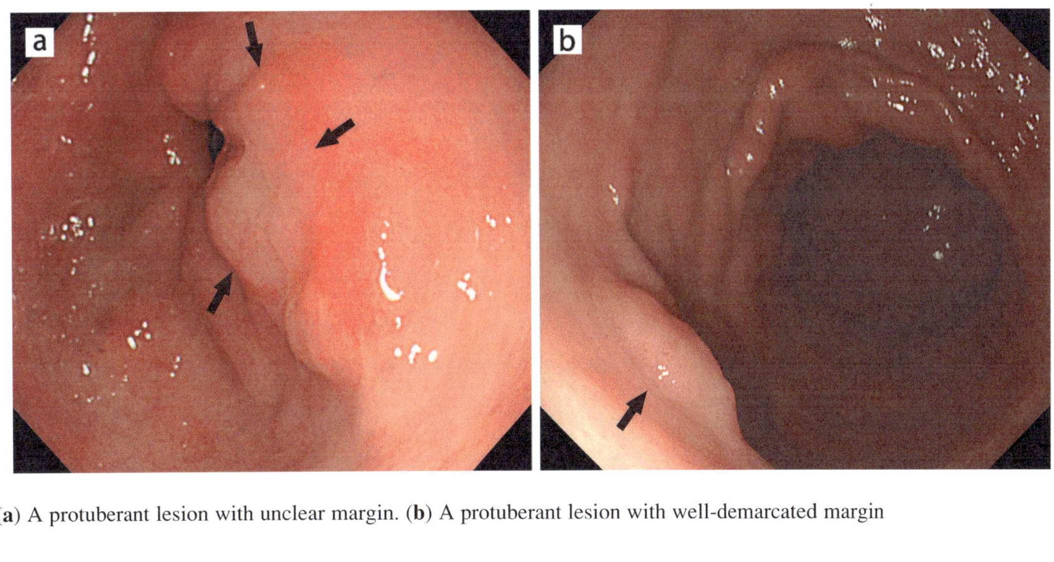

Fig. 2.10 (**a**) A protuberant lesion with unclear margin. (**b**) A protuberant lesion with well-demarcated margin

Differential Diagnosis for Red Protuberant Lesions
Red flat elevated lesions with irregular surface patterns and irregular borders are WDAs. Hyperplastic polyps (HPs), which are also red elevated lesions with well-demarcated borders, are classified as Yamadafied as do red eleva and show large villous patterns on the surface (Fig. 2.11).

Differential Diagnosis for Protuberant Lesions of White or Same Color as Background
Major diseases of whitish protuberant lesions are tubular adenoma (TA), fundic gland polyp (FGP), and IM. Typical TAs show well-demarcated flat protuberant lesions with regular nodular surface. FGPs are well-demarcated protuberant lesions with smooth surface and exist in the fundic gland area. Therefore, when multiple protuberant lesions are observed on or between gastric folds, they are FGPs. Typical endoscopic view of IM shows small white nodules in the antrum. SMTs are also protuberant lesions but are not well demarcated because they are covered by nonneoplastic mucosa (Fig. 2.12).

2.4.3 Depressed Lesions

The most frequent depressed lesions are erosions and focal atrophy. It is important to differentiate these from WDA, PDA, and MALT lymphoma. Key points for differential diagnosis are color, demarcation, and shape. Basically

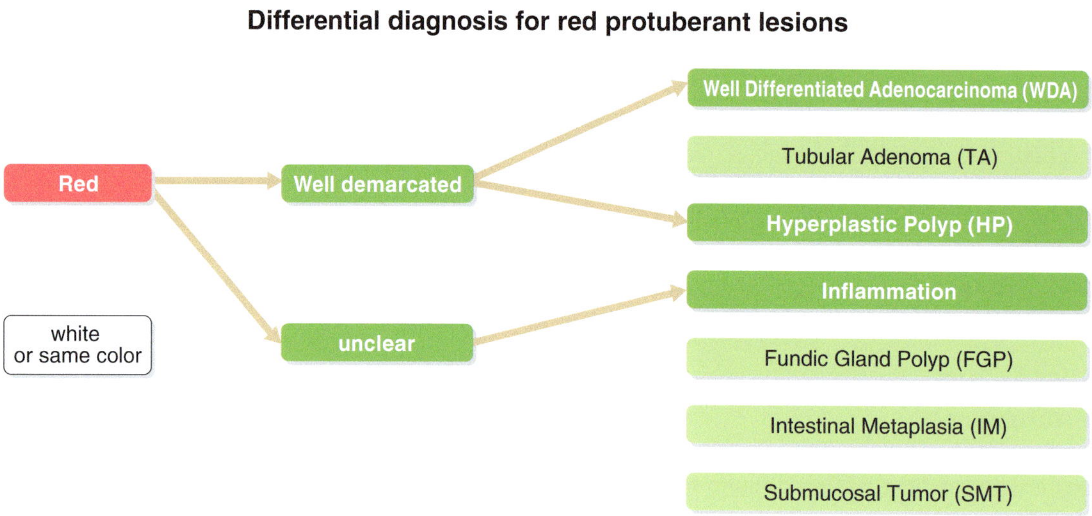

Fig. 2.11 Differential diagnosis for red protuberant lesions

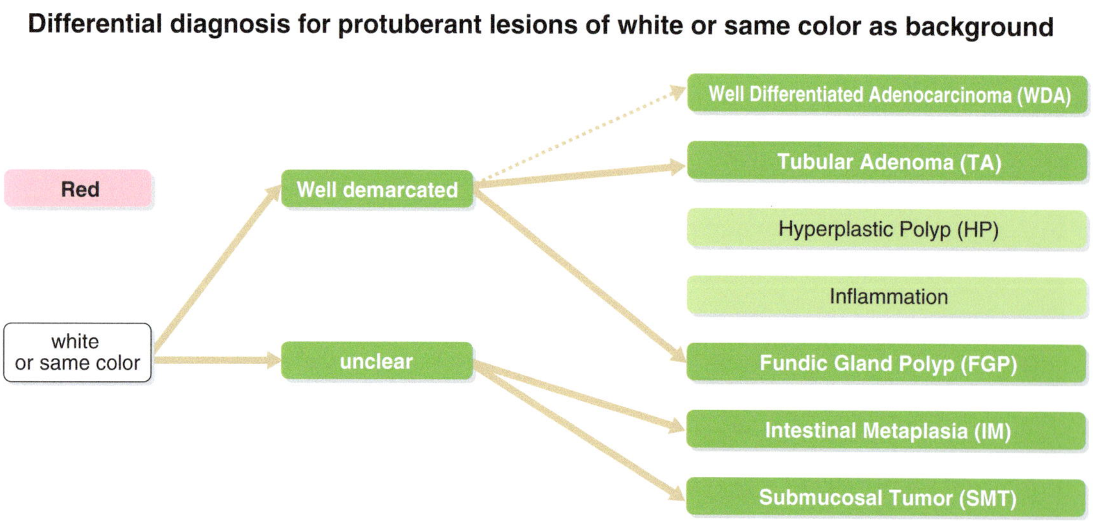

Fig. 2.12 Differential diagnosis for protuberant lesions of white or same color as background

adenocarcinomas have well-demarcated irregular and jagged shapes, and erosions or atrophied areas show regular, smooth shapes with unclear demarcation.

2.4.3.1 Color

Generally, WDAs have glandular structures with proliferated vessels in parenchyma. Therefore, the color is reddish. On the other hand, PDAs spread through the parenchyma destroying vessels. Therefore, the color is whitish. Careful observation of color is very important for early detection of cancers.

2.4.3.2 Shape and Demarcation of Depressed Lesions

Red Depressed Lesions

If a lesion is a well-demarcated reddish depressed lesion, WDA must be suspected first and differential diagnoses of erosion and MALT lymphoma must be considered. When lesions show irregular and well-demarcated depressions, the risk of WDA is high. If the shape of the lesion is round and regular or with unclear margin, erosion must be suspected first and differential diagnosis of MALT lymphoma should be considered (Fig. 2.13).

Whitish Depressed Lesions

When whitish irregularly shaped depressions are observed, the risk of PDA is high. And, when multiple depressed lesions with unclear borders are found, focal atrophy should be considered (Fig. 2.14).

Red PDAs?

PDAs usually appear to be of pale whitish color and sometimes form erosions within. When erosive areas regenerate, a nonneoplastic regenerative layer covers the surface and may

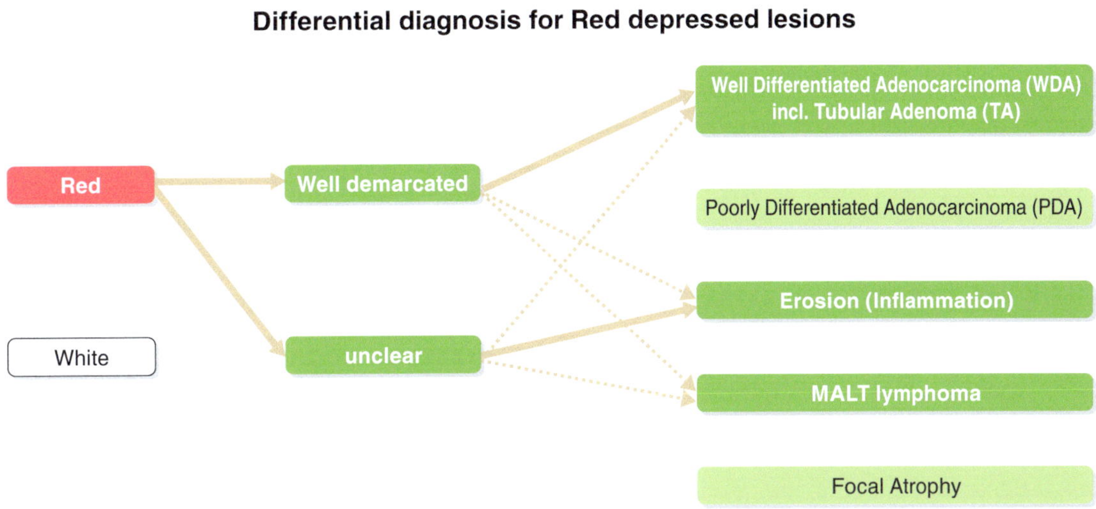

Fig. 2.13 Differential diagnosis for red depressed lesions

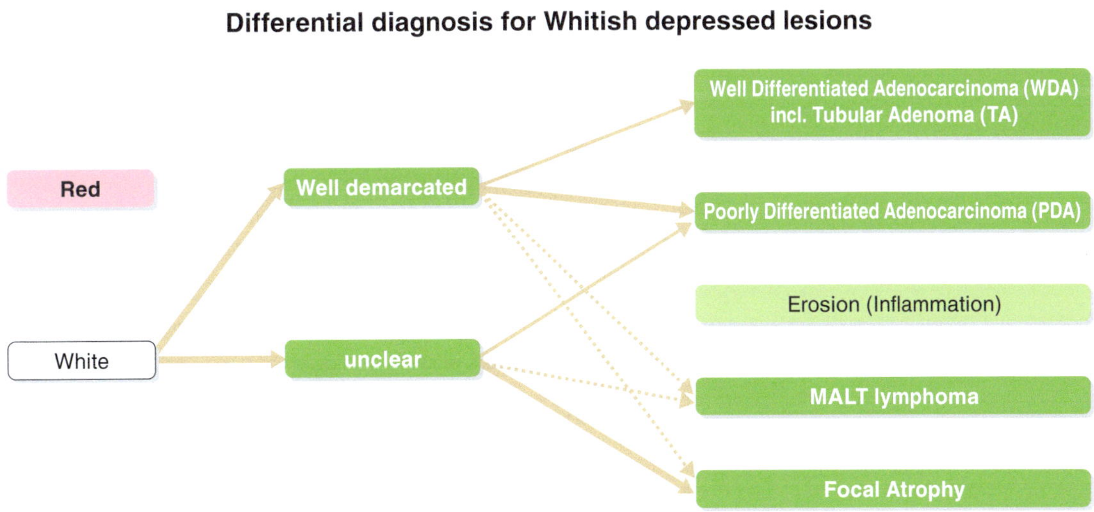

Fig. 2.14 Differential diagnosis for whitish depressed lesions

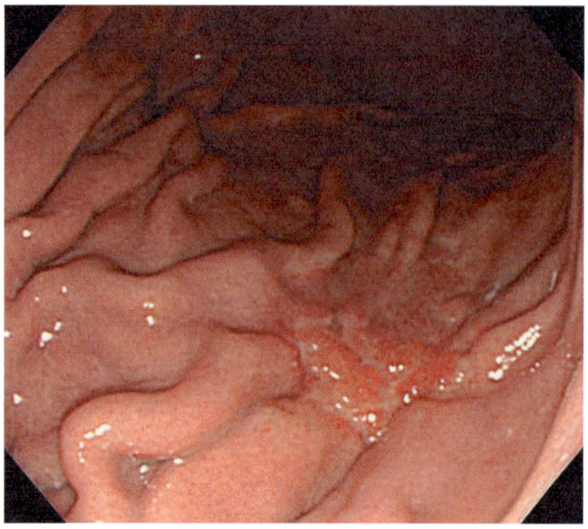

Fig. 2.15 A reddish or whitish lesion?: the color looks like reddish. But, the depressed area showed whitish

appear red. Sometimes, nonneoplastic mucosa may remain within 0-IIc lesions forming "sanctuaries" consisting of islands of nonneoplastic mucosal surface. These nonneoplastic surfaces may appear reddish with inflammation. Beginners may recognize this lesion as a reddish depressed lesion. But if you look carefully, protrusions appear reddish, but depressed areas are pale. Tumors exist only within depressed areas. Therefore, this is not a reddish depressed lesion but a pale depressed lesion (Fig. 2.15).

2.4.4 Vascular Visibility

Since the majority of EGCs are 0-IIc lesions, it is important to search for depressed lesions for detection of EGCs. However, when 0-IIc lesions occur in the atrophied gastric mucosa, detection becomes difficult, as the difference between height of the background mucosa and the depressed lesions becomes less prominent. In these situations, differences in vascular visibility become important clues for detection of EGCs.

While densely present cancer cells interfere with the permeation of light, obscuring visibility of the submucosal vessels, the submucosal vessels in the atrophic gastric areas are easily seen.

When gastric mucosa becomes atrophied, vascular visibility increases making submucosal vessels visible. On the other hand, 0-IIc WDAs have higher cellular density with larger nuclei resulting in poor light permeability and decreased vascular transparency. PDAs, likewise, have cancer cells filling the intracellular space reducing light permeability and vascular transparency. Transparency of submucosal vessels focally decreases with EGCs. When atrophied areas with unclear submucosal vessels are noted, these areas must be carefully observed for EGCs (Fig. 2.16).

2.4.5 Information from the Gastric Folds

Gastric folds exist only within the fundic areas. Therefore, the presence of gastric folds shows where fundic glands exist. Gastric folds provide additional information regarding submucosa, such as "bridging folds" or "fold convergences."

2.4.5.1 Bridging Fold

SMT gradually rise and are covered by nonneoplastic mucosa. Therefore, when SMTs exist within the fundic gland areas, the gastric folds are lifted over the SMTs. These folds lifted over the SMTs look like bridges and are called "bridging folds." EGCs, on the other hand, exist within the mucosa, obliterating the gastric folds. Therefore, the presence of "bridging folds" helps differentiate SMTs from EGCs (Fig. 2.17).

2.4.5.2 Fold Convergence

Fold convergences are caused by fibrosis of the submucosal layer. Proliferation of collagenous fibers within the submucosal layer makes contraction of overlying mucosal lesions, resulting in fold convergences. The major causes of submucosal fibrosis are ulcers and PDAs.

Fold Convergences Caused by Ulcers

When gastric ulcers occur, mucosal layers are eroded exposing the submucosal layers to gastric acids. Proliferation of collagenous fibers within the submucosal layer causes contraction of the ulcer bases assisting with their healing. Fold convergences thus formed generally show smooth shapes.

Fold Convergences Caused by PDAs

When PDAs infiltrate into submucosal layers, proliferated collagenous fibers create contractions and fold convergences result. In such cases, PDAs get mixed with collagenous fibers forming submucosal mass, resulting in fusions of the converging folds (Fig. 2.18).

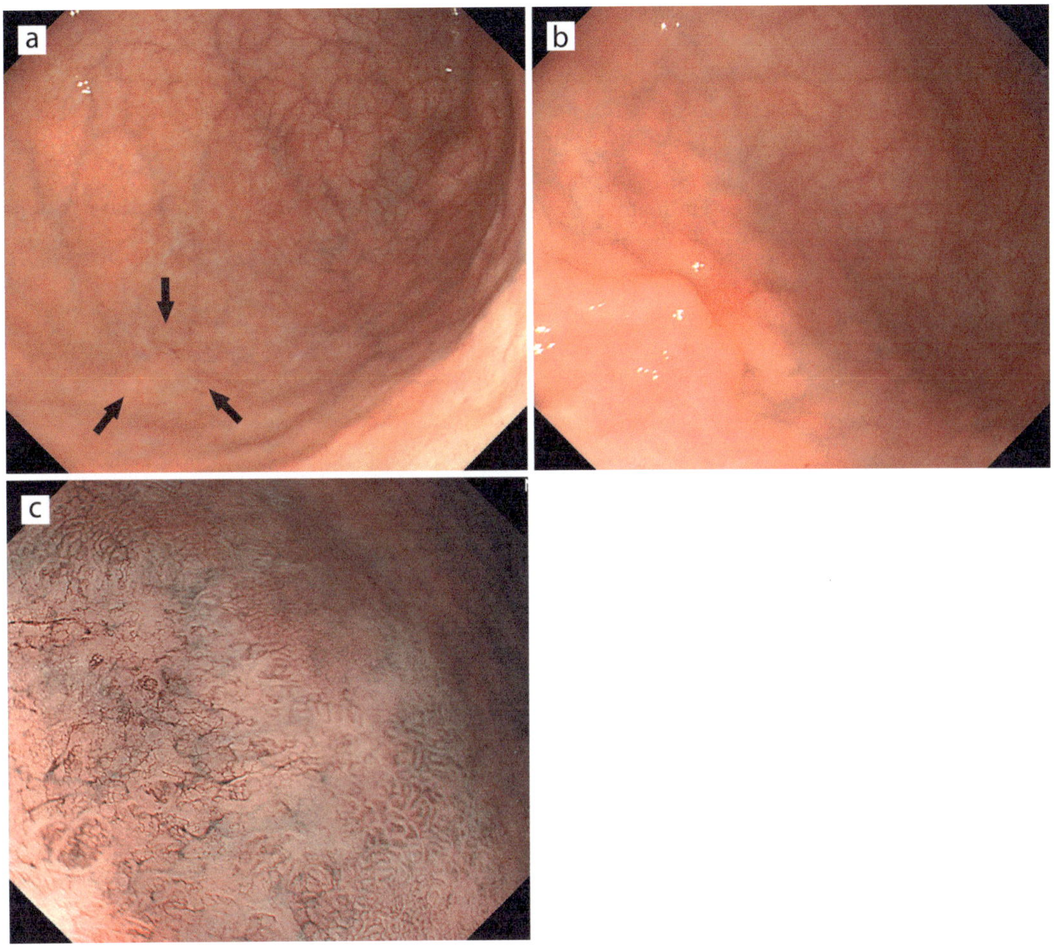

Fig. 2.16 Permeability of submucosal vessels. (**a**) Submucosal vessels were not seen in the arrowed area. (**b**) The lesion became depressed when deflated. (**c**) The surface pattern was unclear, and an irregular vascular pattern was observed. Therefore, the lesion was diagnosed as adenocarcinoma

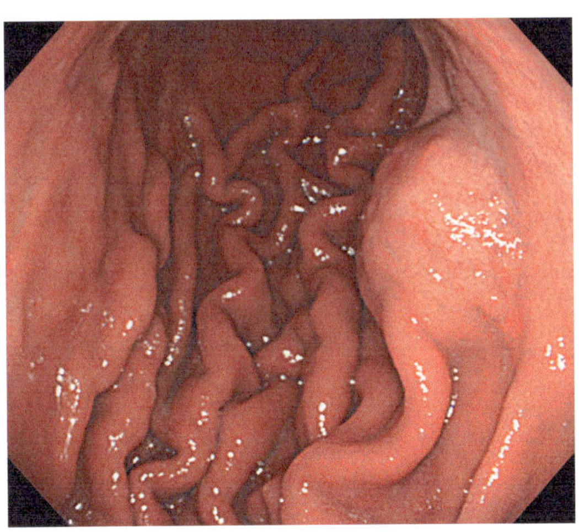

Fig. 2.17 Bridging fold

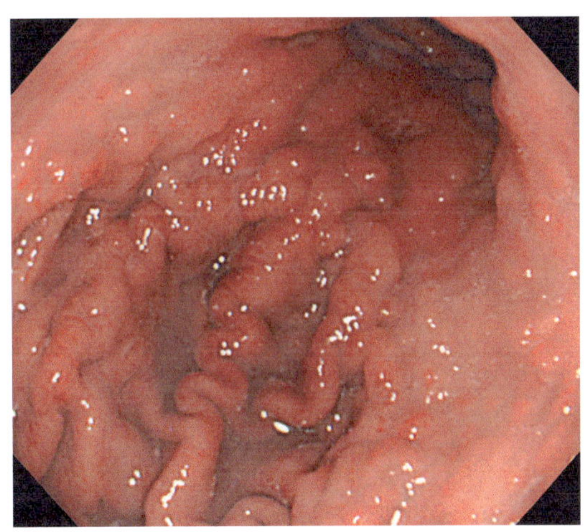

Fig. 2.18 Fold convergence caused by deep invasion of PDA

2.4.5.3 Diagnosis of Invasion Depth by Fold Convergence

0-IIc adenocarcinoma with ulcer scar shows fold convergence. And the folds will show contraction or tapering of convergent folds for intramucosal cancers. On the other hand, 0-IIc adenocarcinomas with submucosal involvements may cause fusion of folds because submucosal infiltration lifts the folds up from the submucosa. Fusion of folds is a finding not seen with minimal submucosal infiltrations, but when seen, it strongly indicates massive submucosal infiltrations.

Reference

1. Yagi K, Nakamura A, Sekine A. Characteristic endoscopic and magnified endoscopic findings in the normal stomach without Helicobacter pylori infection. J Gastroenterol Hepatol. 2002;17:39–45.

3 Diagnosis of Invasion Depth

Akihisa Tomori and Tsuneo Oyama

Gastric cancer arises within the mucosa and infiltrates down to the submucosa. The risk of lymph node metastasis of T1a, AC (adenocarcinoma) is rare. However, the incidence of lymph node metastasis of T1b, SM, AC is around 15 %. Therefore, accurate diagnosis of invasion depth is important for treatment decision making. In this chapter, key points for accurate endoscopic diagnosis of invasion depths are described.

3.1 Surface Patterns of T1a Mucosal Cancer

Intramucosal cancers occur as elevated, flat, or depressed lesions but in general have flat surface. The surface pattern of T1a mucosal AC is flat and regular (Fig. 3.1a). 0-IIa type shows a well-demarcated protrusion (Fig. 3.1b) and 0-IIc type shows a well-demarcated flat depression (Fig. 3.1c).

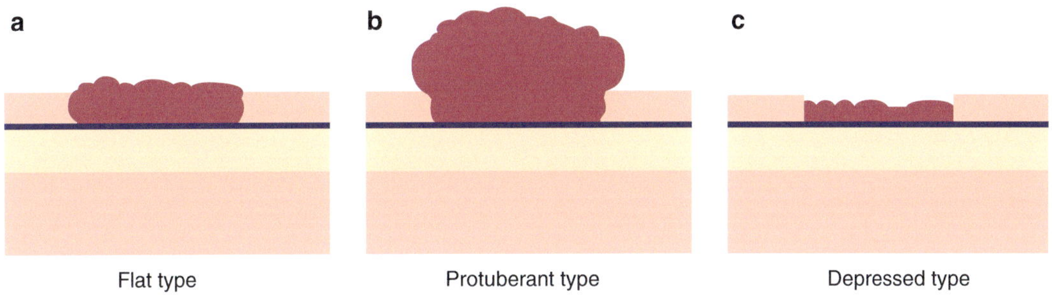

Fig. 3.1 Surface pattern of mucosal adenocarcinoma: (**a**) flat type, (**b**) protuberant type, and (**c**) depressed type

A. Tomori
Department of Gastroenterology, Saku Central Hospital, 197 Usuda, Saku, Nagano 384-0301, Japan

T. Oyama (✉)
Division of Endoscopy, Saku Central Hospital, 197 Usuda, Saku, Nagano 384-0301, Japan
e-mail: oyama@coral.ocn.ne.jp

T. Oyama (ed.), *Endoscopic Diagnosis of Superficial Gastric Cancer for ESD*, DOI 10.1007/978-4-431-54469-2_3

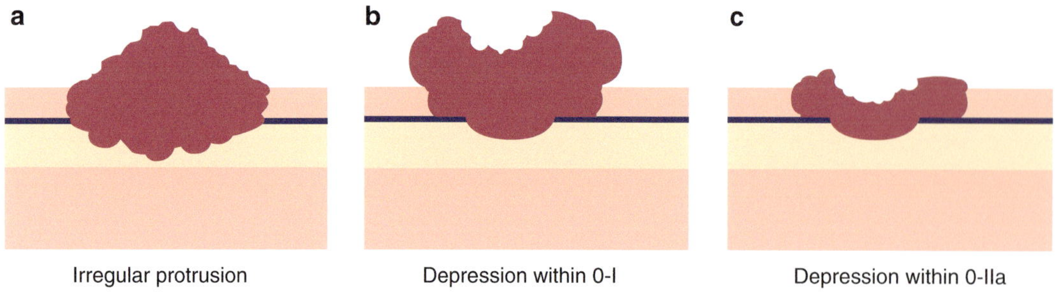

Fig. 3.2 Principle 1. Elevation: (**a**) irregular protrusion and (**b**) depression within 0-I (**c**) depression within 0-IIa

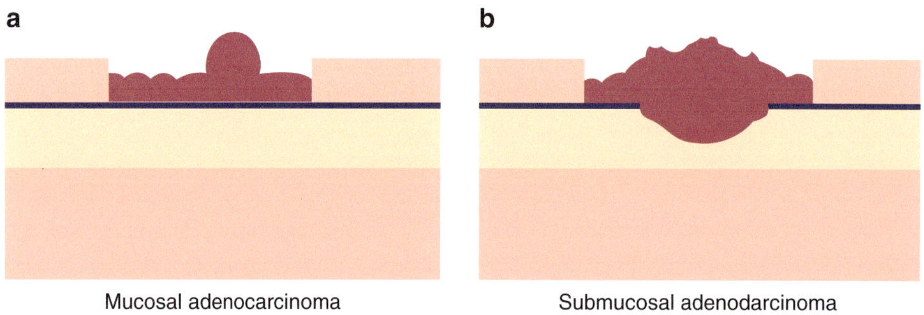

Fig. 3.3 Disappearance of areal patterns: (**a**) mucosal adenocarcinoma and (**b**) submucosal adenocarcinoma

3.2 When Cancer Invades into the Submucosal Layer

3.2.1 Principle 1. Elevation

When cancer invades into the submucosal layer, the submucosal mass invasion characteristically forms a smooth SMT-like elevation (Fig. 3.2a). As the muscularis mucosa gets destroyed, areal patterns disappear and the mucosal surface becomes irregular (Fig. 3.2b, c).

Sometimes, there is an elevation within a 0-IIc lesion. When it is mucosal cancer, the elevation is well demarcated with a sharp rise (Fig. 3.3a). However, if cancer has invaded into the submucosal layer and formed a mass, it causes an SMT-like elevation with a smooth rise, but with an irregular surface (Fig. 3.3b).

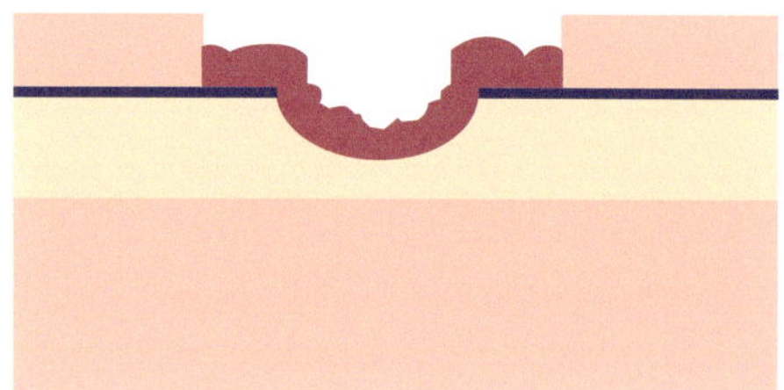

Fig. 3.4 Principle 2. Depression

3.2.2 Principle 2. Depression

Sometimes a deep depression is observed when cancer invades into the submucosal layer. If you find a deep depression within a 0-IIc lesion, submucosal invasion should be suspected (Fig. 3.4).

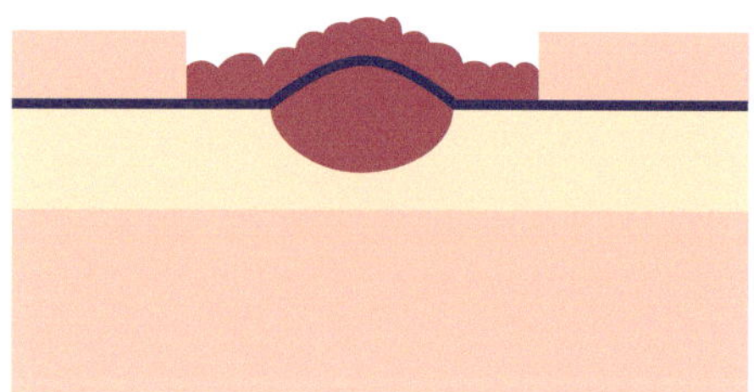

Fig. 3.5 Principle 3. Disappearance of areal patterns

3.2.3 Principle 3. Disappearance of Areal Patterns

Formation of gastric areal patterns requires intact muscularis mucosa. If the surface layer is destroyed by cancer and submucosal cancer is exposed, gastric areal patterns cannot be seen. Observation of surface patterns helps determine if the submucosal cancer is exposed to the surface. If cancer infiltrates into the submucosa without destroying the muscularis mucosa, the surface layer becomes covered by intramucosal cancer and gastric areal patterns remain visible. Even in such situation, observation of the thickness within the 0-IIc area helps determine the presence of submucosal involvements by cancer (Fig. 3.5).

3.2.4 Principle 4. Fusion of the Folds

Gastric folds are composed of muscularis mucosa and mucosa, protruding into the gastric lumen (Fig. 3.6a). Folds within mucosal cancers show thinning or swelling of gastric folds (Fig. 3.6b, c). However, when the cancer has invaded into the submucosal layer and has made a mass lesion, the mass may lift the muscularis mucosae between two folds and fusion of folds may occur (Fig. 3.6d). Therefore, fusion of folds indicates the presence of submucosal invasion.

Principles 1–4 are findings seen when cancer has invaded into the submucosa. These findings help confirm diagnosis of a submucosally invading cancer, but lack of these findings do not negate possibilities of minimal submucosal invasions.

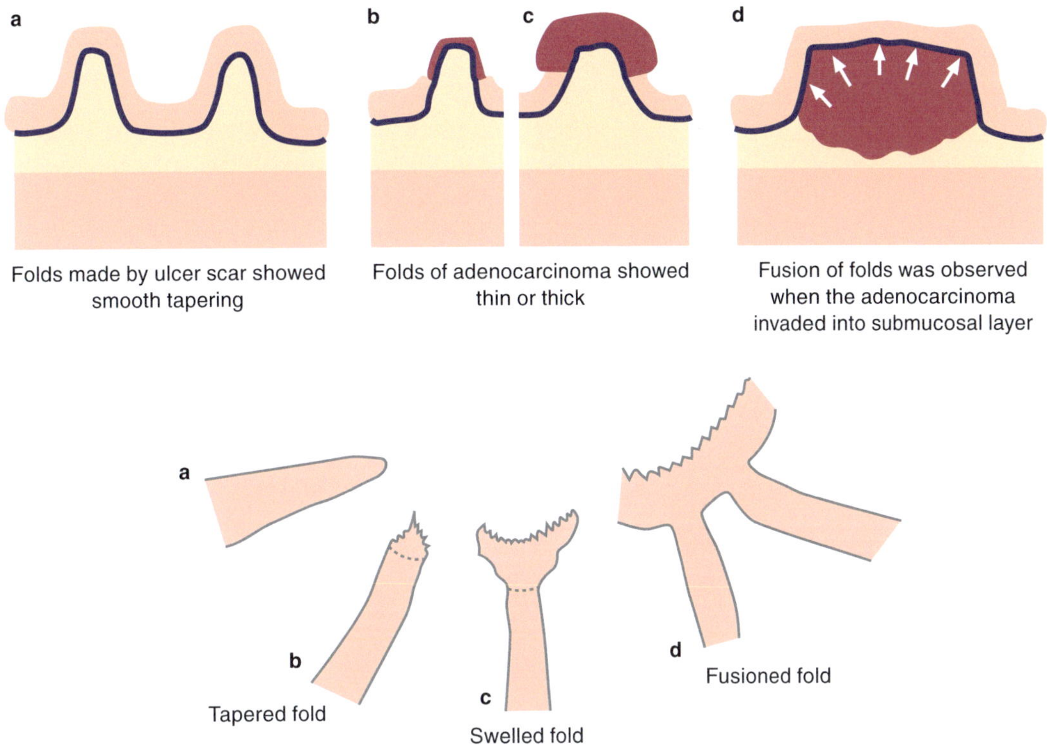

Fig. 3.6 Principle 4. Fusion of the folds. (**a**) Folds made by ulcer scar showed smooth tapering. (**b**, **c**) Folds of adenocarcinoma showed thin or thick (**d**): Fusion of folds was observed when the adenocarcinoma invaded into submucosal layer

3.3 Diagnosis of Invasion Depth, 0-I Type

3.3.1 Case 1. 0-I, T1a, M Cancer

A well-demarcated reddish 0-I lesion is observed in the anterior wall of the gastric antrum (Fig. 3.7a). The surface pattern is irregular with close-up observation (Fig. 3.7b). Irregularly nodular gastric areas are observed by indigo carmine spraying (Fig. 3.7c). Therefore, the lesion can be diagnosed WDA.

A well-demarcated protuberant lesion like in this case with gastric areal patterns on its surface can be diagnosed as mucosal cancer.

3.3.2 Case 2. 0-I, T1a, M Cancer

A well-demarcated 0-I lesion is observed at the posterior side of the lower gastric body. The surface is lobular (Fig. 3.8a) and well demarcated (Fig. 3.8b). An irregular

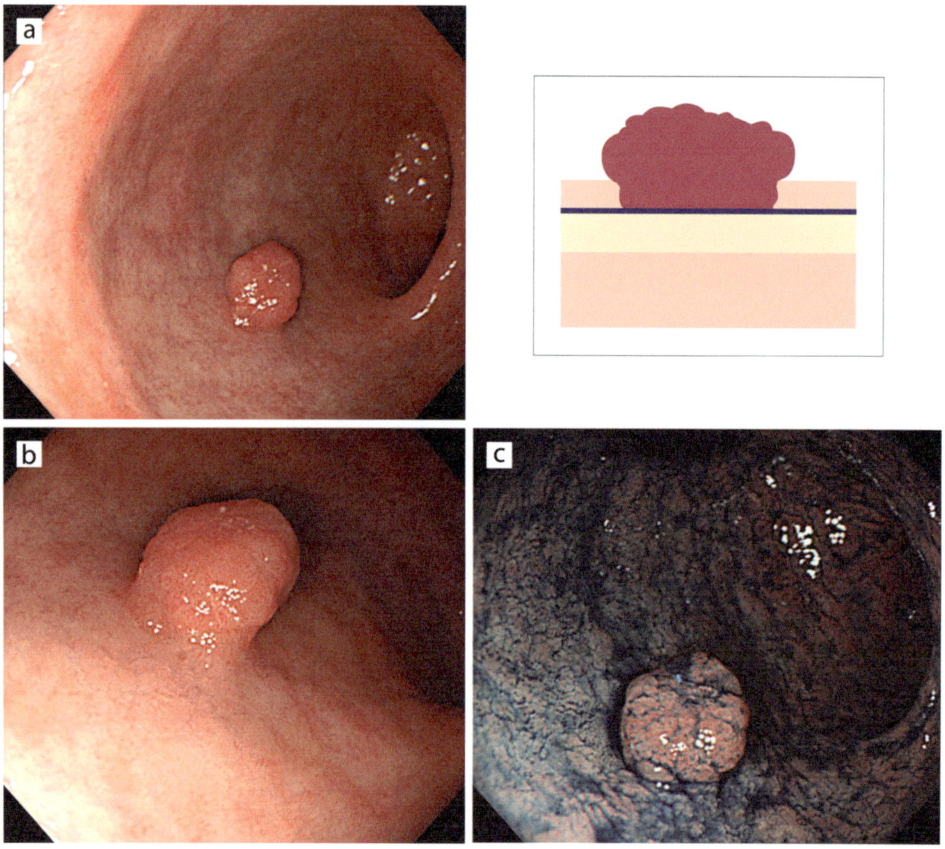

Fig. 3.7 Case 1. 0-I, T1a, M cancer

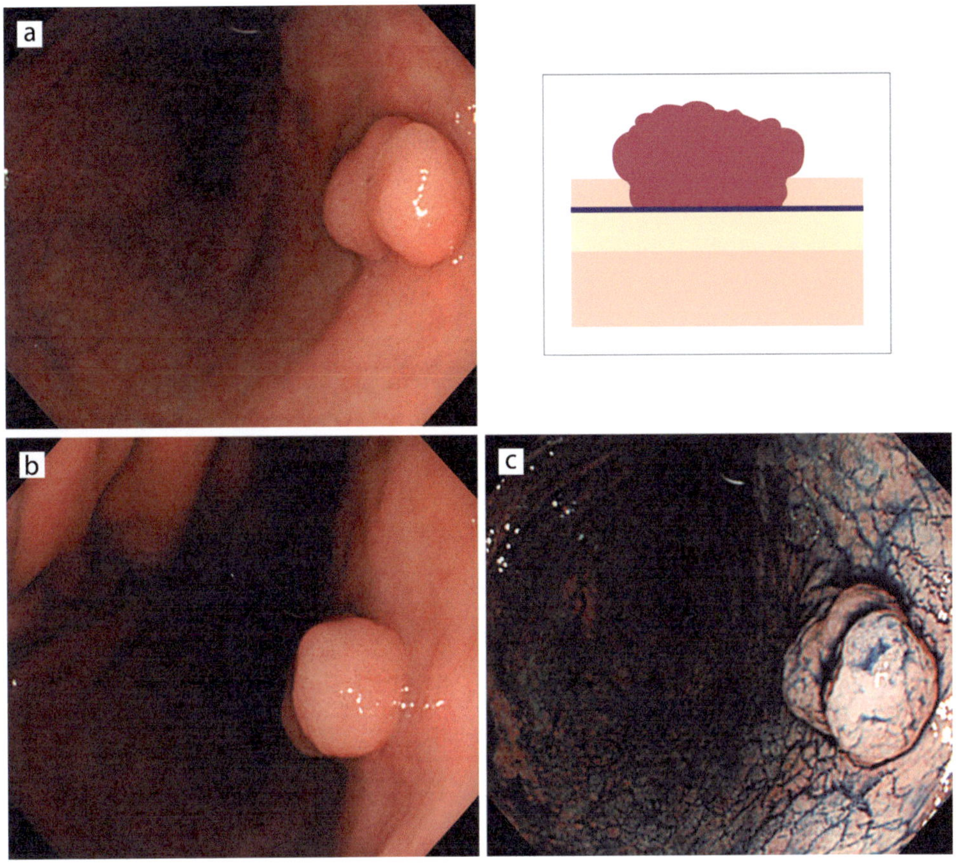

Fig. 3.8 Case 2. 0-I, T1a, M cancer

nodular pattern is observed by indigo carmine spraying (Fig. 3.8c). It is a tall lesion. But, it is a well-demarcated lesion (not SMT-like) with a nodular surface pattern. Therefore, it is diagnosed as mucosal cancer.

3.3.3 Case 3. 0-I, Tb, SM2 Cancer

A reddish protuberant lesion is observed at the anterior side of the gastric body. The background mucosa shows highly visible submucosal vessels due to extensive atrophy of the mucosal surface. The demarcation is clear, except on its lesser curvature side (Fig. 3.9a). Nodular gastric areal patterns are observed in the greater curvature side, but the surface pattern of the lesser curvature side is unclear with no visible gastric areal structures (Fig. 3.9b). Therefore, this lesion is diagnosed as having submucosal invasion (T1b, SM) on its lesser curvature side.

3.3.4 Case 4. 0-I, T1b, SM Cancer

A well-demarcated protuberant lesion is observed at the greater curvature side of the lower gastric body. The surface pattern is irregular and a depression is noted on the surface of 0-I lesion (Fig. 3.10a). The surface pattern of the protuberant lesion is irregular and unclear while the surrounding mucosa shows usual areal patterns with indigo carmine spreading. There is a 0-IIc spreading in the posterior side (Fig. 3.10b). Based on thickness and irregular surface patterns without areal patterns, submucosally invasive cancer (T1b, SM) can be diagnosed. It is important to note differences in surface patterns compared with cases 1 and 2.

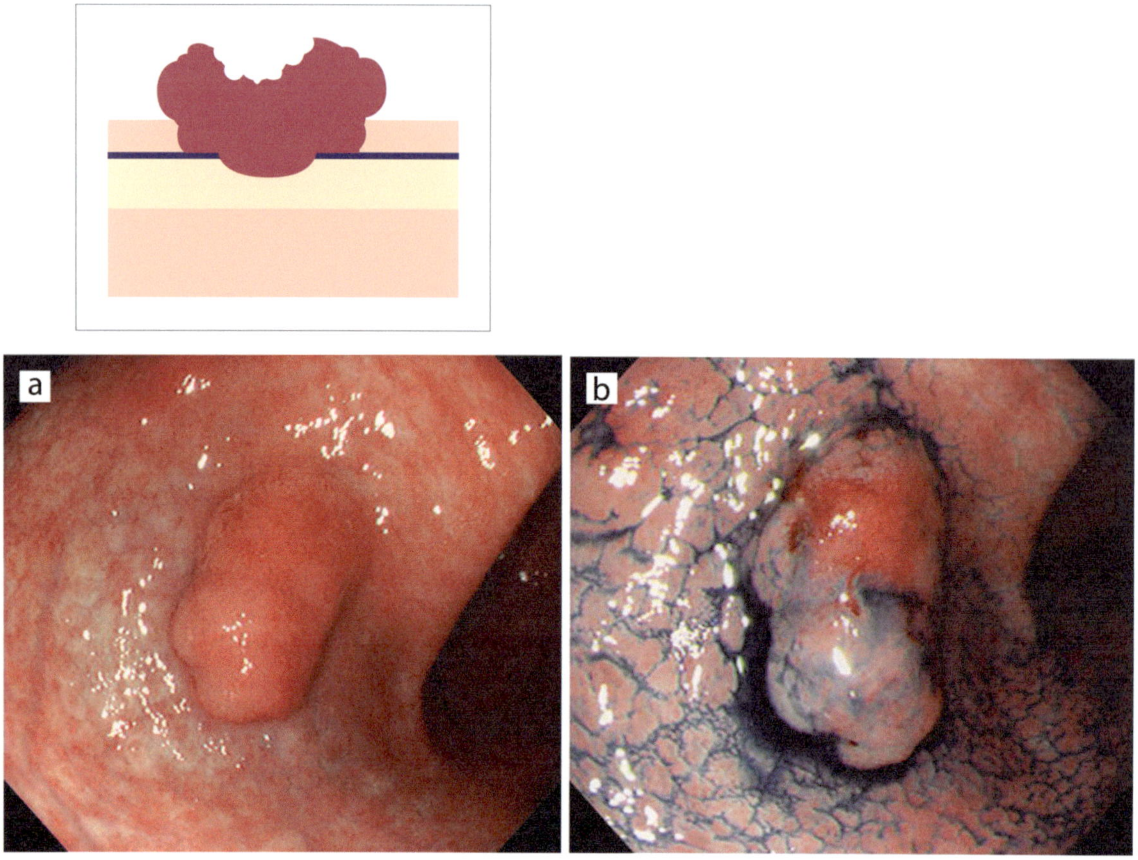

Fig. 3.9 Case 3. 0-I, Tb, SM2 cancer

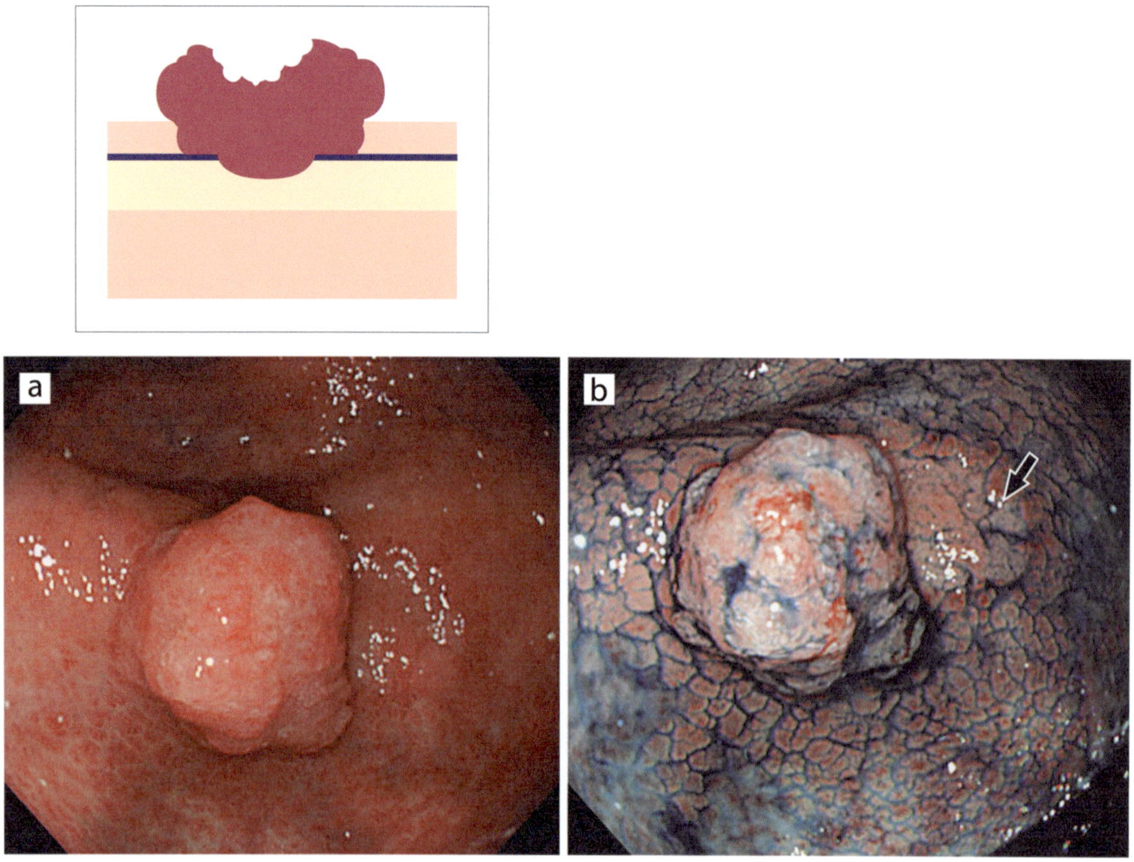

Fig. 3.10 Case 4. 0-I, T1b, SM cancer

3.3.5 Case 5. 0-IIa, T1a, M Cancer

A flat protuberant lesion is observed at the lesser curvature side of the lower gastric body. The background mucosa shows atrophic gastritis with highly visible submucosal vessels due to thin atrophied mucosa (Fig. 3.11a). An evenly nodular pattern is observed after indigo carmine spreading without significant surface elevation or depression. Therefore, this lesion is diagnosed as mucosal (T1a, M) cancer (Fig. 3.11b).

3.3.6 Case 6. 0-IIa, T1b, SM Cancer

A well-demarcated 0-IIa lesion is observed at the anterior side of the gastric midbody. It is a well-demarcated protuberant lesion with a central depression (Fig. 3.12a). Gastric areal patterns are observed at the peripheral area, but the surface pattern becomes unclear in the central part (Fig. 3.12b). A central depression with an unclear surface pattern on a 0-IIa lesion like in this case suggests submucosal invasion (T1b, SM).

3.3.7 Case 7. 0-IIa, T1b, SM Cancer

A 0-IIa lesion is observed at the posterior side of the cardia. It is a well-demarcated protuberant lesion with peripheral constriction suggesting intramucosal cancer on the periphery. But the anal side is a step higher (Fig. 3.13a). This elevation within the 0-IIa lesion is clearly observed by indigo carmine spraying (Fig. 3.13b). Submucosal invasion (T1b, SM) should be diagnosed from such findings.

3.3.8 Case 8. 0-IIc, T1a, M Cancer

A well-demarcated reddish depressed lesion is observed at the anterior side of the gastric antrum (Fig. 3.14a). The surface is flat with usual areal patterns, without significant elevations or

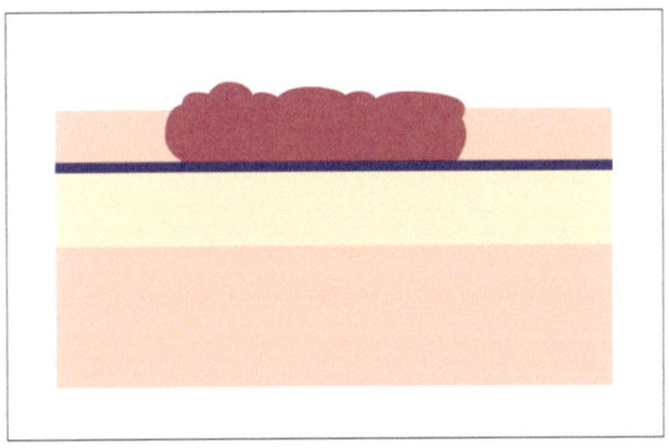

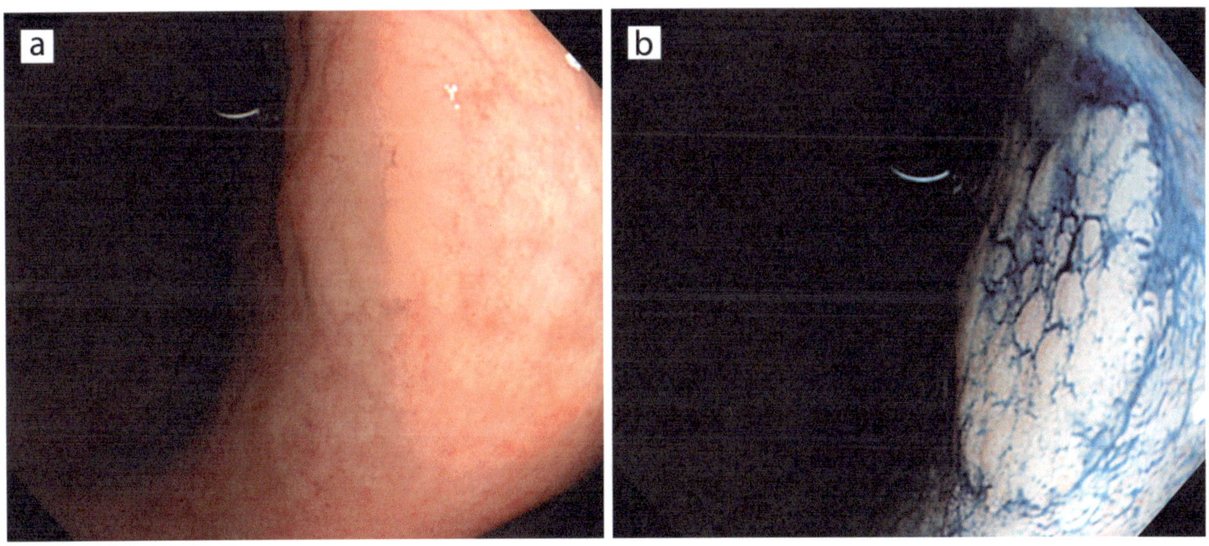

Fig. 3.11 Case 5. 0-IIa, T1a, M cancer

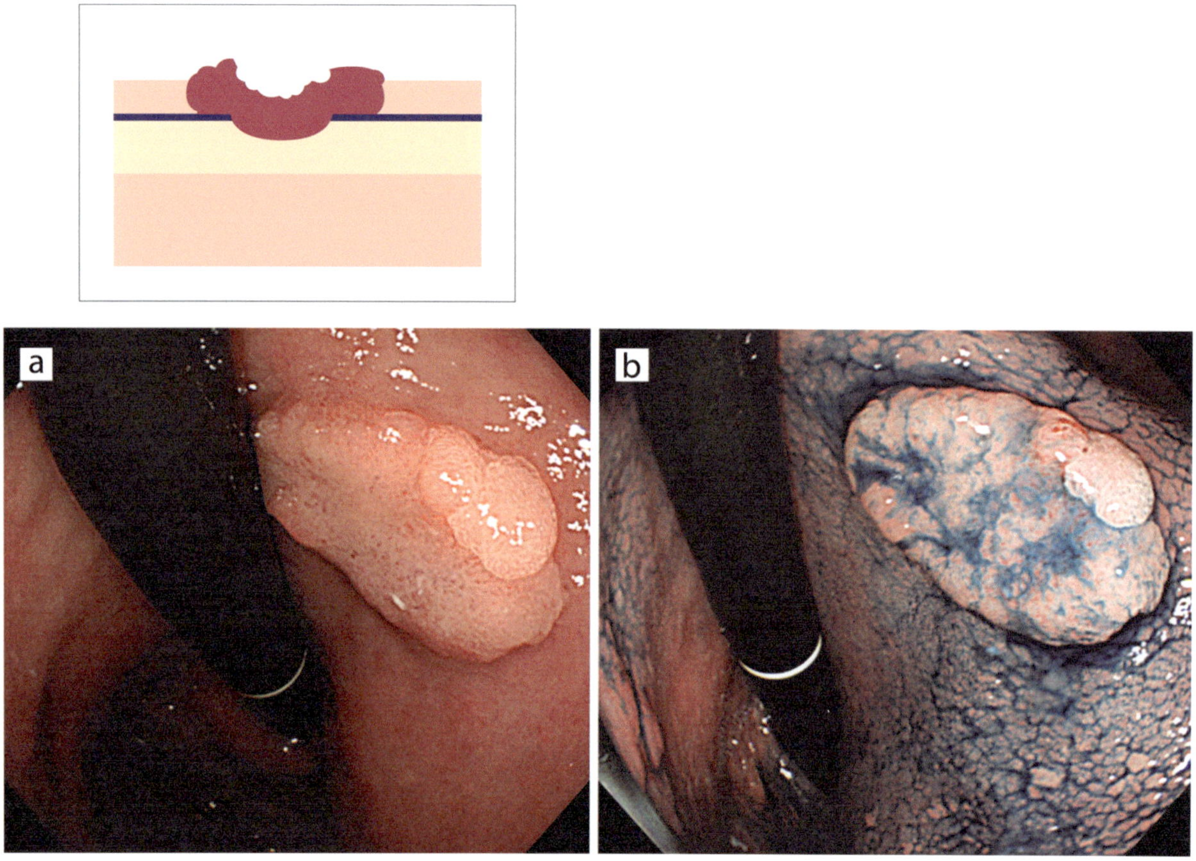

Fig. 3.12 Case 6. 0-IIa, T1b, SM cancer

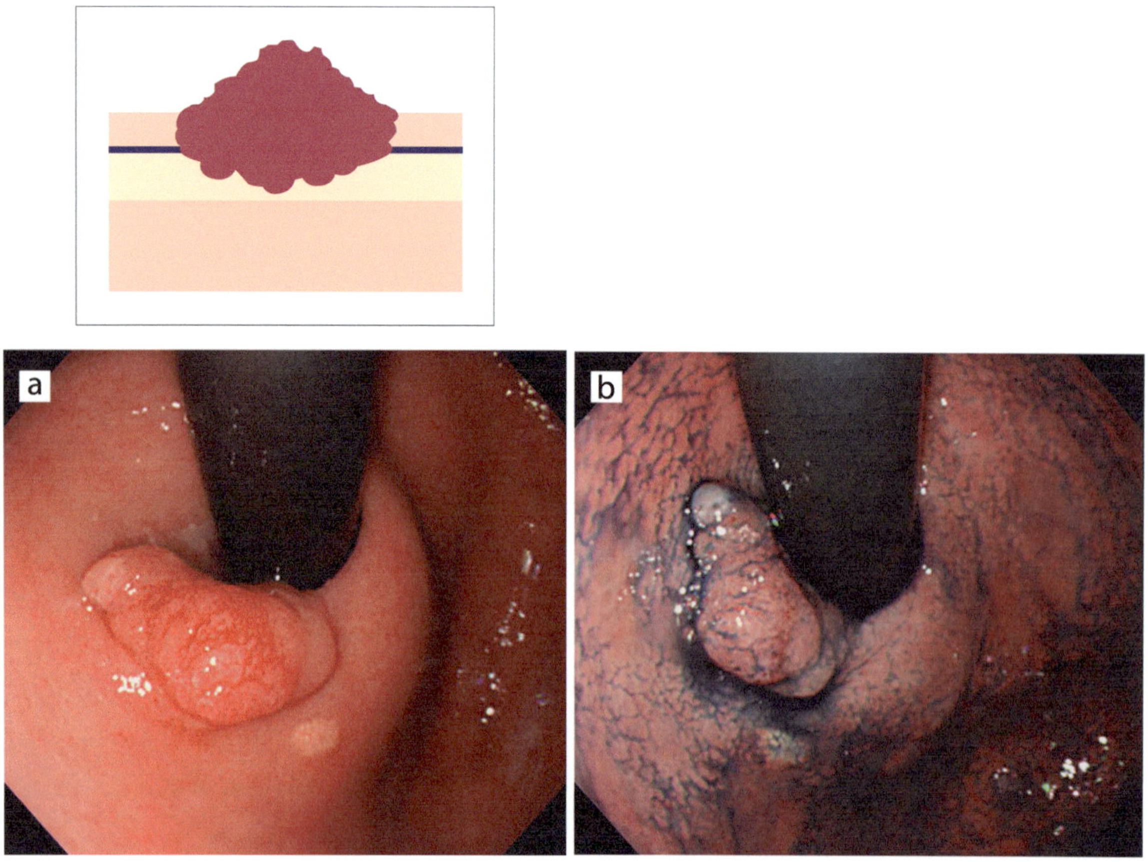

Fig. 3.13 Case 7. 0-IIa, T1b, SM cancer

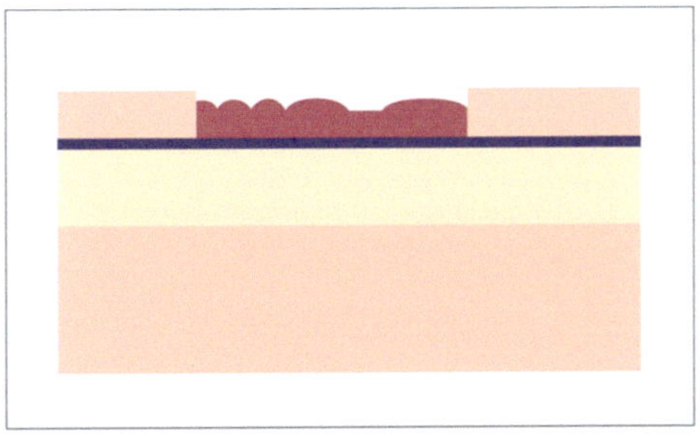

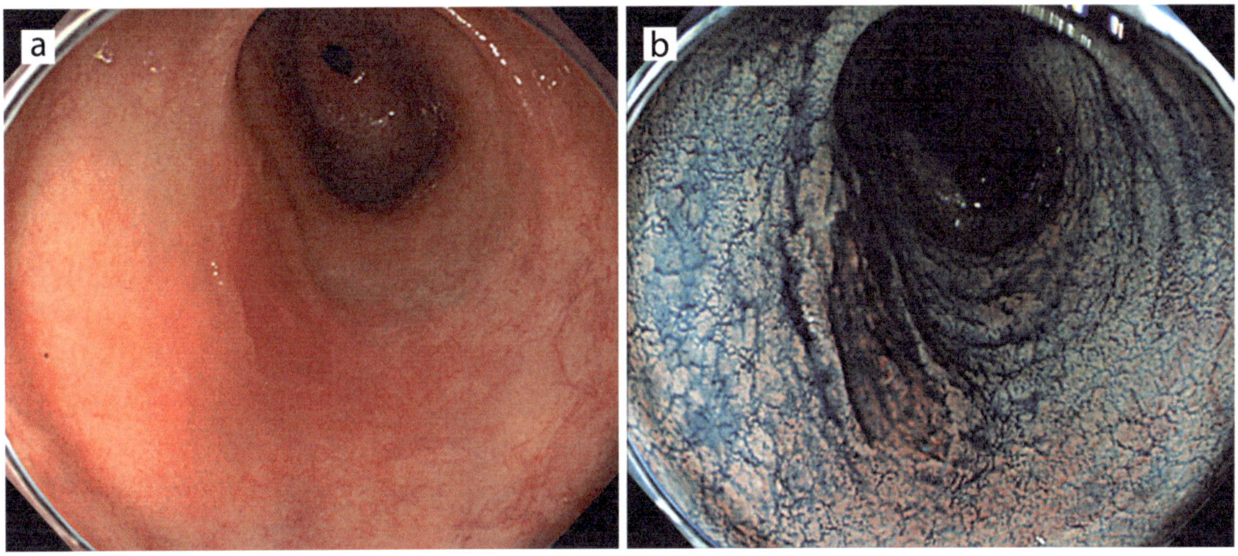

Fig. 3.14 Case 8. 0-IIc, T1a, M cancer

depressions by indigo carmine spraying (Fig. 3.14b). Therefore, the invasion depth is mucosal (T1a, M).

3.3.9 Case 9. 0-IIc, T1b, SM Cancer

A shallow depressed lesion with marginal elevation is observed at the greater curvature of the lower gastric body (Fig. 3.15a). The surface of the depressed lesion is flat, with a focal protrusion within (arrow) (Fig. 3.15b). The protrusion is not well demarcated by indigo carmine spraying (Fig. 3.15c). Almost all of this cancer is intramucosal (T1a, M), except for focal submucosal invasion at the protuberance.

3.3.10 Case 10. 0-IIc, T1b, SM Cancer

A shallow depressed lesion is observed at the greater curvature of the middle gastric body (Fig. 3.16a). A smooth low protrusion is observed at the anal part of the depressed lesion after indigo carmine spraying as this area is noted to be repelling the dye (Fig. 3.16b). This lesion is basically mucosal, except for the thickened area anally with submucosal invasion.

3.3.11 Case 11. 0-IIc, T1b, SM Cancer

A depressed lesion (0-IIc) with fold convergence is observed at the greater curvature of the lower gastric

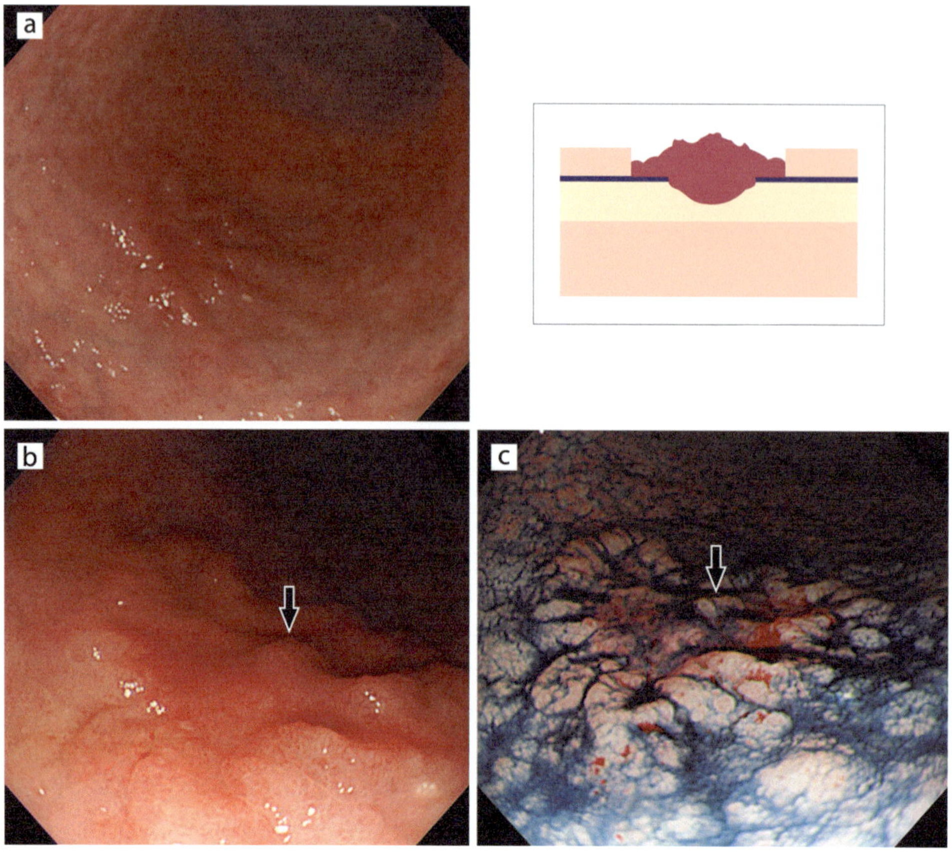

Fig. 3.15 Case 9. 0-IIc, T1b, SM cancer

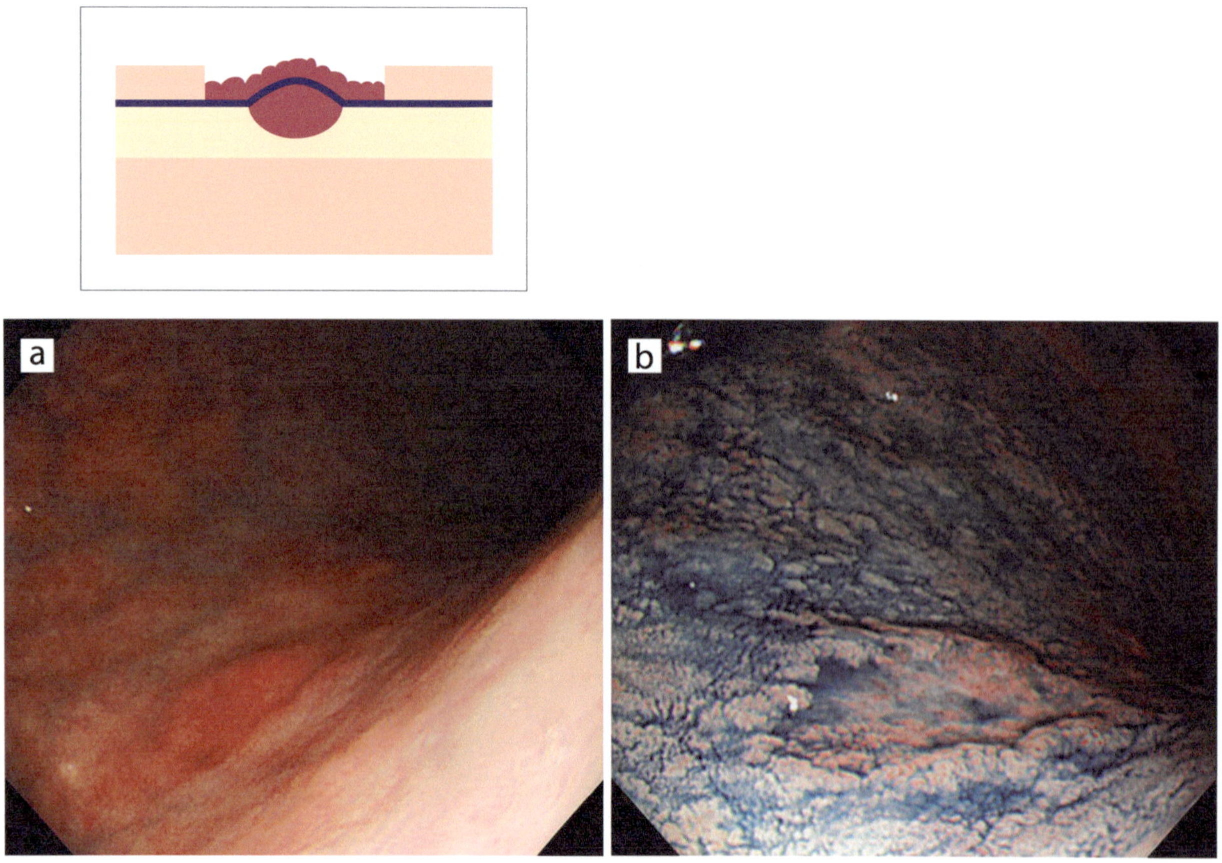

Fig. 3.16 Case 10. 0-IIc, T1b, SM cancer

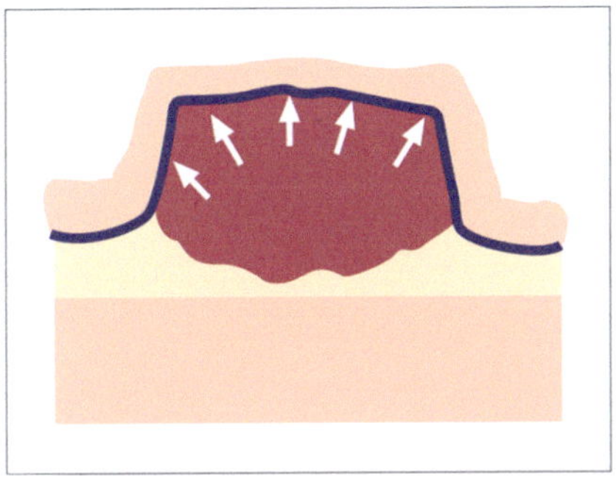

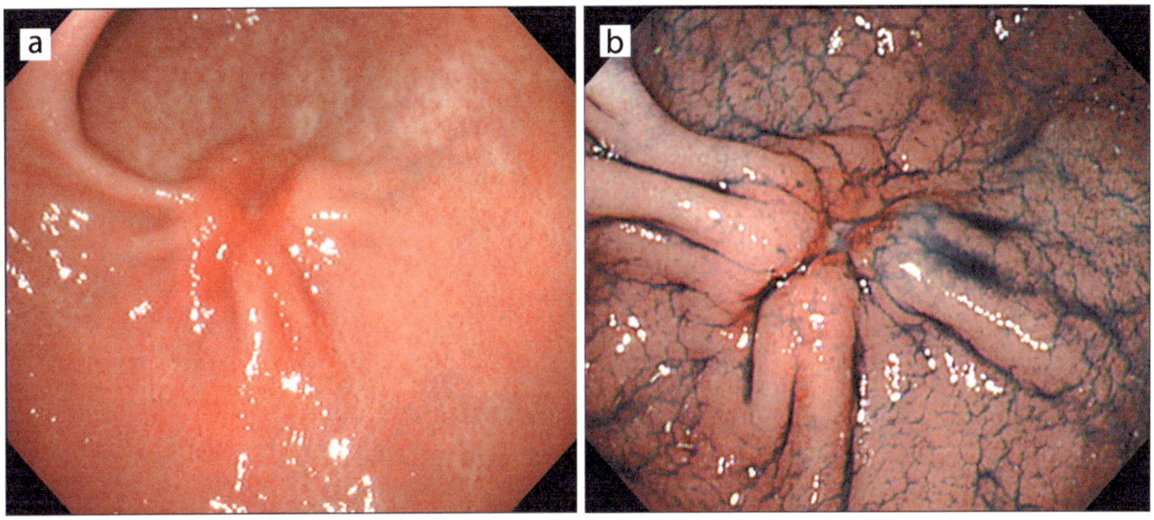

Fig. 3.17 Case 11. 0-IIc, T1b, SM cancer

body (Fig. 3.17a). In cases with fold convergence, finding of fusion of folds becomes a very important key to diagnosis of invasion depth. In this lesion, fusion of gastric folds can be observed by carefully examining after indigo carmine spraying. Fusion is formed as the result of submucosally invasive cancer lifting the mucosal crease between the gastric folds. Based on this finding, this lesion is diagnosed as submucosally invasive cancer (T1b, SM) (Fig. 3.17b).

4 Diagnosis of Lateral Extensions

Akiko Takahashi

ESD is an excellent therapy, because it allows en bloc resections of targeted lesions. However, if preoperative determination of lateral extensions is inaccurate, postoperative pathological evaluation may result in positive lateral margins. Therefore, accurate preoperative diagnosis of lateral extensions is imperative. It is possible to observe surface and microvascular patterns in detail by combination of narrow band imaging (NBI) and magnified endoscopy. NBI magnified endoscopy is useful for diagnosis of lateral extensions of cancerous lesions [1, 2]. Diagnosis of lateral extensions by white light (WL) endoscopy, chromoendoscopy using indigo carmine, chromoendoscopy with acetic acid-indigo carmine mixture (AIM), and NBI magnified endoscopy are explained next. Limitations of NBI magnified endoscopy are discussed also.

4.1 White Light (WL) Endoscopy

The key point in determining lateral extensions by WL endoscopy is to carefully observe color differences and surface "bumps and dents." Differentiated adenocarcinomas often appear reddish with well-defined demarcations (Fig. 4.1a). However, demarcations may be obscured by inflammation of background mucosa by *Helicobacter pylori* infection or intestinal metaplasia (Fig. 4.1b). On the other hand,

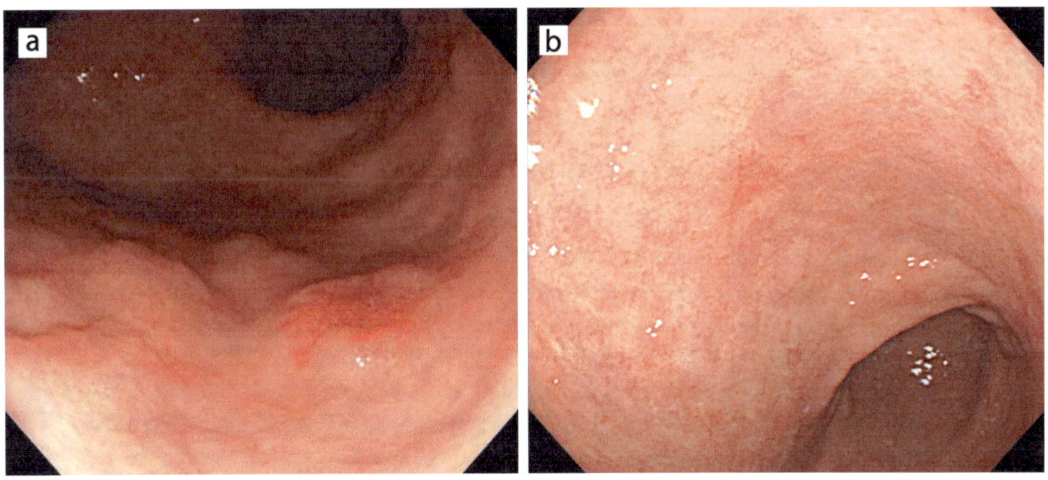

Fig. 4.1 Observation of differentiated adenocarcinoma by WL endoscopy. (**a**) A reddish lesion with clear demarcation. (**b**) A reddish lesion with unclear demarcation

A. Takahashi (✉)
Division of Endoscopy, Saku Central Hospital, 197 Usuda, Saku, Nagano 384-0301, Japan
e-mail: aurevoireurope@yahoo.co.jp

T. Oyama (ed.), *Endoscopic Diagnosis of Superficial Gastric Cancer for ESD*, DOI 10.1007/978-4-431-54469-2_4

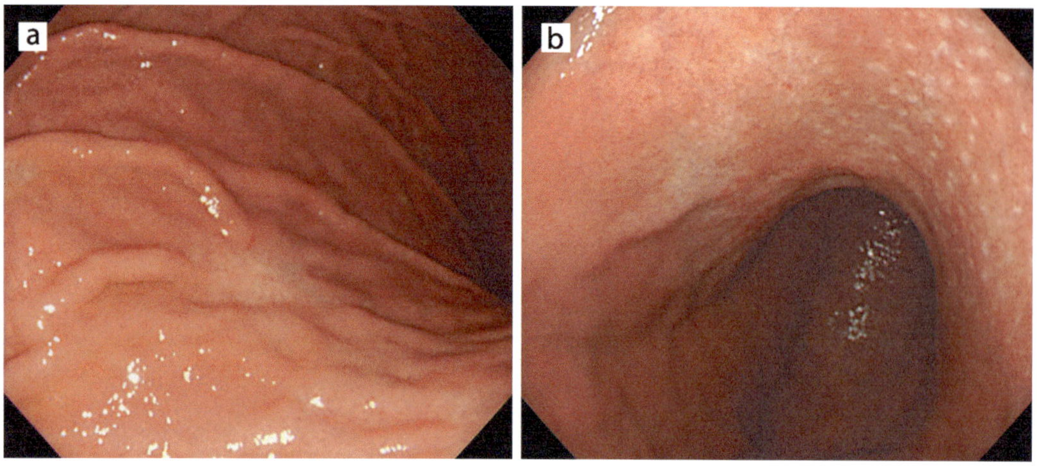

Fig. 4.2 Observation of an undifferentiated adenocarcinoma by WL endoscopy. (**a**) A pale-colored lesion with clear demarcation. (**b**) A pale-colored lesion with unclear demarcation

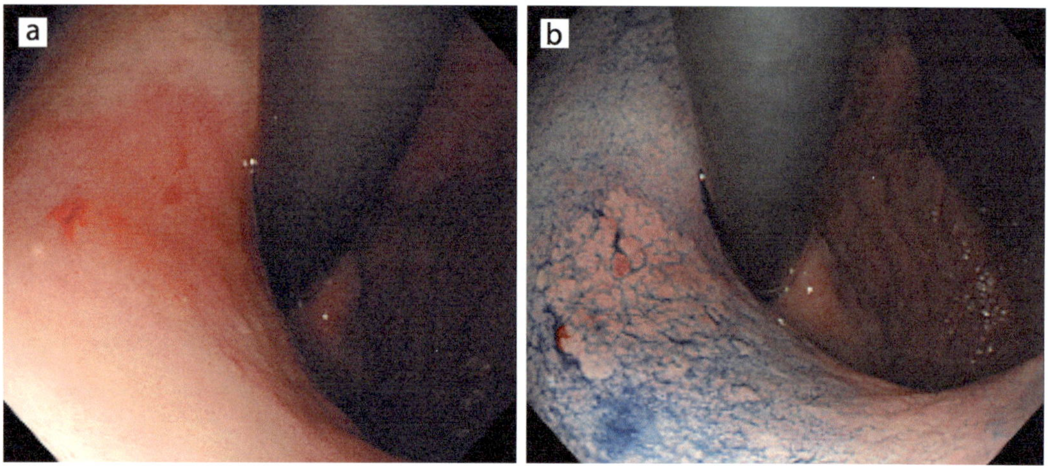

Fig. 4.3 Observation with indigo carmine method. (**a**) WL endoscopy shows a reddish lesion on the lesser curvature of gastric upper body. However, its demarcation is unclear. (**b**) Chromoendoscopy using indigo carmine shows clear demarcation around a lesion. It also shows that the surface pattern is rough

undifferentiated adenocarcinomas often appear pale with well-defined demarcations (Fig. 4.2a). However, demarcations may become less distinct with atrophy of background mucosa (Fig. 4.2b).

Protuberant lesions often are WDAs. Depressed lesions, on the other hand, can be either well-differentiated or undifferentiated adenocarcinomas. Both protuberant and depressed lesions may have flat 0-IIb extensions. And subtle differences in mucosal surfaces must be carefully observed.

4.2 Chromoendoscopy Using Indigo Carmine

The indigo carmine method is one of the "contrast" enhancing methods, in which indigo carmine dye is sprayed to enhance the surface patterns of the lesions by getting pooled in depressed parts of the mucosa (Fig. 4.3). If indigo carmine is sprayed onto lesions covered with mucus, surface patterns cannot be observed clearly. In such cases, the lesions must be rewashed with water to remove mucus. Only then can the lesions be observed well with indigo carmine spray (Fig. 4.4). Some flat lesions may become less distinct with spraying of indigo carmine (Fig. 4.5).

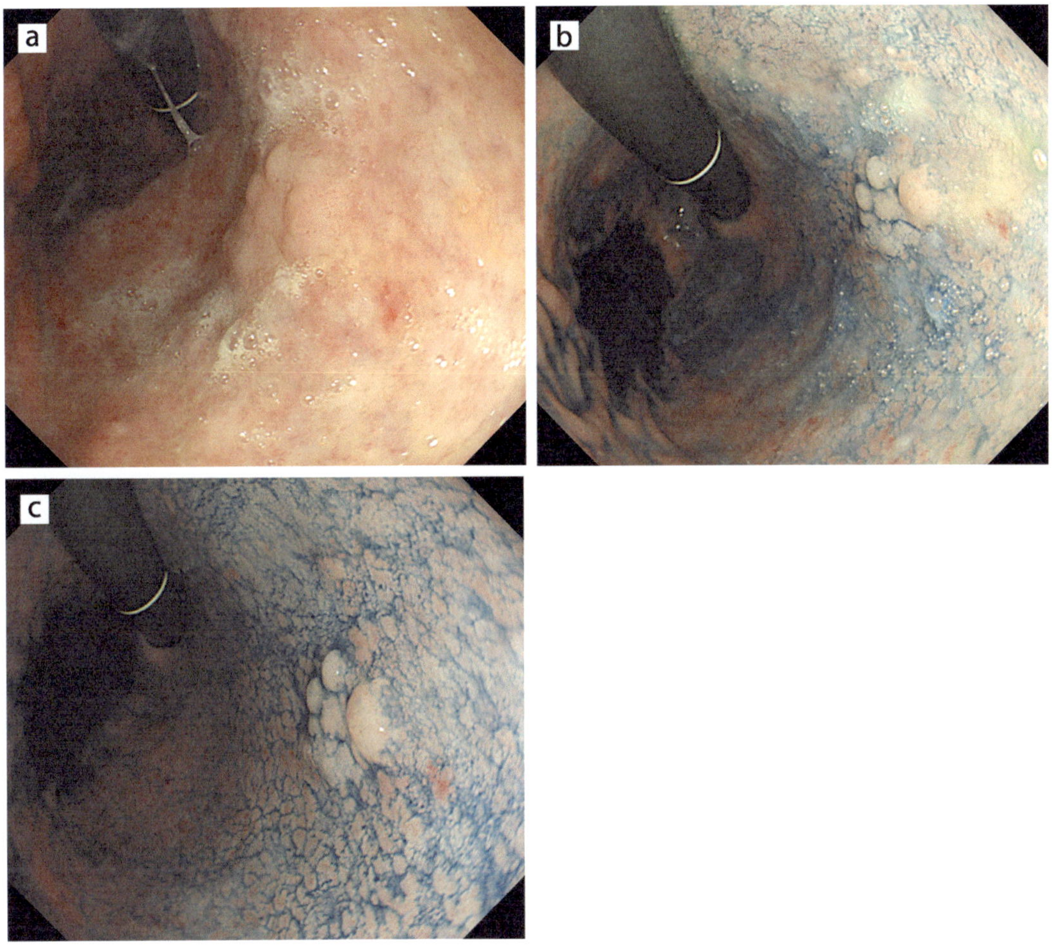

Fig. 4.4 Observation of a lesion with the mucus. (**a**) WL endoscopy before washing of the mucus. (**b**) Chromoendoscopy using indigo carmine without washing of the mucus. (**c**) Chromoendoscopy using indigo carmine after washing of the mucus by water again

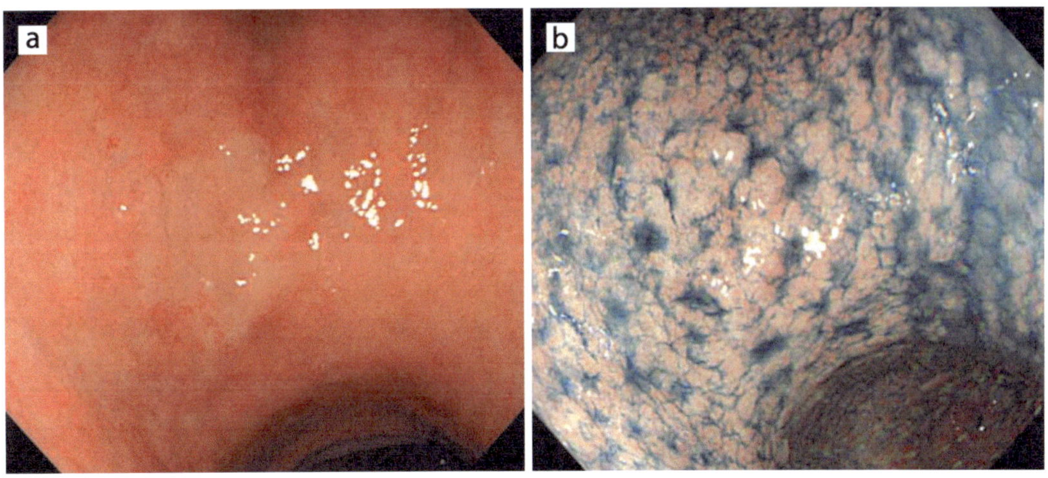

Fig. 4.5 Observation of a flat lesion. (**a**) WL endoscopy shows a whitish lesion with clear demarcation on the lesser curvature of a gastric lower body. (**b**) Chromoendoscopy using indigo carmine shows similar area patterns in both a lesion and its background mucosa. Therefore, the demarcation has become rather unclear with indigo carmine spray

4.3 Acetic Acid and Indigo Carmine Mixture (AIM) Method

The AIM method was developed by Kawahara and others [3] and uses liquid mixed with 0.6 % acetic acid and 0.04 % indigo carmine to be sprayed. Productions of mucus are influenced differently by acid in tumor parts compared with nontumor parts. While indigo carmine sprayed to tumor parts get washed out easily, indigo carmine sprayed to nontumor parts tend to remain unwashed. We can diagnose the borders of the lesions clearly by this mechanism (Fig. 4.6).

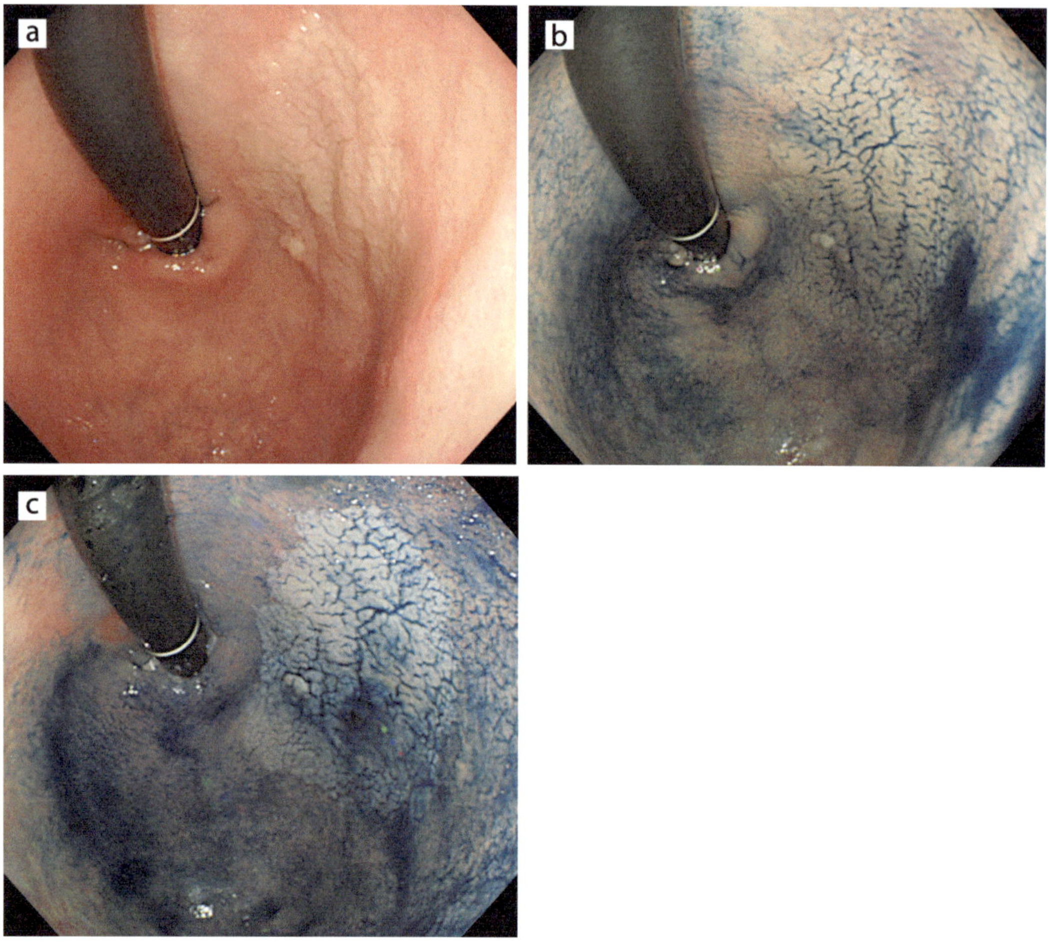

Fig. 4.6 Observation with AIM method. (**a**) WL endoscopy shows a whitish flat protuberant lesion on the anterior wall of a gastric upper body. Its demarcation can be traced almost all the way around by its coloration. However, the demarcation is partially unclear. (**b**) Chromoendoscopy using indigo carmine shows a lesion with rough mucosa as compared with the background mucosa. However, it still shows unclear demarcation without additional information. (**c**) The surface pattern is emphasized with the AIM method, clearly showing the demarcation

4.4 NBI Magnified Endoscopy

Gastric lumens are wide, and nonmagnified NBI images appear too dark for meaningful evaluations. NBI imaging must be combined with magnified endoscopy. It is used for diagnoses of lateral extensions and histological typing by observation of surface patterns and microvascular patterns. A special soft attachment such as black hood attachments™ by Olympus or Elastic touch™ by TOP is recommended for magnified endoscopy.

To better appreciate lateral extensions, background mucosa must be observed first, gradually approaching toward the target lesion to determine the lateral borders. With magnified endoscopy of gastric cancers, it is important to carefully observe the surface patterns and the vascular patterns. Pit-like surface patterns must be observed for their irregularities in shape and variations in size and density (Fig. 4.7a). Villous-like surface patterns must be observed for their irregularities in shape, variations in size, and density and for the presence of "fusions" (Fig. 4.7b).

Vascular patterns must be observed for caliber changes (Fig. 4.8a), for running irregularities (Fig. 4.8b), and for the presence of "network" patterns (Fig. 4.8c). Differences in surface patterns, vascular patterns, and background mucosa must be carefully observed to diagnose lateral extensions of gastric cancers [4–8].

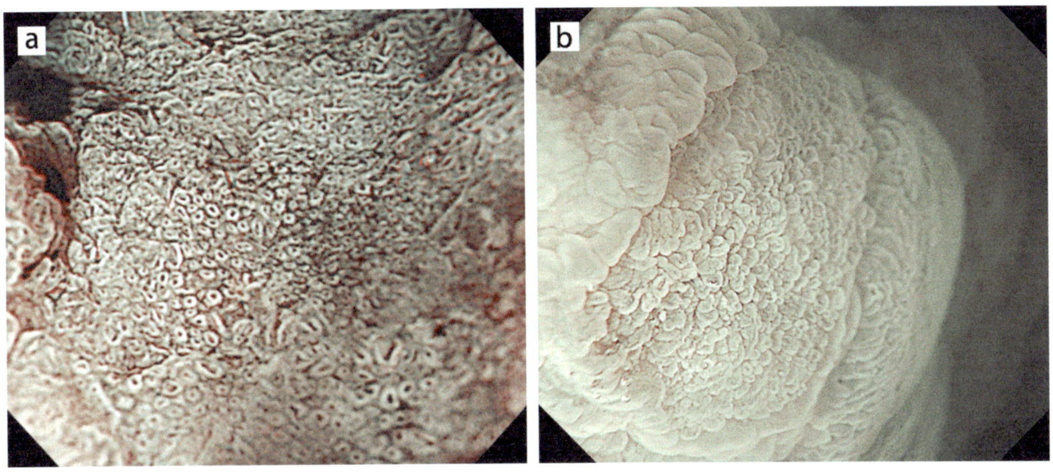

Fig. 4.7 (**a**) Pit-like surface pattern: NBI magnified endoscopy shows an irregular pit-like surface pattern with high density (**b**) Villous surface pattern: NBI magnified endoscopy shows an irregular villous surface pattern with high density and variable sizes. NBI magnified endoscopy shows a slightly irregular villous surface pattern with low density in the background mucosa

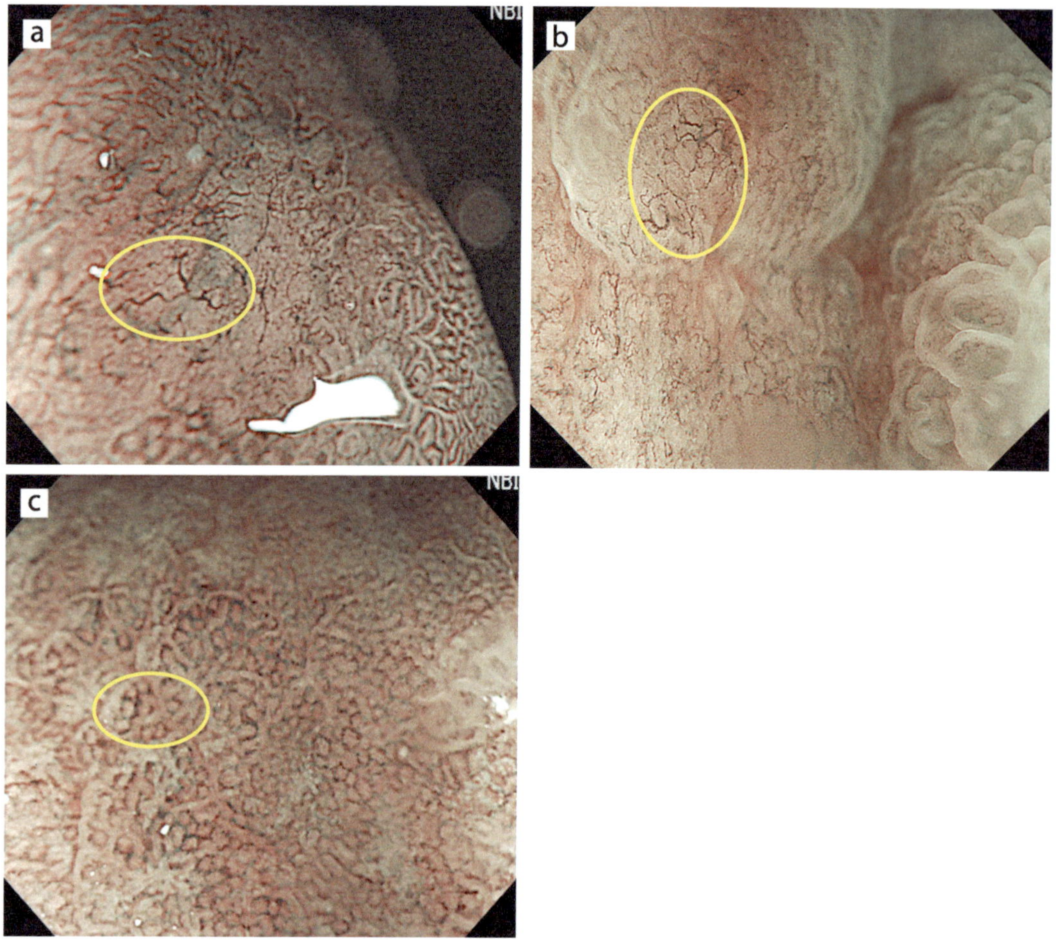

Fig. 4.8 Observation of vascular pattern. (**a**) Caliber change of vessels. (**b**) Running irregularity of vessels. (**c**) Network pattern of vessels

This case is a gastric cancer with 0-IIb that NBI magnified endoscopy was useful for diagnosis of its lateral extensions (Fig. 4.9).

4.5 Limitations in Observation with NBI Magnified Endoscopy

There are some cases in which it is difficult to diagnose the lateral extensions even with NBI magnified endoscopy. One of these cases is undifferentiated adenocarcinoma. The reason is that undifferentiated cancer can laterally extend at the level of the glandular neck zone of the mucosa without exposing itself to the mucosal surface and without causing changes to the vascular and the surface patterns. Therefore, it is necessary in all cases of undifferentiated adenocarcinoma to take biopsies 1 cm away from the margins of the lesions preoperatively to confirm that the biopsied spots are without cancer, allowing for safe margins for ESD.

Diagnosis of lateral extensions becomes difficult when both lesions and their surrounding mucosa have villous-like surface patterns [2, 9]. Therefore, when it is difficult to distinguish neoplastic from nonneoplastic parts even with the use of NBI magnified endoscopy, biopsies from both areas become necessary. It is important to document images of these specific areas before and after biopsies for later confirmation (Fig. 4.10). In addition, the order of which

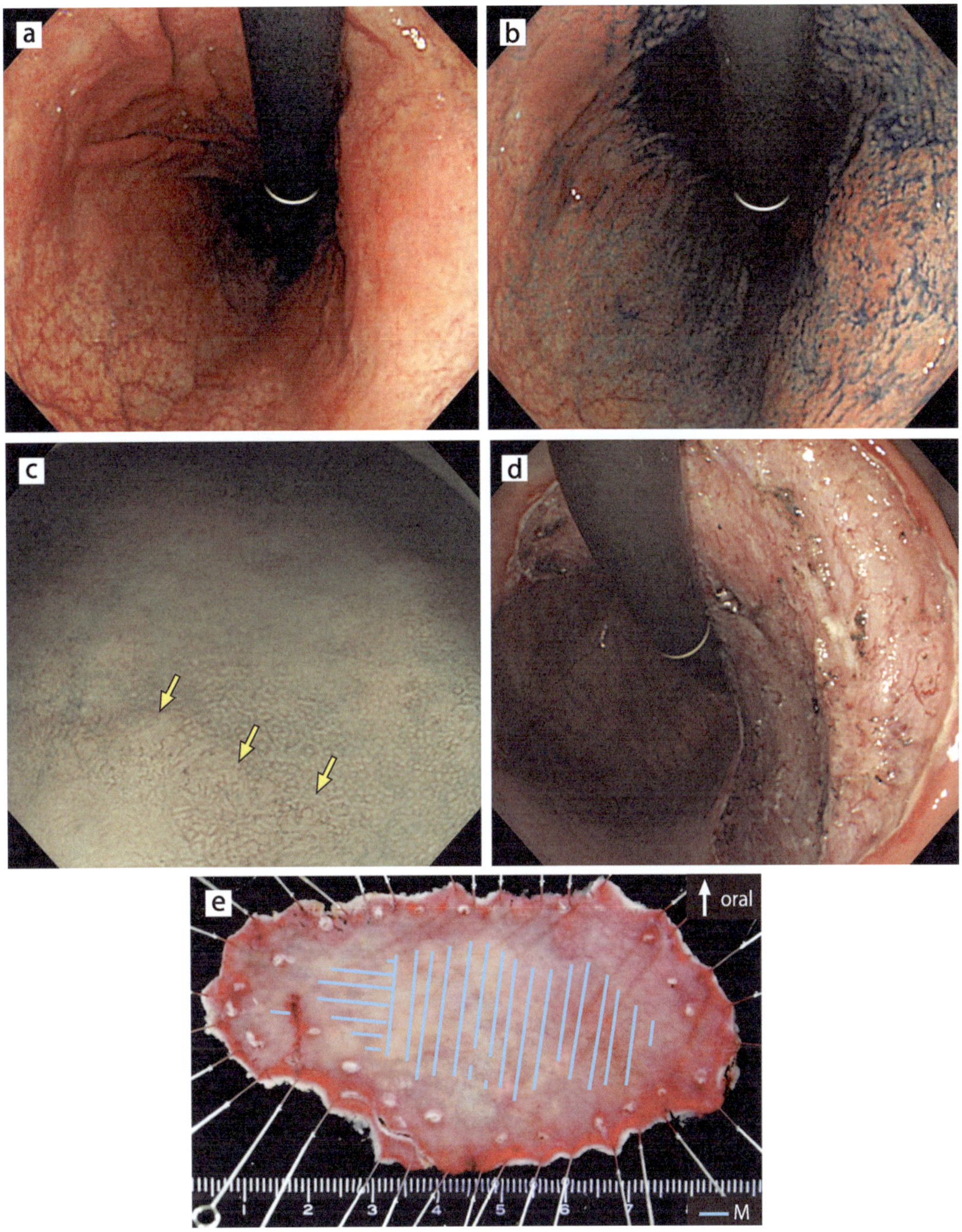

Fig. 4.9 Cancer with a 0-IIb extension. (**a**) WL endoscopy shows a reddish mucosal area without visible submucosal vessels on the posterior wall of a gastric middle body. Its demarcation is unclear. WL endoscopy shows no visible bumps or dents within and no appreciable difference in level with its surrounding mucosa. (**b**) Chromoendoscopy using indigo carmine shows rough surface pattern within the lesion compared with the areal pattern of the background mucosa. Chromoendoscopy using indigo carmine shows clear demarcation on the posterior wall. It shows unclear demarcation on the anal side and the anterior wall, showing a flat surface without bumps or dents. (**c**) NBI magnified endoscopy shows mixed villous and pit-like surface patterns with irregular shape and variable sizes and vascular pattern showing mild caliber changes and running irregularities within the lesion compared with a regular pit-like pattern of the background mucosa. A demarcation line may be drawn between the lesion and its surrounding mucosa by differences in surface and vascular patterns (arrows). (**d**) Therefore, the lesion can be diagnosed to have a wide lateral extension by NBI magnified endoscopy. It was diagnosed as a WDA, T1a-M, 0-IIb+IIa, and was resected en bloc by ESD. (**e**) The final diagnosis was "gastric well-differentiated adenocarcinoma, T1a-M, p Type 0-IIb +0-IIa, 56 × 24 mm, lymph duct and venous invasion negative, lateral, and vertical margins negative"

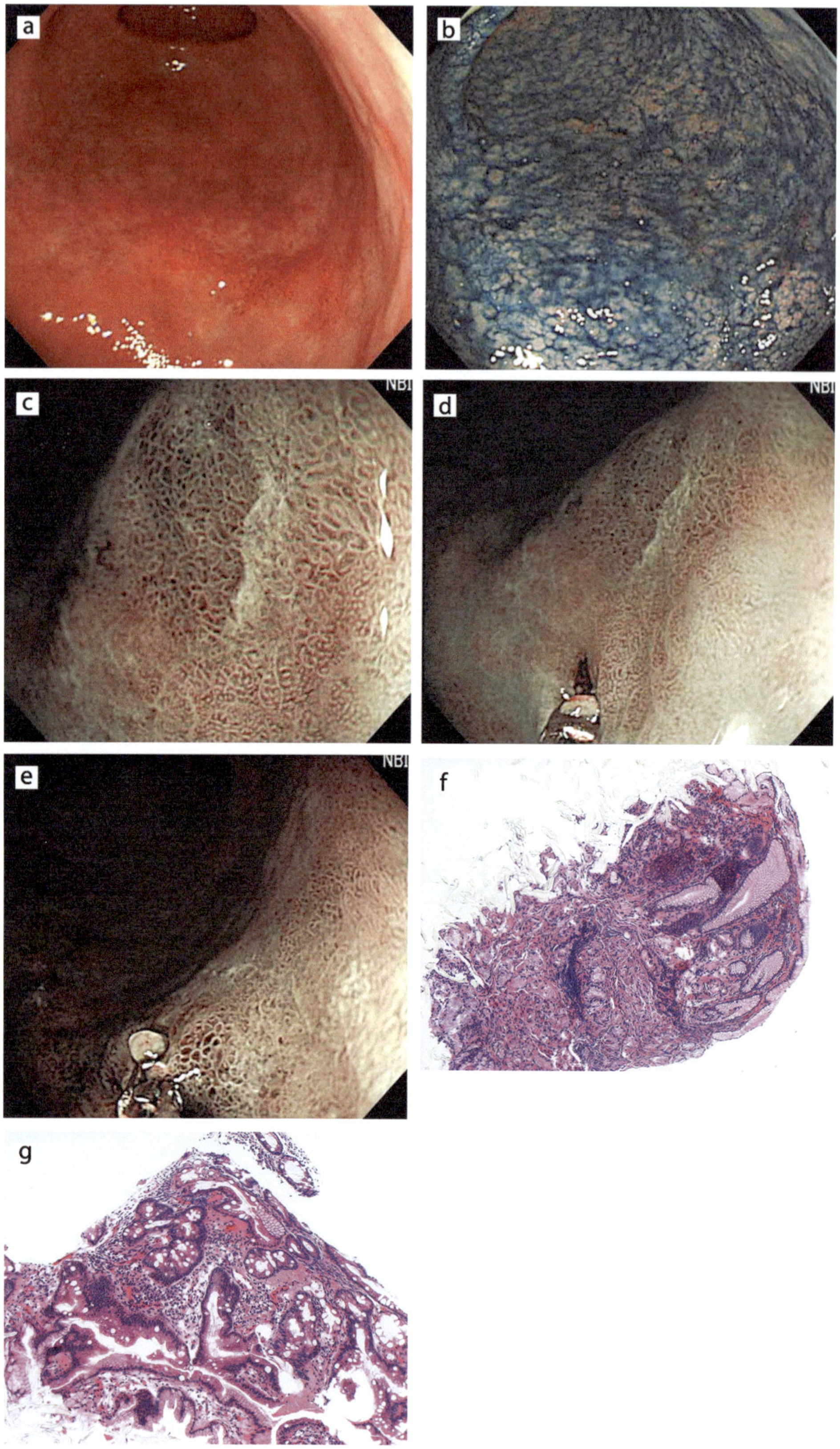

Fig. 4.10 A case in which NBI magnified endoscopy was not effective. (**a**) WL endoscopy shows reddish mucosa with unclear demarcation on the greater curvature of a gastric middle to lower body. (**b**) Chromoendoscopy using indigo carmine shows a lesion with rough mucosa and unclear demarcation compared with the background mucosa. It is difficult to determine whether this is a neoplastic tumor or not by WL endoscopy and chromoendoscopy using indigo carmine. (**c**, **d**, **e**) NBI magnified endoscopy of the oral side of the lesion showed a regular pit-like pattern on the lower right side of the picture (**c**). This area was diagnosed as benign. On the other hand, NBI magnified endoscopy of the oral side of the lesion showed a surface pattern consisting of enlarged villi with irregular shape and variable sizes (**c**). It was suspected that this area was the demarcation. However, biopsies had to be taken from both sides (**d** and **e**) of the demarcation to confirm the diagnosis. (**f**, **g**) Pathologically, a biopsy from the lower area (**d**) showed fundic glands (**f**) and a biopsy from the upper area (**e**) showed WDA (**g**). Therefore, it confirmed that this part was the margin of the lesion

areas to take biopsies from must be decided carefully by taking into consideration the direction of bleeding blood when biopsies are taken, so as not to obscure the areas to be observed with bleeding blood.

Observation with NBI magnified endoscopy is very useful for diagnosis of lateral extensions for gastric cancers. However, use of higher magnification limits its application to observation of very narrow areas. Observation of wider areas by indigo carmine method and AIM method are also essential. Combining these methods with NBI magnified endoscopy is necessary, supplementing its limitations.

References

1. Sumiyama K et al. Narrow band imaging for ESD. Stomach and Intestine. 2005;40:809–16.
2. Takahashi A et al. A case of differentiated early adenocarcinoma that narrow band imaging (NBI) magnified endoscopy was useful in diagnosis of lateral extensions. Endosc Forum Dig Dis. 2006;22:17–21.
3. Kawahara Y et al. Novel chromoendoscopic method using an acetic acid-indigocarmine mixture for diagnostic accuracy in delineating the margin of early gastric cancers. Dig Endosc. 2009;21:14–9.
4. Tomori A et al. Usability of magnifying endoscope in differential diagnosis of a gastric small depressed lesion. Stomach and Intestine. 2006;41:795–803.
5. Nakayoshi T et al. Magnifying endoscopy combined with narrow band imaging system for early gastric cancer: correlation of vascular pattern with histopathology. Endoscopy. 2004;36:1080–4.
6. Kaise M et al. Endoscopic diagnosis of gastric cancer using magnifying endoscopy combined with narrow band imaging system. Clin Gastroenterol. 2006;21:47–53.
7. Fujisaki J et al. Diagnosis of early gastric cancer with magnifying endoscopy, emphasizing use of magnifying narrow band imaging. Clin Gastroenterol. 2006;21:431–40.
8. Kaise M et al. Magnifying endoscopy combined with narrow-band imaging for differential diagnosis of superficial depressed gastric lesions. Endoscopy. 2009;41:310–5.
9. Takahashi A et al. Diagnosis of lateral extensions of gastric cancers by NBI magnified endoscopy. Gastroenterol Endosc. 2006;48 Suppl 2:1873.

5 Diagnosis of Gastric Adenocarcinoma with Magnified Endoscopy

Tsuneo Oyama

Many magnified endoscopic classifications have been reported [1–5]. But a large majority of them are difficult to understand and complicated. The author divided the magnified endoscopic findings into two basic categories of surface and vascular patterns to simplify the diagnostic process [6, 7]. The theory behind this diagnostic approach with magnified endoscopy is explained in this chapter.

5.1 What Does Magnified Endoscopy Show?

In general, observation of vascular structures is emphasized with magnified endoscopy. The vessels are not the cancer itself but they are only affected by the cancer, which could be interpreted as "victims" whose running course are thwarted by the disease. The surface pattern which shows the "villain," the cancer itself, also provides useful diagnostic information. Understanding characteristics of both methods, the method of directly targeting the "villain" (surface structure) and the method of obtaining information from the "victims" (vascular structure), is the key to making a correct diagnosis with magnified endoscopy.

5.2 Surface Patterns

Sakaki classified the gastric surface patterns into seven groups. His classification is the basis of magnified endoscopic diagnosis. The author further simplified to divide the surface patterns into two groups, "villus-like" and "pit-like." "Villi" are finger-like projections, and "pits" are holes in the mucosal surface.

What can one tell from the surface structure? "Theoretical background"

The keys to pathological diagnosis of cancer are structural and nuclear irregularities. Structural irregularities are observed by 40-fold magnification, while nuclear irregularities are observed by 200–400-fold magnification. The maximum magnification by magnified endoscopy is 70–80-fold range. Although not sufficient for observation of nuclear irregularities, its magnification is sufficient for observation of structural irregularities.

5.2.1 Villous Patterns

Villous patterns refer to finger-like projections. Nonneoplastic villi are similar in shape and size and of lower duct density with spaces in between (Fig. 5.1). On the other hand, cancerous villi are densely packed and irregularly shaped (Fig. 5.2).

5.2.1.1 Keys to Observation of Villous Patterns

Nonneoplastic villi are regularly shaped without size variations and are evenly placed with enough spaces in between. They are also surrounded evenly by white zones (Fig. 5.1). In contrast, cancerous villi have various shapes and are densely packed. They are surrounded by uneven white zones (Fig. 5.2).

T. Oyama (✉)
Division of Endoscopy, Saku Central Hospital, 197 Usuda, Saku, Nagano 384-0301, Japan
e-mail: oyama@coral.ocn.ne.jp

T. Oyama (ed.), *Endoscopic Diagnosis of Superficial Gastric Cancer for ESD*, DOI 10.1007/978-4-431-54469-2_5

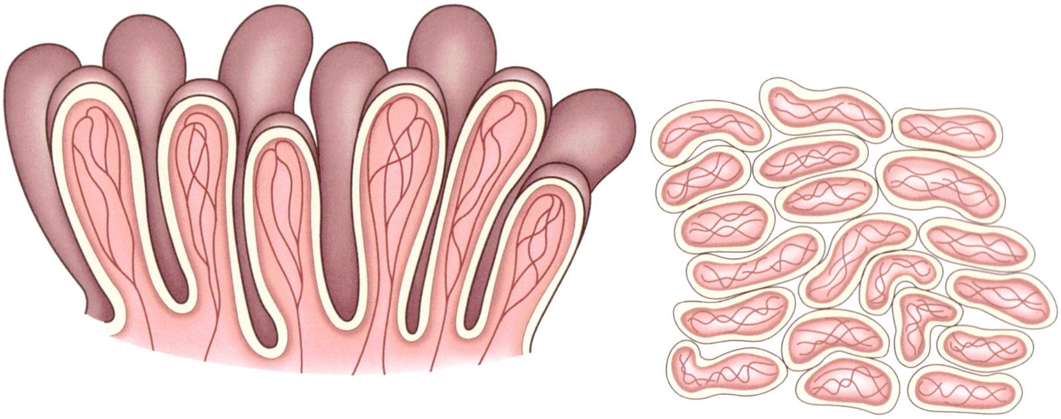

Fig. 5.1 Villous pattern (nonneoplastic)

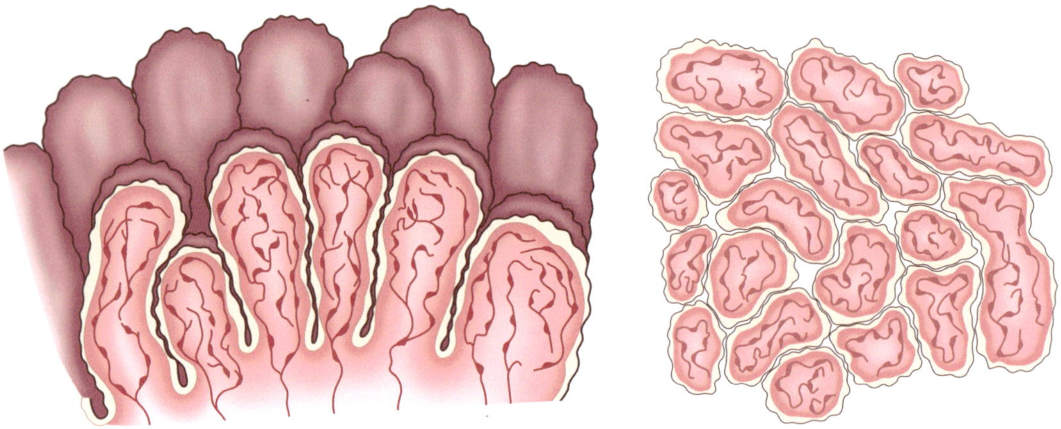

Fig. 5.2 Villous pattern (cancer)

5.2.1.2 Villous Patterns Observed with NBI Magnified Endoscopy

Figure 5.3 shows a case of villous pattern. Finger-like elongated structures are observed. All villi are regularly shaped and evenly spaced. Each villus is independent, and the lesion was diagnosed as nonneoplastic glands. The edge of villi looks like whitish line by NBI. Yagi and his colleagues named his phenomenon as white zone [8].

Figure 5.4a shows a cancer with a villous pattern. Regular villous pattern is noted on the upper side. However, irregular villous pattern is observed in the center part surrounded by a yellow dotted line (Fig. 5.4b). The shape of villi is irregular and their size uneven. The demarcation is recognized by the difference of surface pattern.

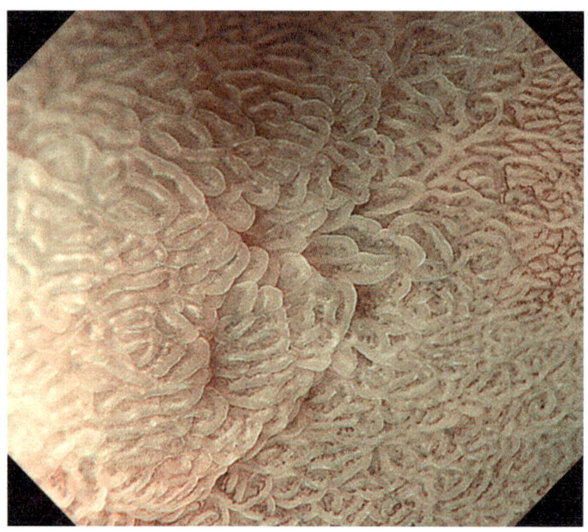

Fig. 5.3 Villous pattern (nonneoplastic case)

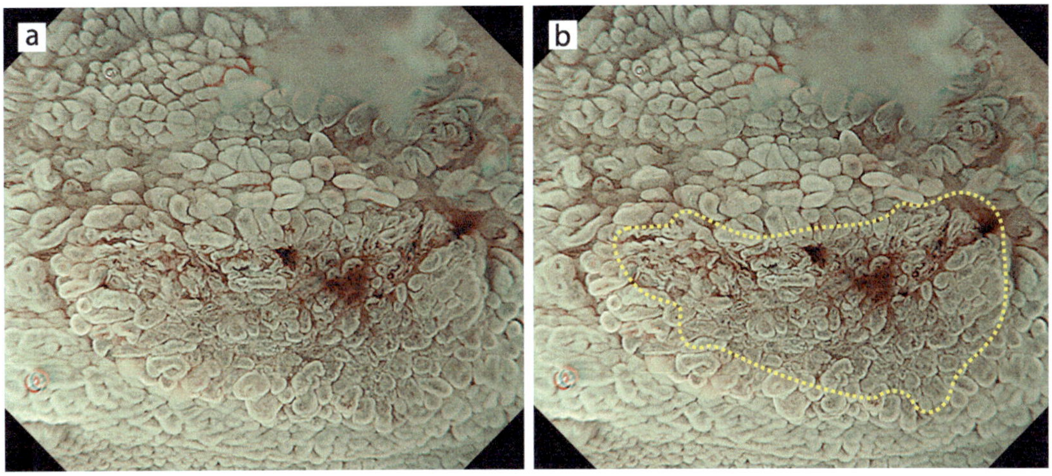

Fig. 5.4 Villous pattern (cancer case)

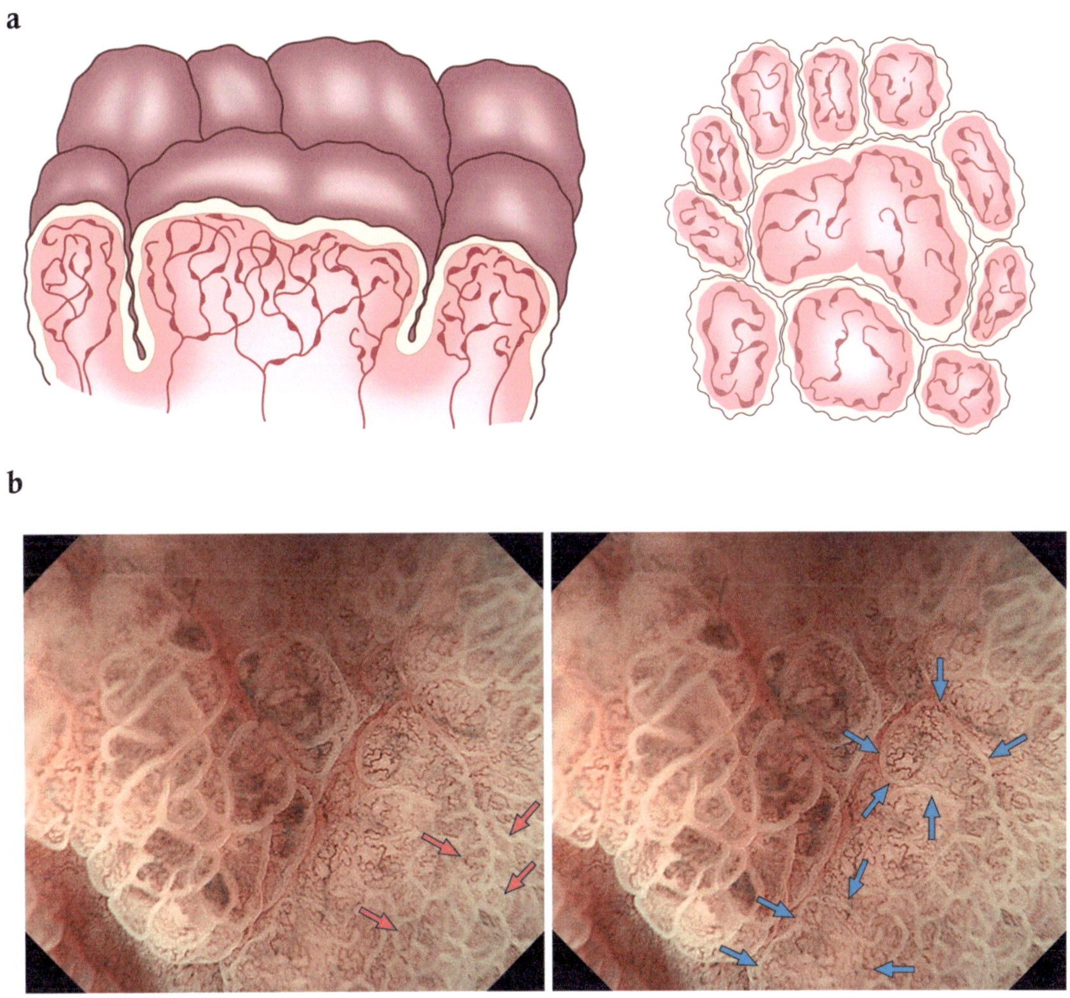

Fig. 5.5 Fusion of villi. (**a**) Irregularly shaped variable-size villi are noted (*red arrows*). (**b**) Fusion of villi is noted (*blue arrows*)

5.2.1.3 Fusion of Villi

WDA usually shows a villous pattern. Fusion of villi, seen with highly irregular villous patterns, may represent a case of moderately differentiated adenocarcinoma (MDA). The red arrows show a villous pattern while the blue arrows show fusion of villi (Fig. 5.5a, b).

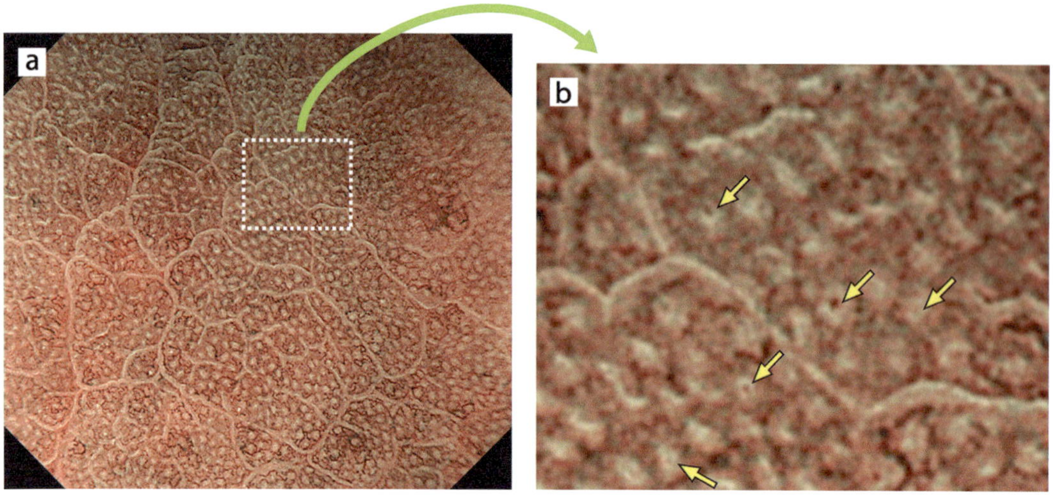

Fig. 5.6 Pit pattern in fundic gland area

> **Key Points in Diagnosis of Villous Patterns**
>
> - Shape
> - Size
> - Density
> - Width of white zone

5.2.2 Pit Patterns

A pit-like structure is a hole-like burrowed structure. The shape of nonneoplastic pit is round and surrounded by a network of regular vessels. A pit should be seen as a black circle by NBI. However, the size of these holes is too small to be identified with moderate magnification power. Pits are surrounded by glandular epithelia which appear white by light reflection. Therefore, a pit is seen as a white circle by low or moderate power magnification,

Figure 5.6a is a magnified endoscopic image of the fundic glands. There are many white spots. But black holes are observed inside the white circles with maximum magnification (Fig. 5.6b). Therefore, pits appear black when carefully observed with maximum magnification.

Pits are surrounded by glandular epithelia, which appear white when observed with NBI. With low to moderately magnified NBI, black pits are too small to be recognized, but the surrounding glandular epithelia are recognized as white round structures. Therefore, structures represented by white dots seen with low to moderate magnification represent the pit-like structures.

Pits seen in nonneoplastic mucosa are represented by pit-like structures noted in fundic gland areas (Fig. 5.6a). They are small circles regularly spaced without size variations. In contrast, pit-like structures noted in cancer are irregularly shaped, varied in size, and densely placed.

5.2.2.1 Structure of Nonneoplastic Pits

Nonneoplastic pits are regularly shaped and surrounded by networks of regular microvessels (Fig. 5.7).

5.2.2.2 Structure of Cancerous Pits

Cancerous pits are densely placed and irregularly shaped with uneven sizes. And irregular microvessels are observed in the interstitial spaces between them (Fig. 5.8).

> **Key Points in Diagnosis of Pit Patterns**
>
> - Shape
> - Size
> - Density

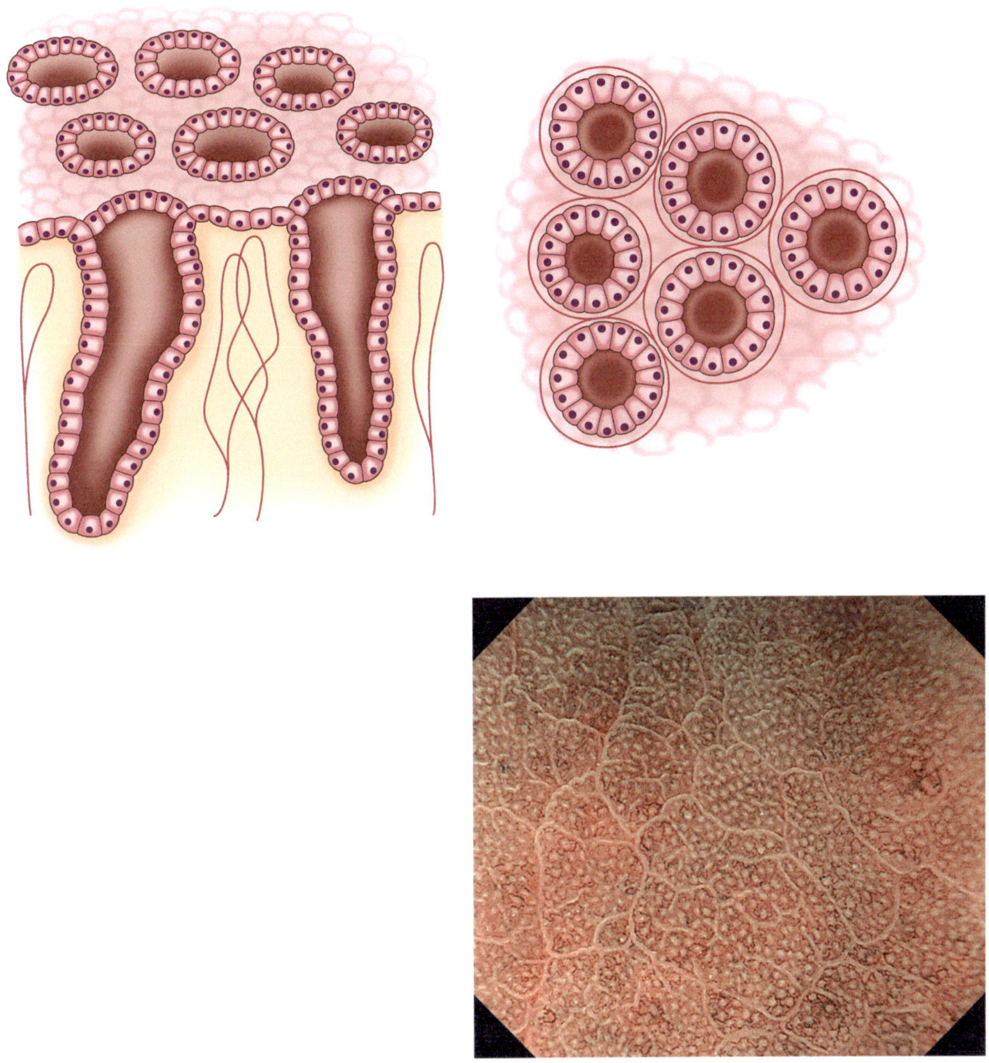

Fig. 5.7 Pit pattern (nonneoplastic)

5.3 Vascular Patterns

Caliber changes, tortuosity, and presence of absence of network formations are the important points to observe in microvessels. Caliber change means the change of diameter. When the diameter of microvessels becomes thicker or thinner abruptly, the microvessels are judged to have a caliber change. When a caliber change greater than the diameter the vessel occurs, the change is judged significant. Tortuosity of vessels however is rather subjective. A network represents a closed-loop formation of a microvessel. When a vascular loop is traced to return to its origin, a network is judged to be present.

5.3.1 Key Points in Diagnosis of Vascular Patterns

The space between glandular ducts is called the parenchyma in which blood vessels run. When the basic structure is a pit pattern, microvessels run around the pits to form networks. When vascular networks are found, a diagnosis of WDA can be made, as reported by Nakayoshi and his colleagues as a good sign of WDA [2].

On the other hand, PDA infiltrates through the parenchyma destroying preexisting glandular structures. Therefore, microvessels, rather than forming networks, branches in complex fashions, running tortuously. Nakayoshi described these irregular microvessels as “corkscrew” vessels. Since the vessels are not forming spirals like corkscrews, the author uses the term of “nonnetwork” to describe these irregular microvessels.

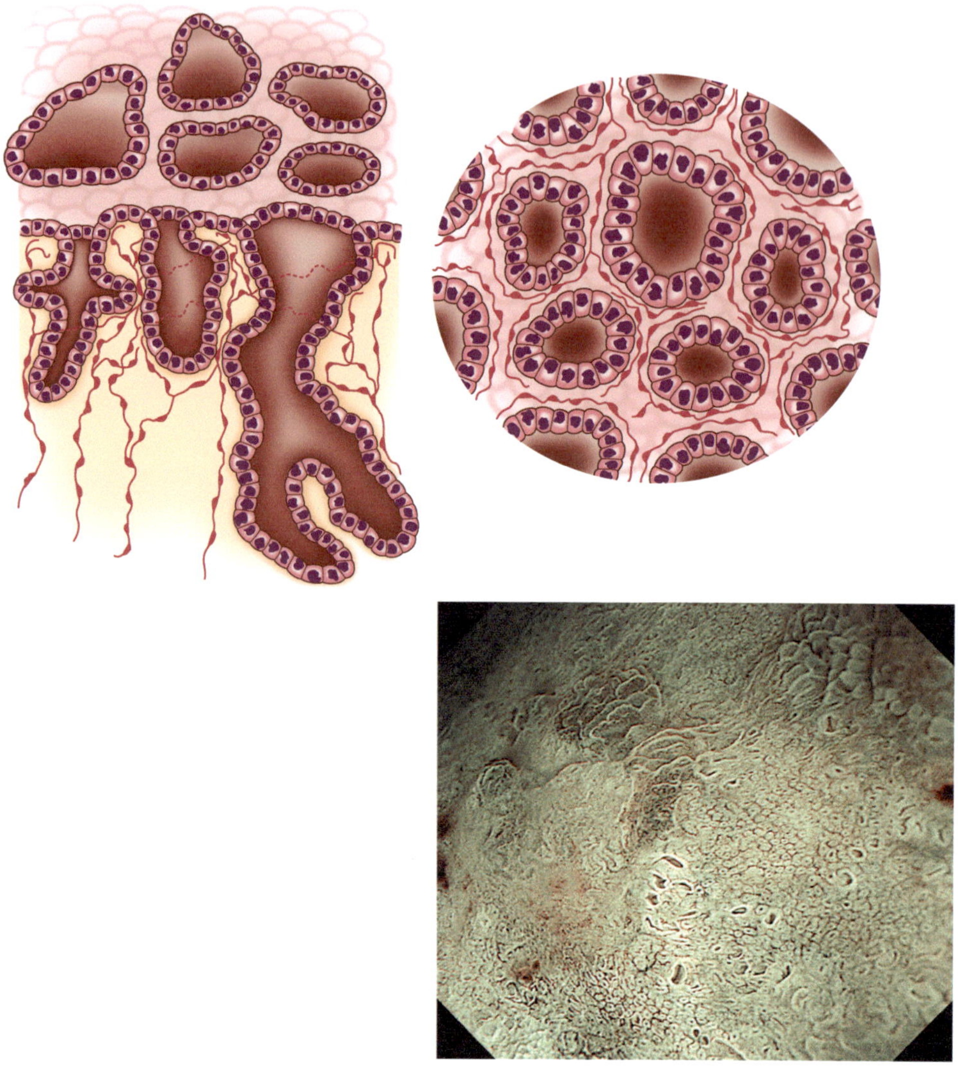

Fig. 5.8 Pit pattern (cancer)

Key Points in Diagnosis of Vascular Patterns

- Caliber change
- Tortuosity
- Presence of absence of network formation

5.4 Relationship Between Surface Pattern and Vascular Pattern

5.4.1 Villous Structure and Vascular Pattern

Vascular running and the surface structure are closely related to each other. When the surface pattern is villi-like, blood vessels can run within each villus but not across villi. Vascular running laterally becomes limited to a short distance. Running irregularities therefore become difficult to judge, and caliber changes are mainly evaluated (Fig. 5.9).

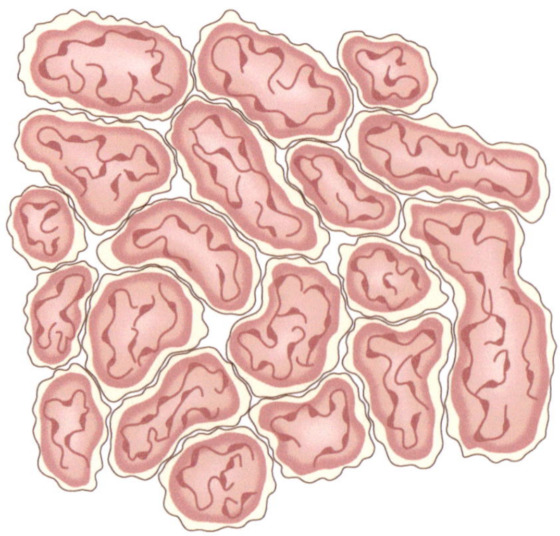

Fig. 5.9 Blood vessels within villi

When duct density is high, villi may be so densely packed to make the surface structure obscure. But for the basic structure of villous pattern, vessels cannot run across adjacent villi and short vessels alone are observed.

Villous structures and irregular microvessel within the villi are observed on the left side of Fig. 5.10a. But the surface structure becomes unclear in the central part. But, since the lengths of visible microvessels appear short, the basic structure can be suggested to be a villous pattern. Figure 5.10b is NBI magnified endoscopy after acetic acid spreading. The surface pattern becomes enhanced and clearly shows a villous pattern in the central part. This was not visible previously with NBI magnified endoscopy but suggested by microvascular observation.

Like this case, it is possible to predict a surface pattern from vascular structures. Also, the use of acetic acid spraying makes more detailed observation of surface structures possible. Sometimes, observations of surface patterns become possible after acetic acid application even for cases where surface patterns appear unclear with NBI magnified endoscopy.

However, if fusion of villi occurs, vessels can run longer distances laterally; their tortuosity and caliber changes become easily observable (Fig. 5.11).

5.4.2 Pit-Like Structure and Vascular Pattern

When the basic structure is a pit pattern, microvessels can run longer, showing running irregularities and caliber changes, at the same time as making a network around each pit (Fig. 5.12). Sometimes, the surface pattern becomes uncertain, when the density of glands is extremely high. However, if a network microvascular pattern is observed, it is possible to predict a pit to exist at the center of the network. Network patterns become a good marker of WDA.

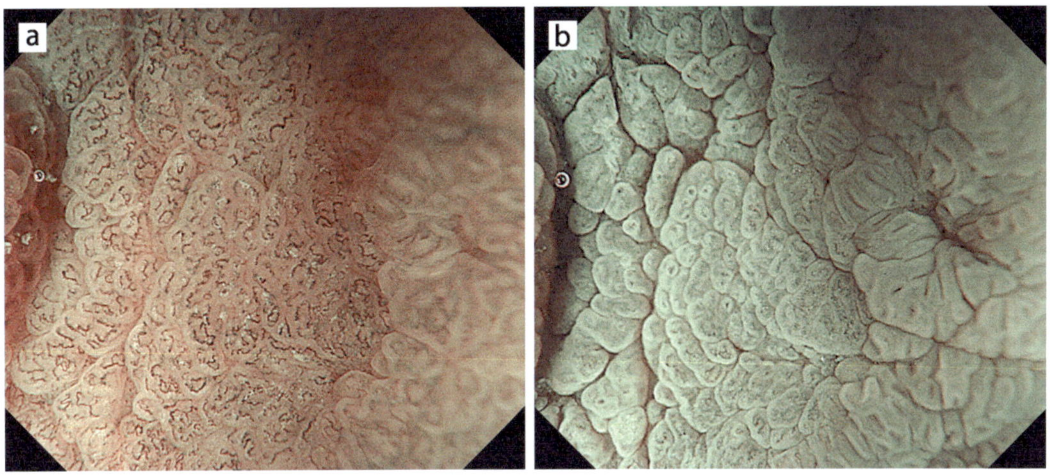

Fig. 5.10 (**a**) NBI magnified endoscopic image. (**b**) Image obtained after acetic acid spraying

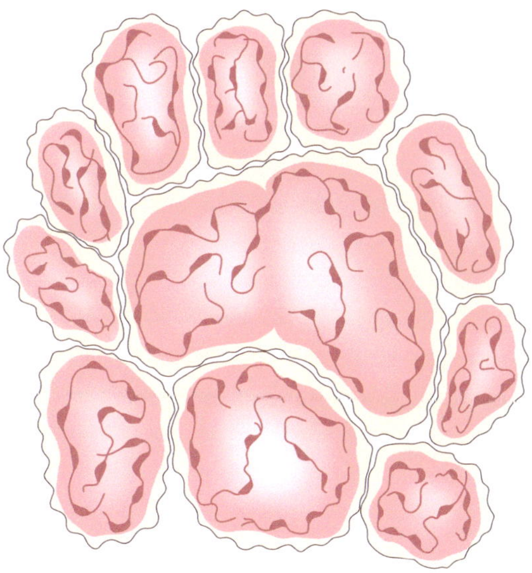

Fig. 5.11 Blood vessels within fused villi

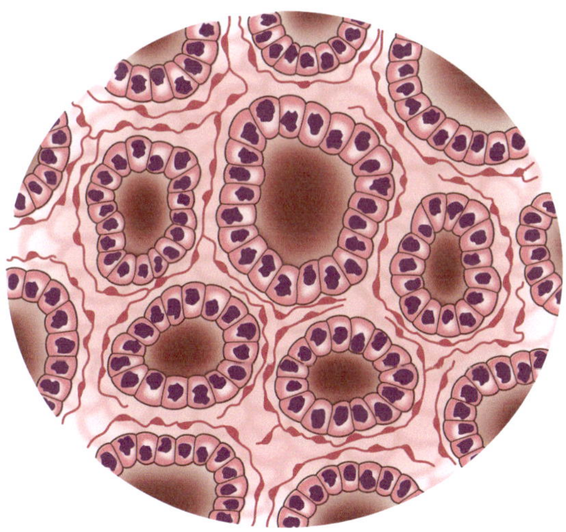

Fig. 5.12 Blood vessels surrounding pits

Microvessels with network are observed on the right side of Fig. 5.13a, but the surface pattern is uncertain without visible pit-like structures. However, pits can be identified as black openings clearly visible within networks after acetic acid spraying (Fig. 5.13b). Acetic acid is very useful for observation of surface patterns. Like this case, pit-like structures may exist even when the surface shows "no structure"; we use the term "uncertain" or "unclear" rather than "no structure" to describe when a surface pattern cannot be determined.

On the other hand, moderately differentiated adenocarcinoma has ducts branching irregularly, modifying the shape of the parenchyma irregularly as well. As the blood vessels must run through the parenchyma, vascular structures become complicated, unable to form networks. Presence or absence of networks, therefore, is useful for pathological diagnosis.

5.5 Diagnosis of Histological Type by Magnified Endoscopy

Basically, WDA grows, replacing the whole layer of nonneoplastic glands, and manifests its surface pattern differently. For example, irregularly shaped pits or villi, as well as uneven sizes, or fusion of villi may be seen. With moderately differentiated adenocarcinomas, the surface structures often become unclear. In general, PDA destroys preexisting glandular ducts, and the surface structure becomes unclear. However, when PDA extends laterally at the level of glandular neck area leaving the glandular ducts intact, the surface pattern may not show atypia. Figure 5.14 shows the findings of magnified endoscopy. Thick line shows the highest incidence, thin line moderate incidence, and dotted line low incidence.

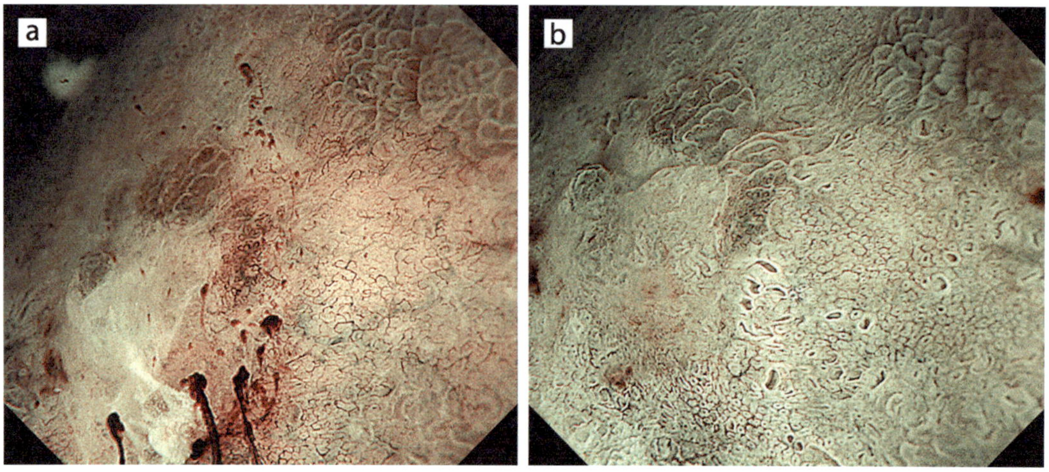

Fig. 5.13 Pit pattern and blood vessels. (**a**) NBI magnified endoscopic image. (**b**) Image obtained after acetic acid spraying

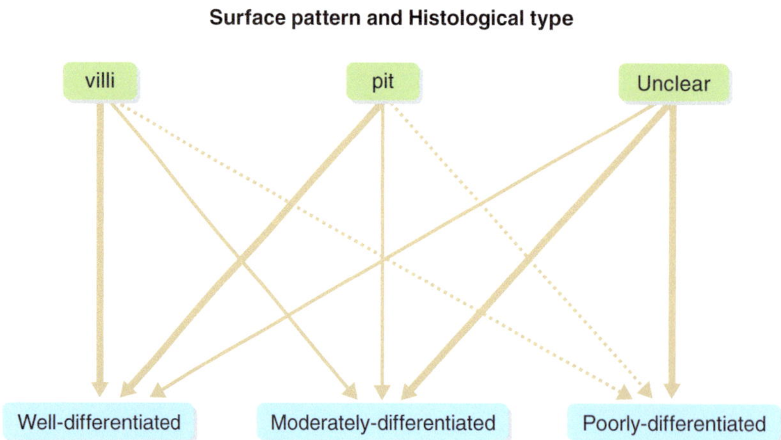

Fig. 5.14 Chart 1 surface pattern and histological type

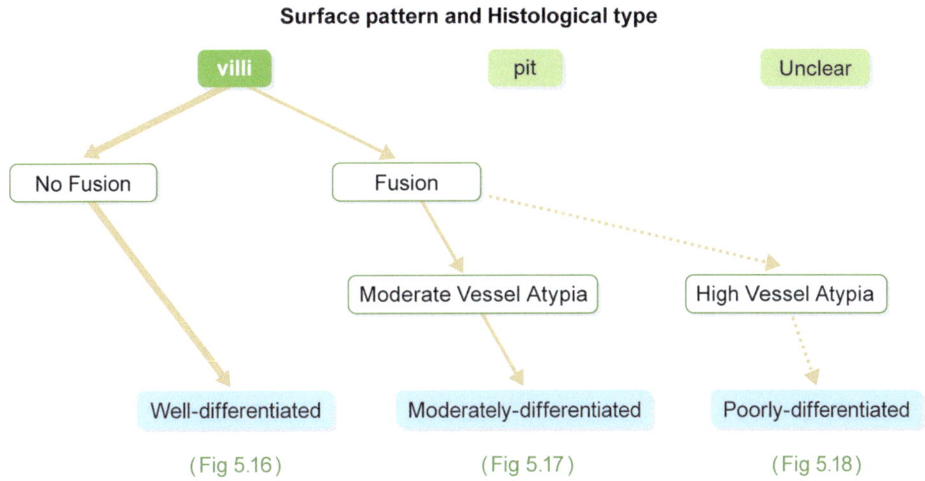

Fig. 5.15 Chart 2 surface pattern and histological type (villous pattern)

5.5.1 Villous Pattern

Irregular villous patterns can confirm diagnosis of WDA regardless of vascular patterns. But, when villous patterns show fusion of villi, moderate to PDA must be distinguished. Therefore, observation of micro vascular pattern and acetic acid spraying become necessary for further examination (Fig. 5.15).

Irregular villi are observed in Fig. 5.16. The density is high, and the size of villi is uneven. The lesion is diagnosed as WDA from such findings.

Irregular villous pattern is observed on the right side of Fig. 5.17a. And the villi are smaller and fused in the central part. The histology of the central part is MDA (Fig. 5.17b).

Figure 5.18a is a NBI magnified endoscopic view of PDA. Villous pattern is observed in the upper part (Fig. 5.18b, red arrow). The shape of villi is regular, and the density low. The surface pattern of the central part is uncertain (Fig. 5.18c, blue arrow). But irregularly running micro vessels with caliber changes and nonnetwork micro vessels is observed supporting the diagnosis of PDA. And the same irregular vascular pattern is also observed in the regular appearing villi of Fig. 5.18b.

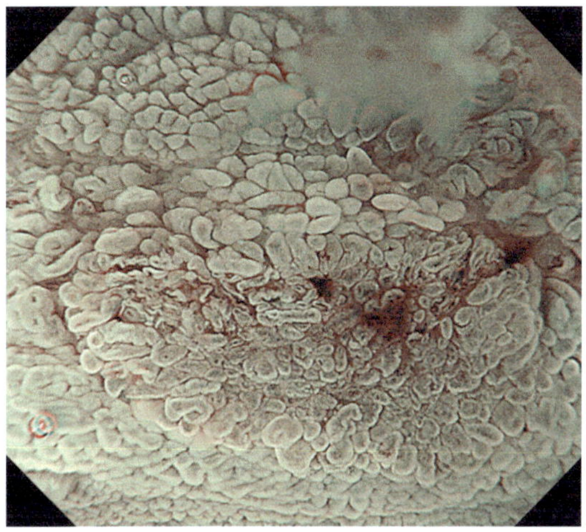

Fig. 5.16 Villous pattern of WDA (without fusion of villi) (same as Fig. 5.4a)

5.5.2 Pit Pattern

Irregular pit means WDA or MDA. The surface pattern becomes unclear when PDA becomes exposed to the surface. However, a regular pit pattern may remain, when the volume of PDA is small and cancer spreads laterally through

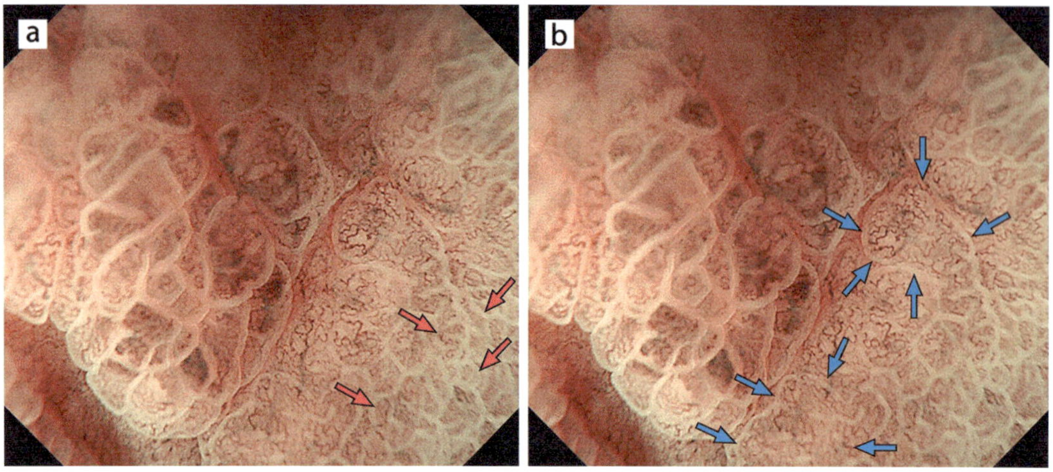

Fig. 5.17 Villous pattern of MDA (with fusion) (same as Fig. 5.5). (**a**) Irregularly shaped variable-size villi are noted (*red arrows*). (**b**) Fusion of villi is noted (*blue arrows*)

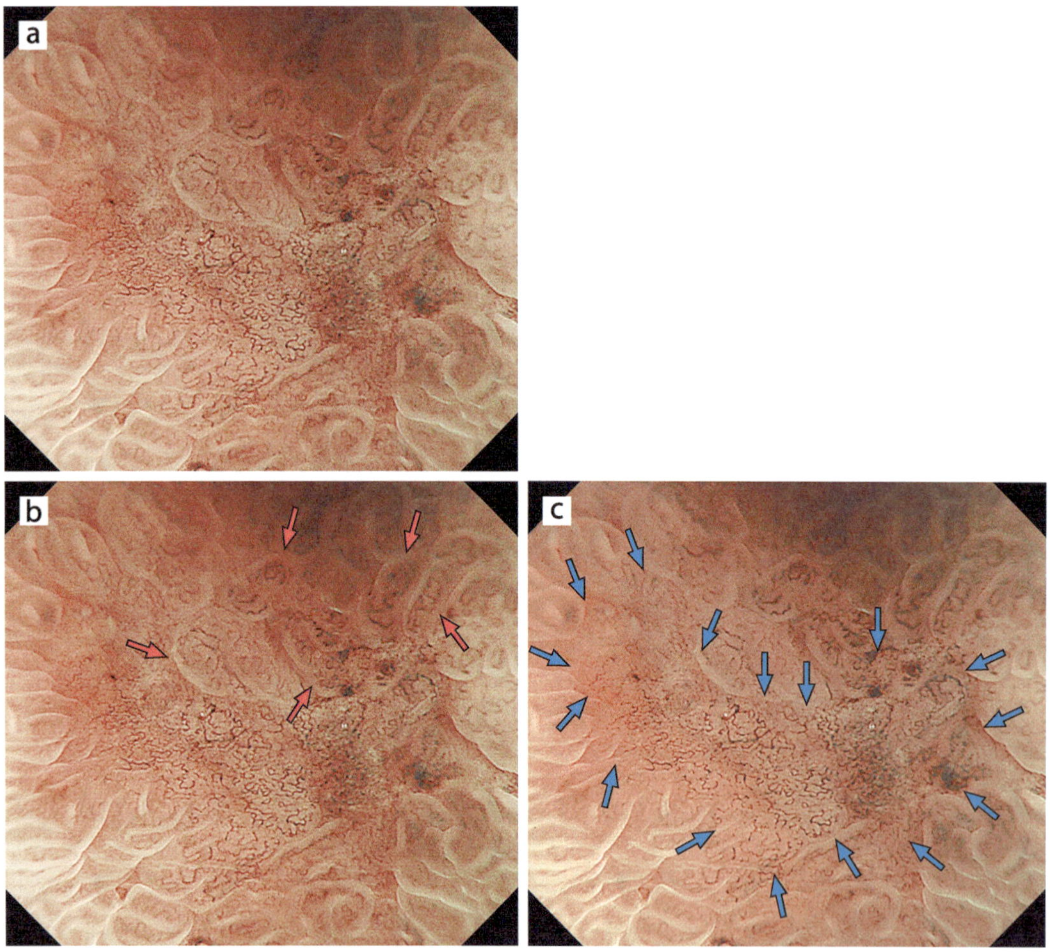

Fig. 5.18 Villous pattern of PDA (with fusion). (**a**) NBI magnified endoscopic image of PDA. (**b**) Irregularly shaped villi are noted (*red arrows*), but with low density. (**c**) The surface pattern has become unclear, and irregularly shaped blood vessels with caliber changes and irregular running are noted (*blue arrows*)

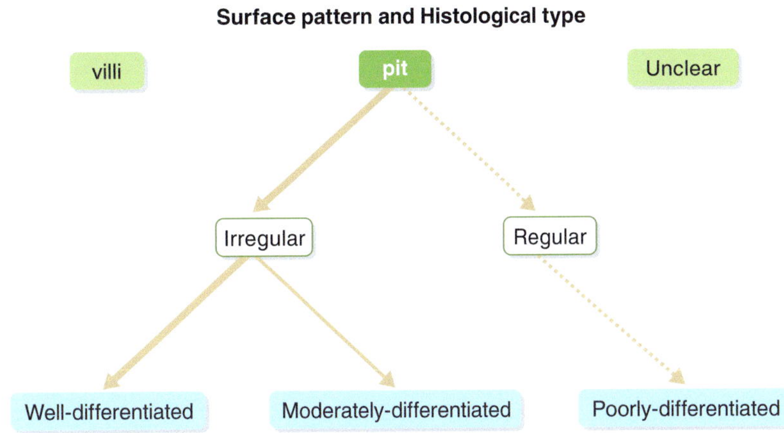

Fig. 5.19 Chart 3

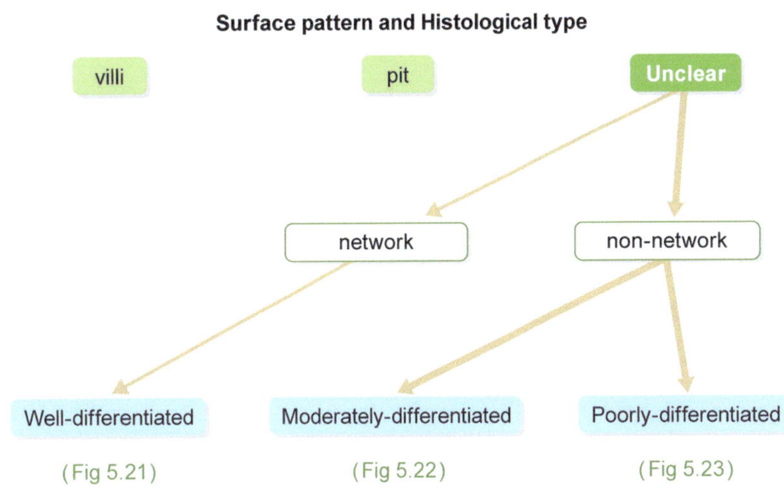

Fig. 5.20 Chart 4

the parenchyma, leaving the preexisting nonneoplastic glandular ducts (Fig. 5.19).

5.5.3 Unclear Surface Pattern

When the surface pattern is unclear, diagnosis of adenocarcinomas ranging from WDA, MDA, and to PDA should be considered (Fig. 5.20). Observation of microvascular pattern, followed by observation of surface pattern with acetic acid spraying, is useful.

Even when the surface pattern is unclear, if vascular networks are observed, diagnosis of WDA can be made. In such cases, pit-like structures can be noted with acetic acid spraying (Fig. 5.21). When the surface pattern is unclear and nonnetwork vessels are observed either MDA or PDA is present, and it is sometimes difficult to distinguish the two (Figs. 5.22 and 5.23).

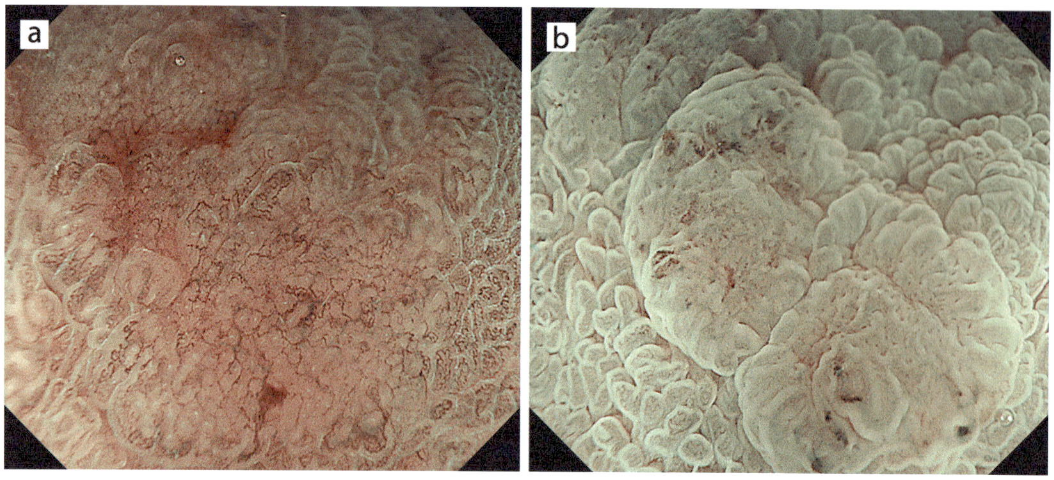

Fig. 5.21 (**a**) NBI magnified endoscopic image of WDA. (**b**) Image obtained after spraying of acetic acid

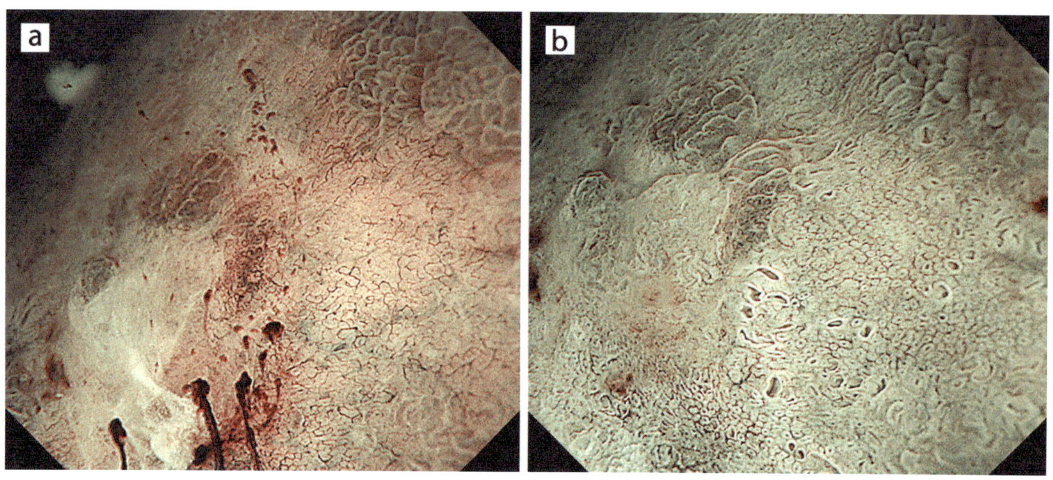

Fig. 5.22 (**a**) NBI magnified endoscopic image. (**b**) Image obtained after acetic acid spraying

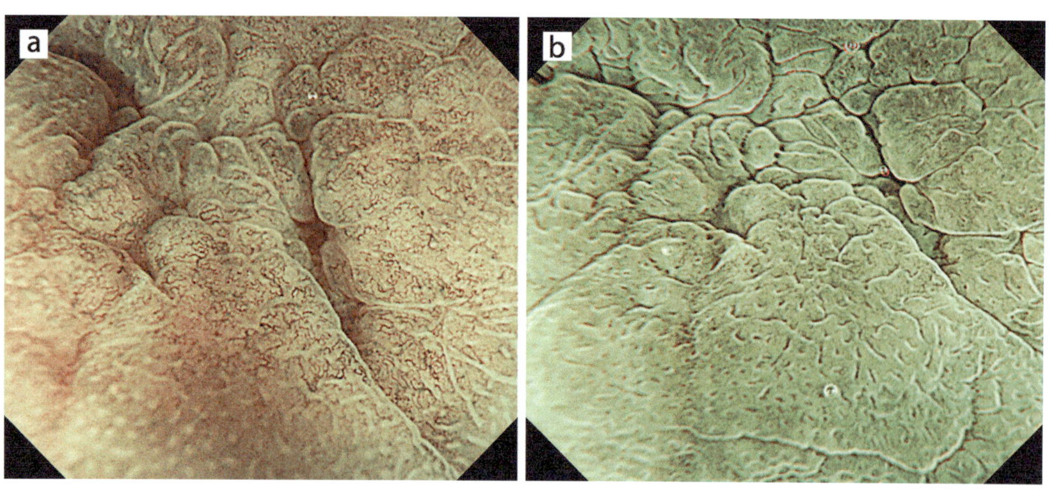

Fig. 5.23 (**a**) NBI magnified endoscopic image. (**b**) Image obtained after acetic acid spraying

References

1. Sakaki N et al. Magnifying endoscopic observation of the gastric mucosa, particularly in patients with atrophic gastritis. Endoscopy. 1978;10:269–74.
2. Nakyoshi T et al. Magnifying endoscopy combined with narrow band imaging system for early gastric cancer: correlation of vascular pattern with histopathology. Endoscopy. 2004;36:1080–4.
3. Yagi K et al. Magnifying endoscopy with narrow band imaging for early gastric adenocarcinoma. Dig Endosc. 2008;20:115–22.
4. Inoue H et al. Diagnosis of gastric cancer with magnifying endoscopy required in the era of endoscopic submucosal dissection (ESD): classification based on glandular structure and vascular pattern diagnosed with crystal violet chromoendoscopy and NBI magnifying endoscopy. Nippon Rinsho (Japanese). 2007;66:1023–7.
5. Yao K et al. Novel magnified endoscopic findings of microvascular architecture in intramucosal gastric cancer. Gastrointest Endosc. 2002;56:279–84.
6. Tomori A et al. Differential diagnosis of depressed small gastric cancers: comparisons of magnified and usual endoscopy. Stomach and Intestine. 2006;41:795–803.
7. Oyama T et al. Magnified endoscopy findings of ulcerative lesions of the stomach and differentiating malignant from benign ulcers. Stomach and Intestine. 2007;42:706–10.
8. Yagi K et al. Detailed examinations for lateral extensions: evaluations with magnified endoscopy. Stomach and Intestine. 2009;44:663–74.

Part II

Endoscopic Diagnosis for Gastric ESD – Diagnosing Typical Cases

Type 0-I Gastric Cancer

6

Tomoaki Shinohara

T. Shinohara (✉)
Department of Gastroenterology, Saku Central Hospital, 197 Usuda,
Saku, Nagano 384-0301, Japan
e-mail: sino4512@yahoo.co.jp

T. Oyama (ed.), *Endoscopic Diagnosis of Superficial Gastric Cancer for ESD*, DOI 10.1007/978-4-431-54469-2_6

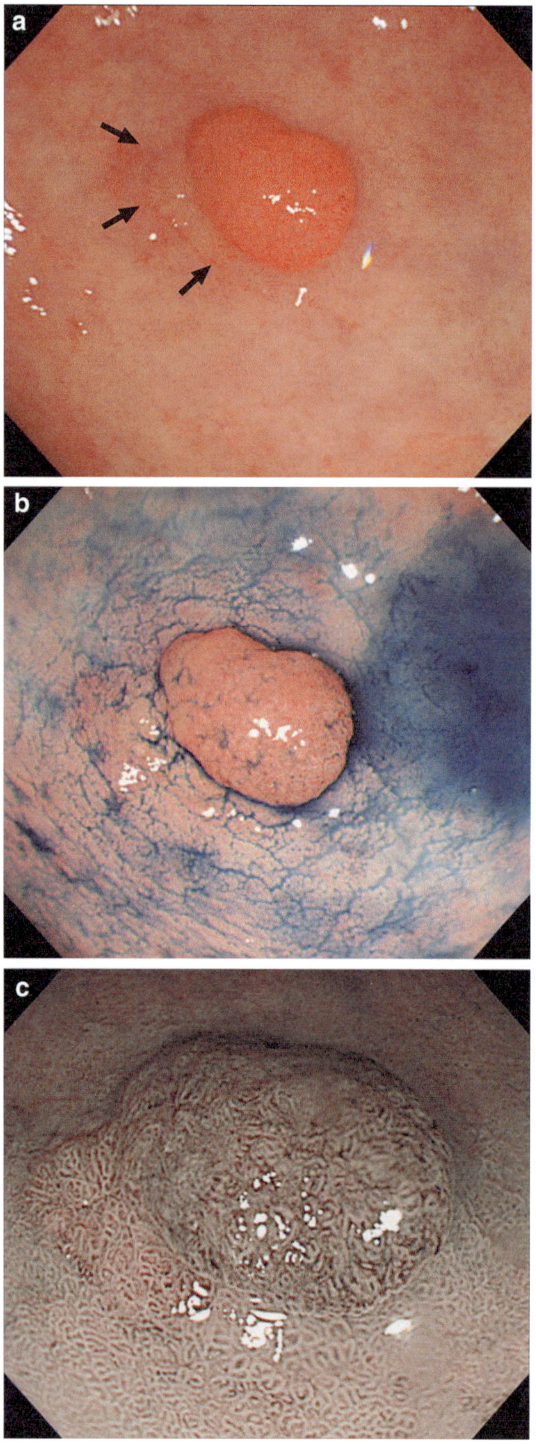

Fig. 6.1 Type 0-I gastric cancer. (**a**) Let's try first to diagnose a lesion with WL endoscopy (**b**) Indigo carmine stained image (**c**) NBI endoscopic image

6.1 Let's Try to Diagnose This Lesion

6.1.1 Let's Try First to Diagnose a Lesion with WL Endoscopy

- A well-demarcated and reddish protuberant lesion is located at the lesser curvature of the gastric antrum. This lesion appears nodular without lobulations. Its mucosal surface pattern is fine, dense, and full, without papillary or coarse gyrous pattern which are usually observed in hyperplastic polyps. Therefore, this lesion is strongly suspected to be an epithelial neoplasm. And more, its reddish color and tall height suggest cancer rather than tubular adenoma (Fig. 6.1a).

6.1.2 Let's Notice the Mucosal Surface Irregularity and Color Changes Around the Protrusion

- A discolored flat elevation devoid of vascular visibility exists at the anal-anterior side of the protrusion as indicated by black arrows (Fig. 6.1a).

6.1.3 Let's Spray with Indigo Carmine

- Spray with indigo carmine and observe the surface irregularity of the protrusion. Shallow grooves are observed on the surface of the reddish protrusion, but no depressed planes are seen. The protrusion repels indigo carmine more than the surrounding mucosa. This finding suggests that the protrusion is covered by more densely glandular surface than its surrounding mucosa.
- Although a flat discolored elevation is suspected to coexist as a 0-IIa component by WL endoscopy, the margin of the elevation is rather unclear by indigo carmine spraying (Fig. 6.1b).

6.1.4 Let's Use NBI

- Try to observe the whole lesion by NBI of low-power magnification. A dark brownish 0-I component and a light brown 0-IIa component of the lesion are observed, and their margins are clearly seen by difference in color (Fig. 6.1c).

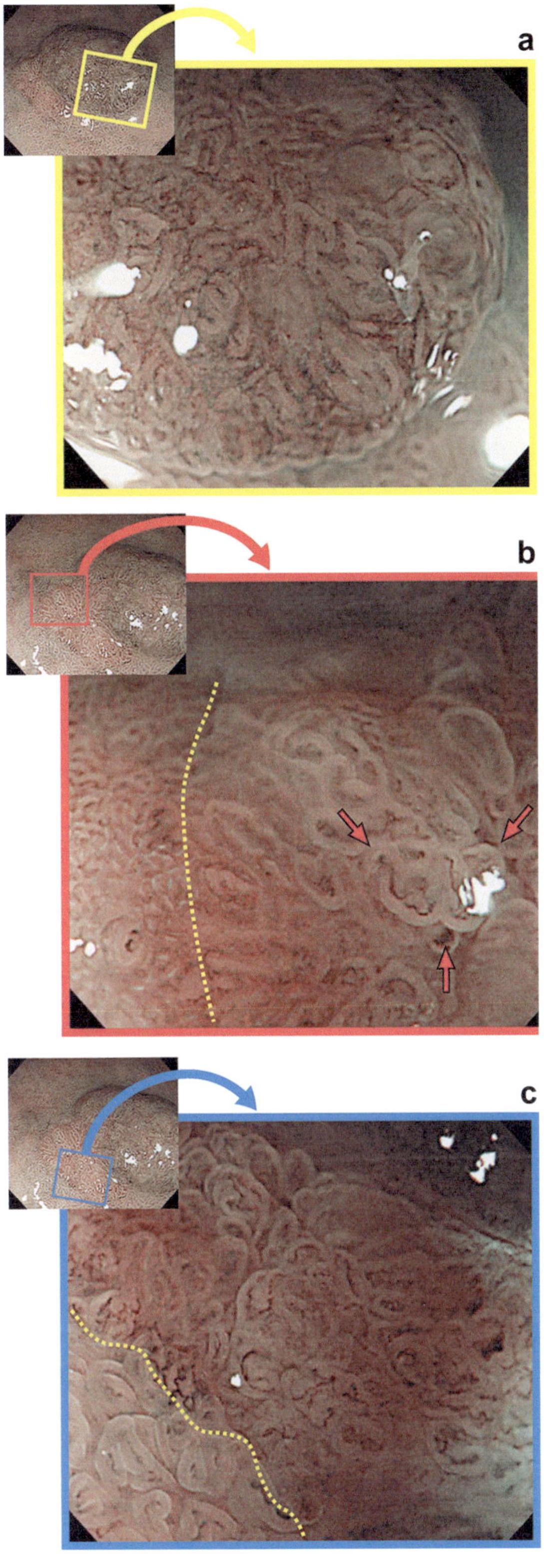

Fig. 6.2 Type 0-I gastric cancer

6.1.5 Let's Note the Different Surface Patterns

- Next, note the differences in surface patterns of the lesion with the surrounding mucosa. The surrounding mucosa shows a regular villous pattern. The 0-I component consists of irregular pitlike pattern. The 0-IIa component consists of villi of variable sizes. The two are not separated by a normal mucosa and are diagnosed as one lesion (0-I + IIa) (Fig. 6.1c).

6.1.6 Let's Observe the 0-I Component Using Magnification

- This is an NBI magnified endoscopic image of the anal margin of the 0-I component.
- The pitlike structures which show irregular branching and anastomosis of variable pit sizes are observed on the surface of the protrusion.
- Thick vessels with caliber changes and running irregularity are observed around the pits (Fig. 6.2a).

6.1.7 Let's Observe the 0-IIa Component Using Magnification

- This is an NBI magnified endoscopic image of the anterior side of the 0-IIa component. Background mucosa shows fine villous structures, while the 0-IIa shows villous structures of variable sizes. So the border of the 0-IIa is clearly seen (yellow dotted line).
- A fusion of villi is observed within the 0-IIa as noted by red arrows. This finding is specific for neoplastic mucosa, never detected in normal mucosa (Fig. 6.2b).

6.1.8 Let's Note Vascular Patterns

- The background mucosa shows villous structures. Each villus is uniform in size and has a thin spiral vessel within.
- The 0-IIa component consists of villi, but they are irregularly shaped and variable in sizes. Dilated blood vessels with caliber changes and irregular running are noted within these villi.
- The border between the 0-IIa component and the normal mucosa is clear as noted by yellow dotted line (Fig. 6.2c).

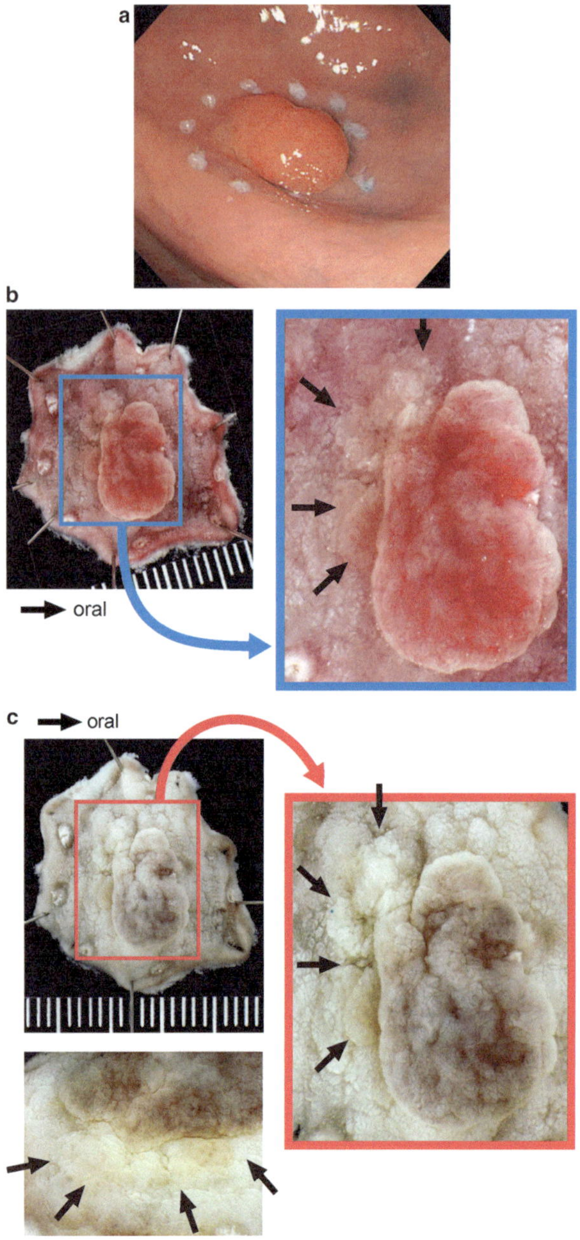

Fig. 6.3 (a) Endscopic image of circumferencial marking before ESD (b) Freshly resected specimen (c) Fixed specimen

6.2 From ESD to the Final Diagnosis

6.2.1 Let's Perform ESD

- Preoperative diagnosis is type 0-I + IIa gastric cancer, WDA, depth M. After marking using NBI-magnifying observation, ESD is performed (Fig. 6.3a).

6.2.2 Let's Observe the Freshly Resected Specimen

- The right side of these images is the oral side. The 0-I component is strongly reddish and its surface is irregular. The 0-IIa component has similar or slightly yellowish color than the normal mucosa and its margin appears irregular. Although the background mucosa shows uniform velvety structure, the 0-IIa component is recognized as a coarse villous structure. On the basis of differences in color and surface structure, the margin of the 0-IIa is diagnosed as noted by black arrows (Fig. 6.3b).

6.2.3 Let's Observe the Fixed Specimen

- After fixation of the specimen, surface irregularity is enhanced, and the surface structure has become more distinct. Irregularly branching, densely distributed pits are observed in the 0-I component.
- Both the 0-IIa and the surrounding mucosa have villous structures, but the 0-IIa has irregularly shaped villi of varied sizes. The margin of the 0-IIa is diagnosed as noted by the black arrows on the basis of differences in surface structure.
- We observed the 0-IIa from the anal side adjusting the viewing angle to match the endoscopic image. The base of the protrusion is recognized clearly (Fig. 6.3c).

Figure 6.4 shows histological images of 0-IIa (yellow box) and 0-I (green box) in section d as noted on the fresh specimen.

Yellow box is a middle-power picture (HE stained) of the surface of 0-IIa. This was diagnosed as WDA because of increased nuclear density and irregularly branching and densely distributed glands.

Green box is a middle-power picture (HE stained) of the surface of 0-I. This was diagnosed as well differentiated to papillary adenocarcinoma based on the tall tubular to papillary growth of glands. Dilated vessels are observed at the inter-cryptal space, which are corresponding to endoscopic and macroscopic reddish color.

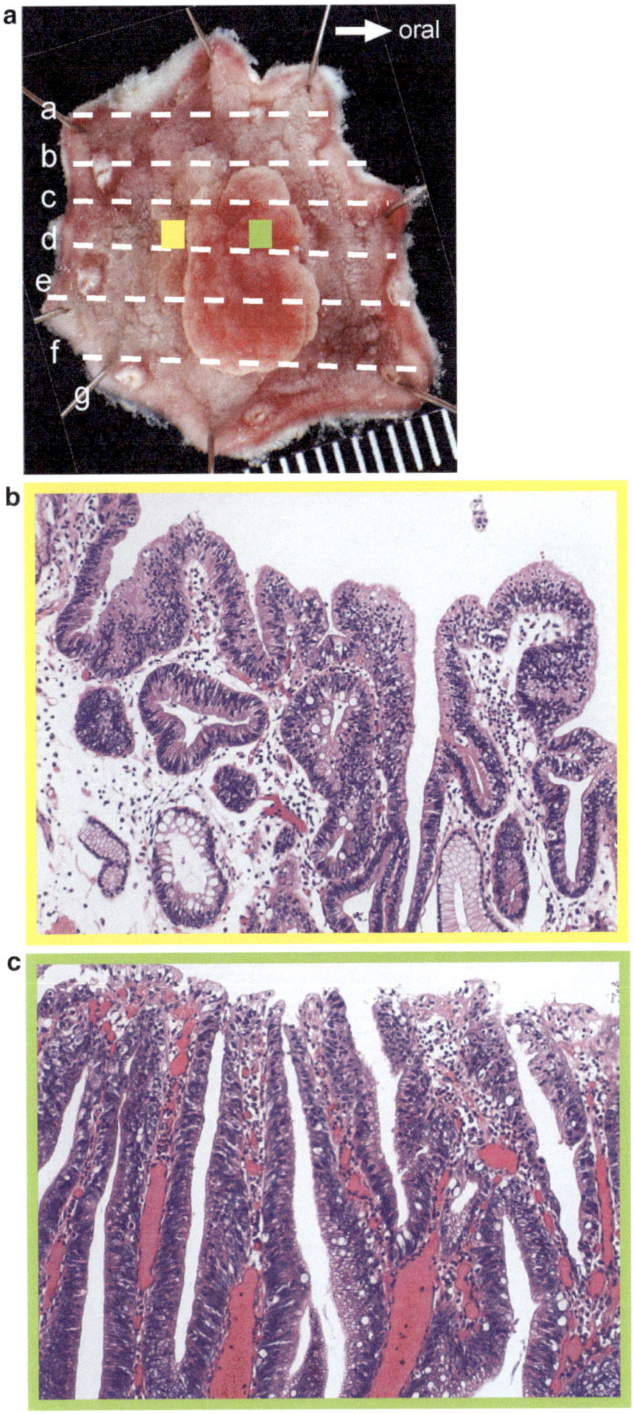

Fig. 6.4 Histological images of 0-IIa and 0-I

Figure 6.5 is a mapping of the cancer distribution projected on the flesh specimen. Intramucosal cancer corresponds to the 0-I and the 0-IIa.

Finally, a comparison of stereomicroscopic picture and NBI low-power view is shown in the Fig. 6.5. The 0-IIa component consisting of irregular villi of varied sizes reflects

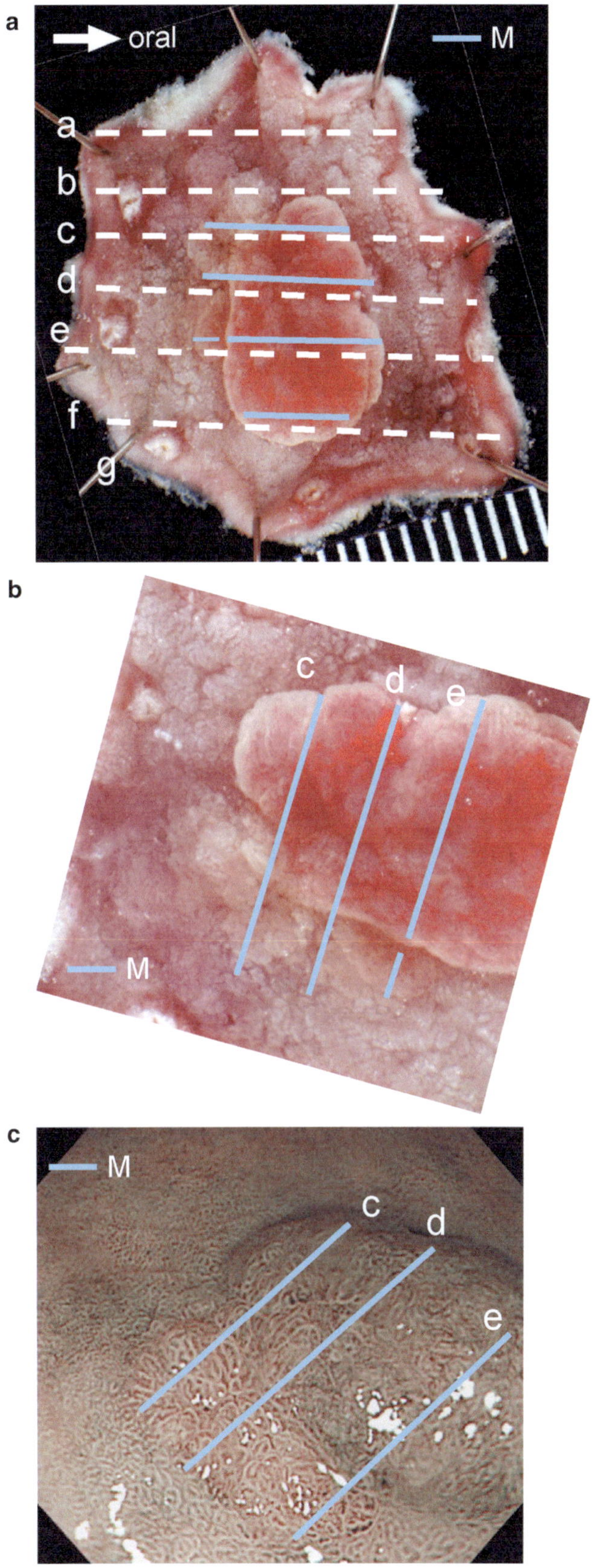

Fig. 6.5 Mapping of the cancer distribution projected on the freshly resected specimen

mucosal spread of WDA. Although the lateral extension of the 0-IIa is unclear under WL and indigo carmine observation, it can be diagnosed correctly by using NBI-magnifying observation.

Conclusive Diagnosis
Gastric adenocarcinoma, tub1 > pap, T1(M), ly0, v0, LM(−), VM(−), pType 0-I + IIa, 12 × 8 mm, L, Less.

Summary
We presented a case of type 0-I + IIa gastric cancer located at the lesser curvature of the antrum. For a simple type 0-I cancer, it is easy to diagnose its lateral extension. However, we must pay careful attention to possibly coexisting 0-IIa or 0-IIa components. In this case, NBI-magnifying observation was useful because it disclosed the lateral extension of the 0-IIa clearly. It is important not to miss slight color changes or irregularities noted around protruded type 0-I lesions.

7 Type 0-IIa Gastric Carcinoma

Tadashi Miike

T. Miike (✉)
Department of Gastroenterology and Hematology (Internal Medicine),
Faculty of Medicine of University of Miyazaki, 5200 Kiyotakecho,
Kihara, Miyazaki, Miyazaki 889-1692, Japan
e-mail: tadashi_miike@med.miyazaki-u.ac.jp

T. Oyama (ed.), *Endoscopic Diagnosis of Superficial Gastric Cancer for ESD*, DOI 10.1007/978-4-431-54469-2_7

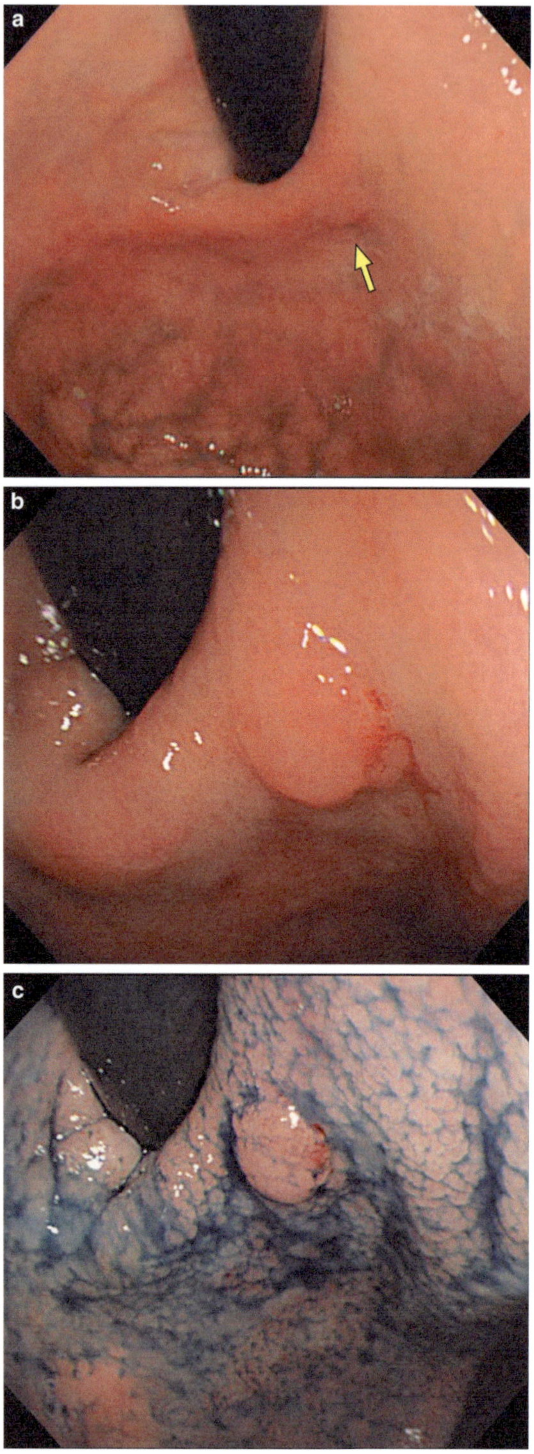

Fig. 7.1 (**a**, **b**) WL endoscopic image (**c**) Indigo carmine stained image

7.1 Let's Try to Diagnose This Lesion

7.1.1 At First, Let's Wash Out the Mucus Completely

- Since the fornix of a stomach is a likely location to have adherent mucus, it is important to wash out the mucus completely to be able to fully observe the mucosa.
- After carefully washing out the adherent mucus, a reddish protruding lesion (as indicated by the yellow arrow) on the anterior wall of the upper gastric body is observed (Fig. 7.1a).

7.1.2 Let's Closely Observe the Lesion

- On closer observation, a slightly reddish protruding lesion with a smooth surface is noticed on the anterior wall of the upper gastric body.
- Since the lesion is an isolated protruding lesion, an adenoma is suspected.
- The demarcation of the protruding lesion can be mostly traced, but the demarcation on its oral edge is unclear (Fig. 7.1b).

7.1.3 Let's Spray the Lesion with Indigo Carmine

- When sprayed with indigo carmine, a detailed observation of both the borderline and the surface pattern of this lesion has become possible.
- The demarcation of the lesion has become distinct by height differences of the protuberance and the surrounding mucosa.
- Compared with the regular gastric areal patterns noted in the background mucosa, the surface of the protruding lesion repels indigo carmine and shows irregular gastric areal patterns (Fig. 7.1c).

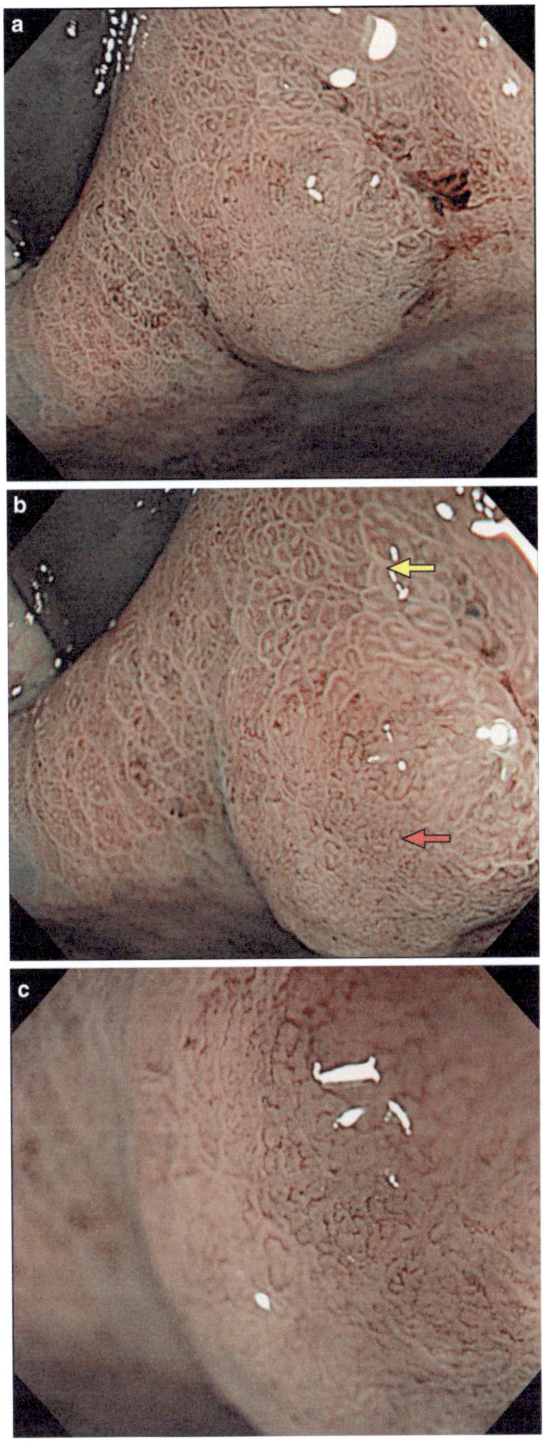

Fig. 7.2 (**a**) Lower magnification NBI endoscopic image (**b**) Medium range magnification NBI endoscopic image (**c**) Full zoom magnification NBI endoscopic image

7.1.4 Let's Use NBI

- NBI allows observation of both surface and vascular patterns.
- The surface pattern can be observed with lower magnification NBI.
- Mixed regular pit and villi-like patterns are noticed in the background mucosa, but the surface pattern of the protruding lesion is obscured (Fig. 7.2a).

7.1.5 Let's Observe Carefully the Surface Pattern

- The surface pattern can be observed in detail with a medium range magnification NBI.
- The area indicated by the yellow arrow is nonneoplastic because of the mixed regular pit and villi-like patterns.
- On the other hand, the protruding surface area indicated by the red arrow is obscured. The surface, however, shows irregular vascular patterns (Fig. 7.2b).

7.1.6 Let's Observe Carefully the Vascular Pattern

- With full zoom magnification NBI, vascular patterns can be observed in detail.
- Based on irregular running and caliber changes of blood vessels, as well as partially present vascular networks, the lesion can be thought of as a WDA (Fig. 7.2c).

7.2 From ESD to the Final Diagnosis

7.2.1 Let's Observe the Freshly Resected Specimen

- The right side of the image is the oral side.
- A round protruding lesion is noted in the center, and its border can be traced by difference in height.
- Irregular and coarse "bumps and dents" are noted on the surface of the protruding lesion.
- The color of the protruding lesion is mostly pale and focally reddish (Fig. 7.3a).

7.2.2 Let's Observe the Pathological Specimen

- Histology of the protruding lesion (HE stained).
- Dense proliferation of irregular tubular glands through the whole layer of mucosa is noted with structural atypia (Fig. 7.3b).

7.2.3 Let's Observe Under Higher Magnification

- Histology of the protruding lesion (HE stained) at higher magnification.
- Proliferation of neoplastic cells with irregularly shaped large nuclei is noted.
- Based on increased N/C ratio, irregularly arranged nuclei, and loss of polarity, diagnosis of a WDA (tub1) can be made (Fig. 7.3c).

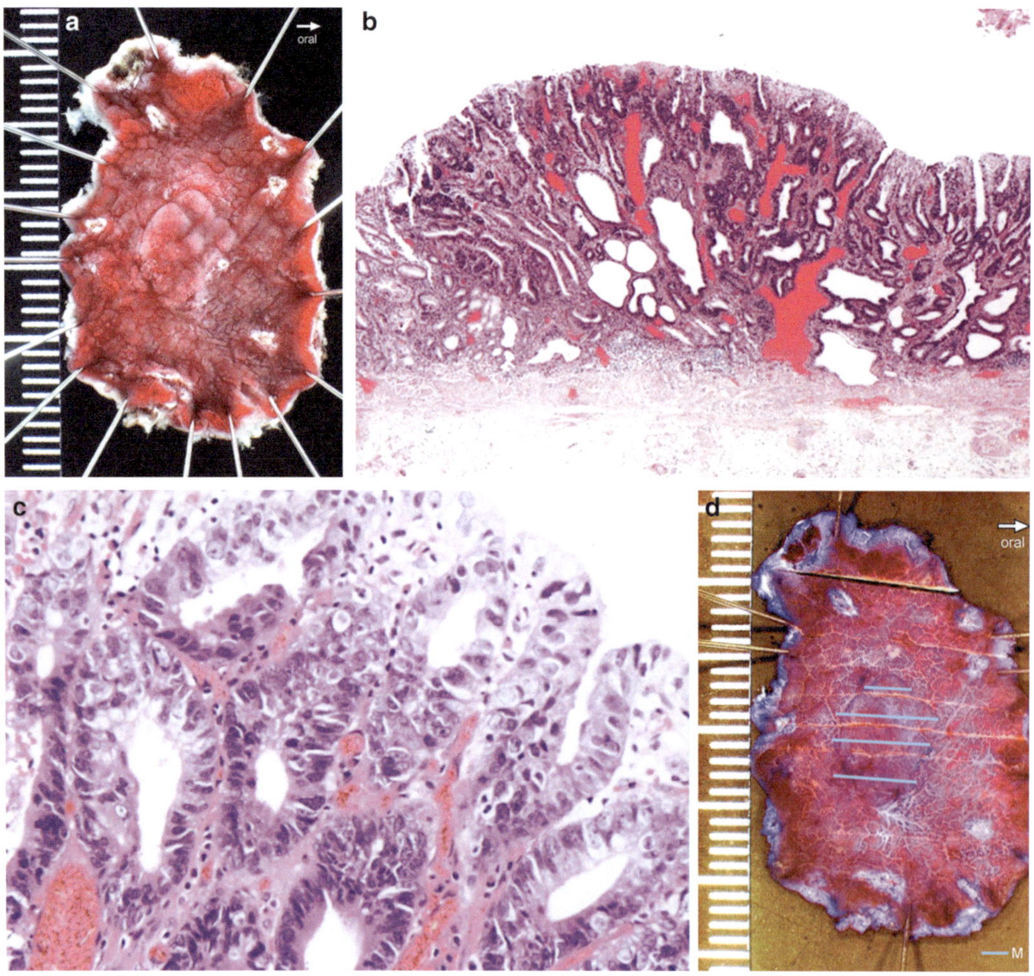

Fig. 7.3 (a) Freshly resected specimen (b, c) Histlogy image of the protruding lesion (d) Mapping of the cancer distribution projected on the freshly resected specimen

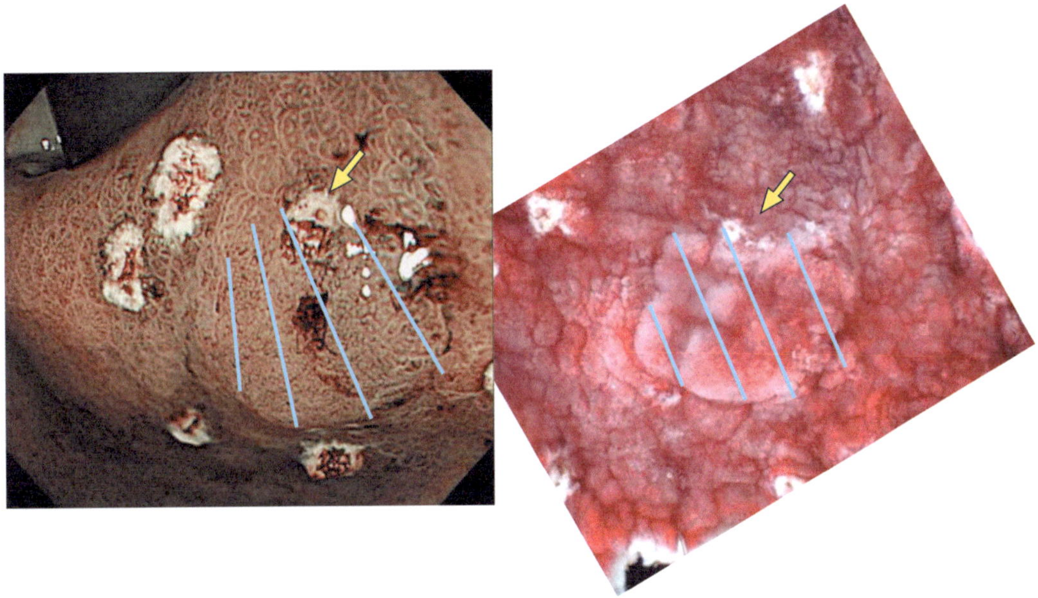

Fig. 7.4 Comparison between the NBI endoscopic image and the freshly resected specimen. Mapping of the cancer distribution projected on both images

7.2.4 Let's Compare the Fresh Specimen with the Endoscopic Image

- The endoscopic view of the protruding lesion is compared with the freshly resected specimen by rotating the image of the resected specimen to have the oral marks indicated by the yellow arrows in the same orientation (Fig. 7.4).

Conclusive Diagnosis (Fig. 7.3d)

Gastric adenocarcinoma, tub1, T1(M), ly0, v0, LM (−), VM(−), pType 0-IIa, 9 × 7 mm, U, Ant.

Summary

The anterior wall of the upper gastric body tends to have adherent mucus. Careful washing of mucus allowed a lesion to be recognized in this area. Observation with WL and with indigo carmine spray showed an isolated well-demarcated flat raised lesion suspected to be an adenoma. But, observation with NBI using gradually higher magnification showed on the surface of the protruding lesion an area of obscure surface pattern and irregular runs and caliber changes of dilated blood vessels as well as focally present vascular networks. Diagnosis of a well-differentiated tubular adenocarcinoma (tub1) was made.

8 Early Stage Type 0-IIa Gastric Cancer

Kenji Kunieda

K. Kunieda (✉)
Division of Oncology, Saku Central Hospital, 197 Usuda, Saku,
Nagano 384-0301, Japan
e-mail: kunieda.kenji@sakuhp.or.jp

T. Oyama (ed.), *Endoscopic Diagnosis of Superficial Gastric Cancer for ESD*, DOI 10.1007/978-4-431-54469-2_8

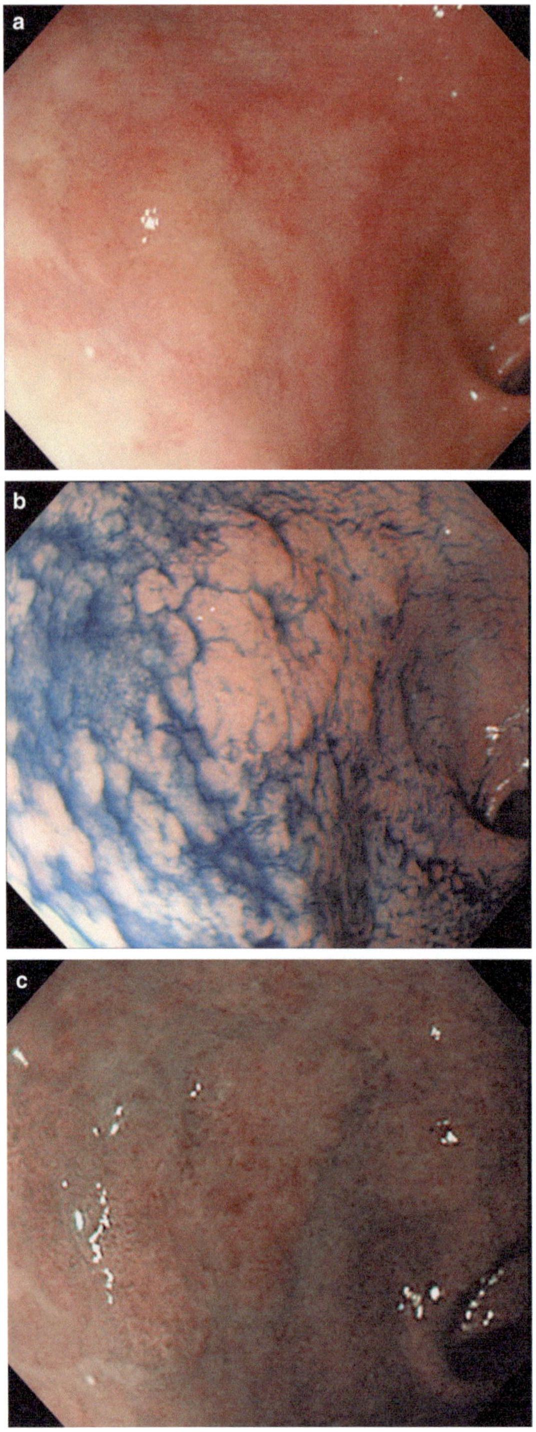

Fig. 8.1 (**a**) WL endoscopic image (**b**) Indigo carmine stained image (**c**) NBI endoscopic image

8.1 Let's Try to Diagnose This Lesion

8.1.1 Let's Pay Attention to Mucosal Irregularities and Color Variations

- The background is atrophic mucosa consisting of a mixture of discolored and inflamed mucosa.
- In the anterior wall of the antrum, an irregularly shaped, smooth, gently sloping, protruding lesion is seen.
- The color of the lesion is a mixture of discoloration and inflammation, with a shallow depression observed on the top.
- The boundary of the lesion can be recognized partly on the anterior wall but is mostly indistinct (Fig. 8.1a).

8.1.2 Let's Spray with Indigo Carmine

- When sprayed with indigo carmine, the anal side of the margin becomes distinct, but the oral side of the margin remains indistinct.
- When compared with the surrounding gastric areal structures, indigo carmine is repelled from the surface of the protruding lesion, and narrow grooves are observed within the coarse areal structures (Fig. 8.1b).

8.1.3 Let's Use NBI

- Using NBI, the entire lesion is captured in one field of vision for observation.
- Compared with the background mucosa, this lesion can be recognized as a slightly reddish area.
- The margin between the lesion and the background mucosa is recognized by the difference in color.
- However, non-magnified observation with NBI is not suited for screening because of insufficient light intensity, making images to be generally dark (Fig. 8.1c).

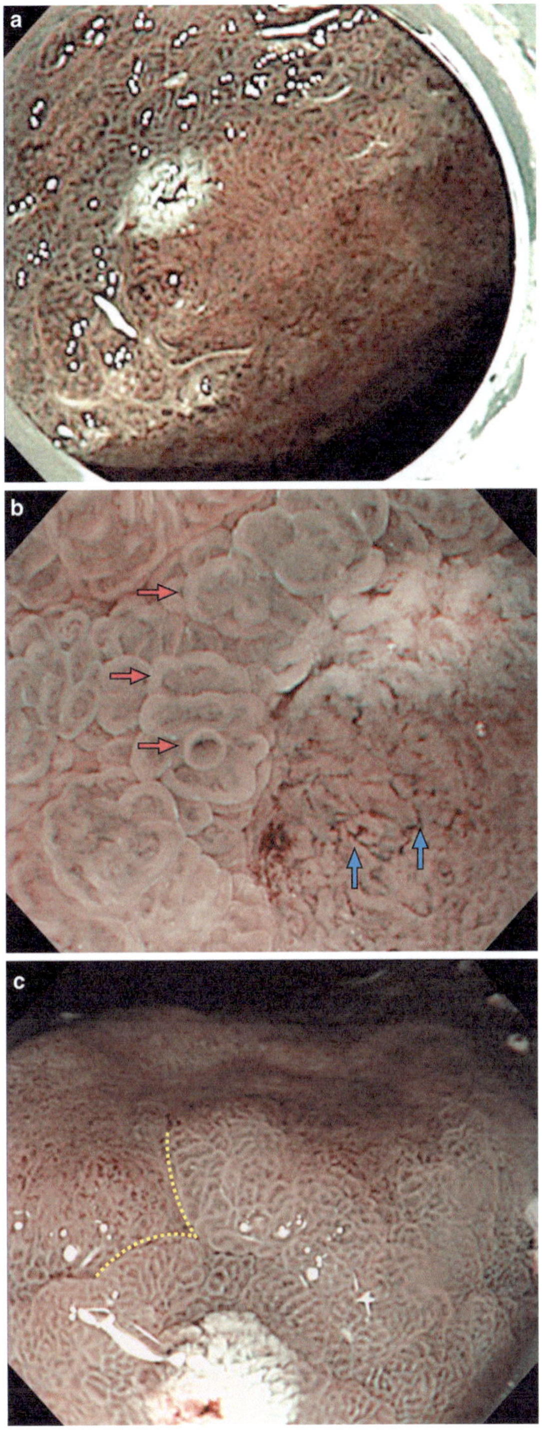

Fig. 8.2 (a) Medium magnification NBI endoscopic image (b) High-power magnification NBI endoscopic image (c) NBI magnified endoscopic image

8.1.4 Let's Examine at Medium Magnification

- This is from a margin of a 0-IIa lesion.
- In the background mucosa, non-irregular, rounded villous structures and, in part, regular pit structures are seen.
- In contrast, villous structures of variable sizes are observed within the lesion, and although unclearly, some irregular villous structures are seen in part.
- Based on the difference in surface structures, the demarcation line is determined and a marking is placed on it (Fig. 8.2a).

8.1.5 Let's Examine at High-Power Magnification

- This is an image of the area surrounding the marking at high-power magnification.
- The rounded villous structures without irregularities marked by the red arrows are observed in the mucosa surrounding the lesion.
- By contrast, in the area marked by the blue arrows within the lesion, the surface structures are indistinct and abnormal blood vessels following irregular routes and varying diameters can be seen.
- In addition, vascular networks are observed in part (Fig. 8.2b).

8.1.6 Let's Determine the Margin of the Anterior Wall by Using NBI

- This is a NBI magnified endoscopic image of the anterior wall.
- Rounded villous structures without irregularities are observed in the surrounding background mucosa.
- In contrast, high density of differently sized, irregularly arranged villous structures is observed within the lesion, and both boundaries (yellow dotted line) are clear from the difference in structures.
- Based on the above, the lesion was classified as a 0-IIa lesion, and diagnosed as a WDA with an invasion depth is intra-mucosa. The entire circumference marking was conducted, and en bloc resection was performed with ESD (Fig. 8.2c).

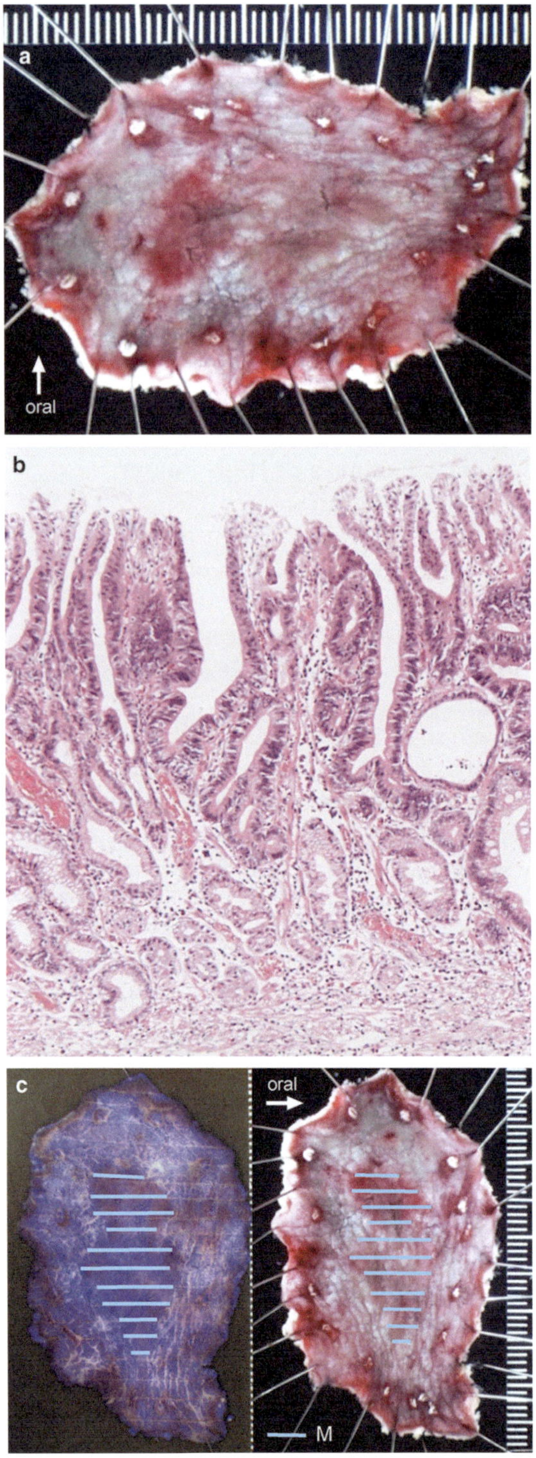

Fig. 8.3 (**a**) Freshly resected specimen (**b**) Histlogy image of the lesion (**c**) Mapping of the cancer distribution projected on the freshly resected specimen

8.2 From ESD to the Final Diagnosis

8.2.1 Let's Examine the Freshly Resected Specimen

- The upper part of the image is the oral side.
- A flat, protruding lesion can be seen in the center.
- The surface is smooth.
- The margin of this lesion is recognizable by redness and protrusion (Fig. 8.3a).

8.2.2 Let's Examine Histopathology of This Lesion

- This is a high magnification of a hematoxylin and eosin staining image of the discolored area of the protruding lesion.
- Based on high density of nuclei and irregular glands with abnormal branching, the lesion can be diagnosed as a WDA (tub1).
- Oval-shaped nuclei and stratification of nuclei are noted.
- Highly dense glandular tubes with nuclear atypia are noted with narrowed stroma containing decreased numbers of blood vessels.
- This histological finding supports pale coloration of the lesion.
- These pathological findings supported the discoloration of the lesion (Fig. 8.3b).

8.2.3 Let's Place a Mapping of the Lesion on the Specimen

- The right side is the oral side.
- The extent of a WDA is consistent with this 0-IIa protruding lesion.
- Diagnosis of lateral extensions by endoscopic findings is almost consistent with the extent of tumor (Fig. 8.3c).

8.2.4 Let's Compare the Pathological Specimen with the Endoscopic Image (1)

- In Fig. 8.4a, a mark had been placed on the boundary between the surrounding mucosa and the lesion. Well-ordered villous structures are seen to the left side of the mark. By contrast, the surface structure within the lesion is indistinct, and abnormal vascularization exhibiting a partial network, varied diameters, and irregular routes is observed.
- The histopathology corresponding to the area marked with the yellow dotted line in Fig. 8.4a is shown in Fig. 8.4b. On the right side of the boundary mark, there are tumor ducts with structural abnormalities and swollen nuclei. And, intestinal metaplasia is observed on the left side of the mark.

8.2.5 Let's Compare the Pathological Specimen with the Endoscopic Image (2)

- The boundary of the lesion is clearly seen in Fig. 8.5a.
- There are morphologically villous structures without irregularities surrounding the mark. By contrast, highly dense slightly irregular villous structures are observed within the lesion.
- The histopathology corresponding to the area marked with the blue line in Fig. 8.5a is shown in Fig. 8.5b. On the left side of the Fig. 8.5b, there are tumor ducts with structural abnormalities. By contrast, there are glandular ducts without irregularities between the lesion and the mark.

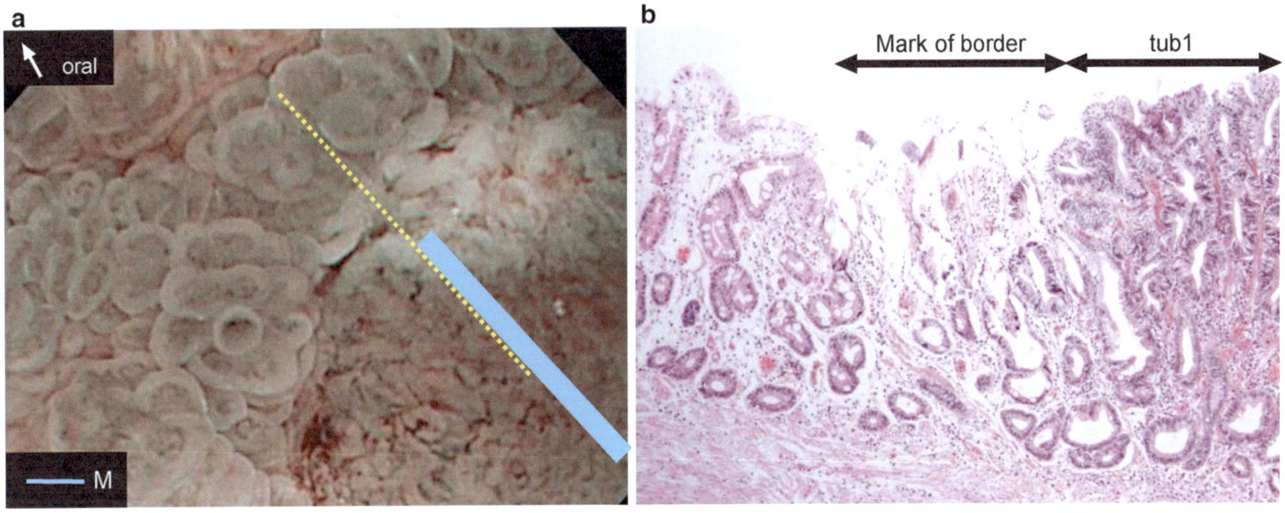

Fig. 8.4 Comparison between the NBI endoscopic image and the histology image (1)

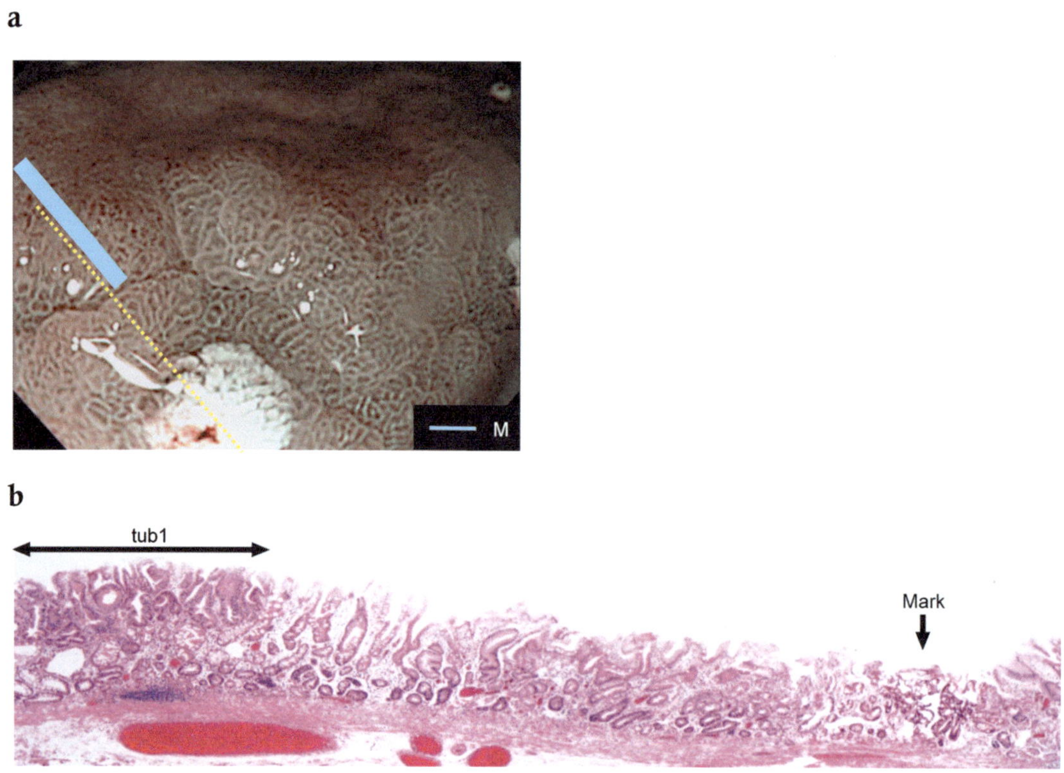

Fig. 8.5 Comparison between the NBI endoscopic image and the histology image (2)

Conclusive Diagnosis (Fig. 8.3c)
Gastric adenocarcinoma, Tub1, T1(M), ly0, v0, LM (−), VM(−), pType 0'IIa, 25 × 12 mm, L, Ant.

Summary
The boundary around this 0-IIa lesion existing on the anterior wall of the antrum is indistinct by white light (WL) imaging. However, the boundary with the surrounding mucosa can be clearly identified from differences in the surface structures with magnified NBI. Furthermore, diagnosis of WDA (tub1) can be made because villous structures and vascular networks are observed by magnified NBI.

9 Type 0-IIb Gastric Cancer

Koichi Okamoto

K. Okamoto (✉)
Department of Gastroenterology and Oncology, University of Tokushima, 2-24, Shinkura-cho, Tokushima 770-8501, Japan
e-mail: tagayasu33jp@yahoo.co.jp

T. Oyama (ed.), *Endoscopic Diagnosis of Superficial Gastric Cancer for ESD*, DOI 10.1007/978-4-431-54469-2_9

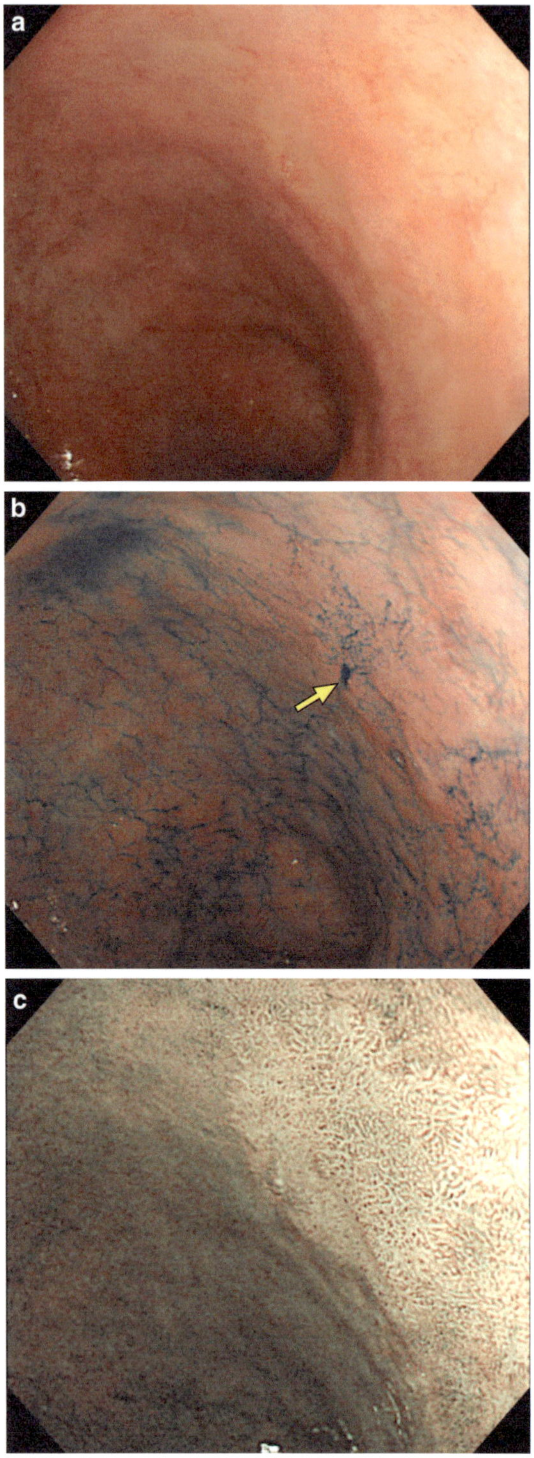

Fig. 9.1 (**a**) WL endoscopic image (**b**) Indigo carmine stained image (**c**) Low magnification NBI endoscopic image

9.1 Let's Try to Diagnose This Lesion

9.1.1 Pay Attention to the Color Tone

- **Focus on discoloration.**
  An area of discoloration is recognized on the posterior side of the lesser curvature of the gastric antrum. It is possible to observe the boundary circumferentially, and no similar lesion is observed around it. Therefore, an epithelial tumor is suspected. It is difficult to determine whether it is an elevated or a depressed lesion by WL imaging.
- **Focus on the color tone inside the lesion.**
  This is a lesion with whitish discoloration, but it is mixed with a slightly reddish area in the lesion (on the oral side), which suggests cancer rather than adenoma.
- **Focus on the background mucosa.**
  The adjacent mucosa is heterogeneous in color with a mixture of redness and whitish discoloration. Therefore, atrophic gastritis is diagnosed (Fig. 9.1a).

9.1.2 Let's Spray Indigo Carmine

- It will be easier to compare images with and without indigo carmine spraying when a picture is taken before and after indigo carmine dye is sprayed while maintaining the same visual field.
- **Focus on the boundary of the lesion.**
  In this case, a well-demarcated lesion by WL imaging unexpectedly becomes obscure after indigo carmine spraying. Lesions with little undulation may become ill delineated by spraying of indigo carmine and result in misdiagnosis.
- **Focus on the surface of the lesion.**
  The area with a mixture of redness (at the oral side of the lesion) by WL imaging is recognized as an area repelling the dye a little, while the dye gets pooled at the anal side of the lesion as a fine gutter-like structure. The gutter-like pooling of the dye demonstrated by yellow arrow is a biopsy scar (Fig. 9.1b).

9.1.3 Points for NBI Magnifying Observation

- With NBI magnifying observation, it is easier to identify an area at a higher magnification when a picture of the whole lesion is first taken at a low magnification.

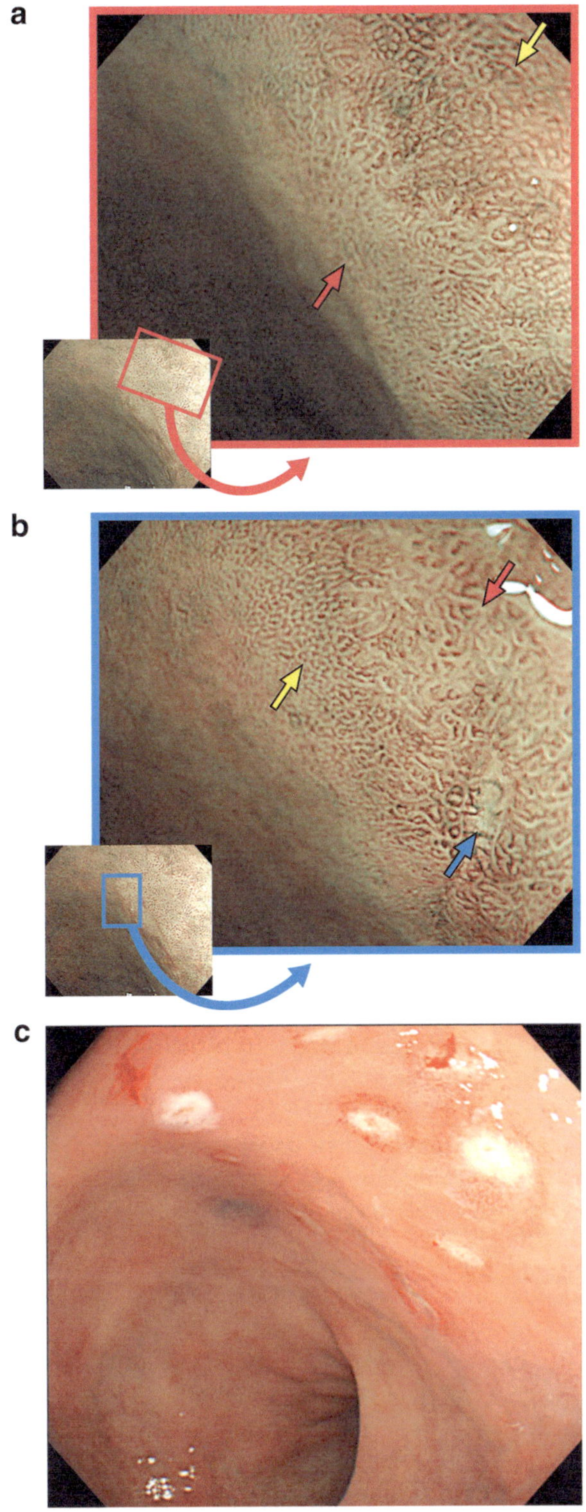

Fig. 9.2 (a, b) Moderate magnification NBI endoscopic images (c) Endscopic image of circumferencial marking before ESD

9.1.4 Let's Look at NBI Images at a Low Magnification

- Compared with the image by WL imaging, the boundary is better delineated as the difference in color and structure by spraying of indigo carmine dye (Fig. 9.1c).

9.1.5 Let's Observe the Oral Side

- When the lesion is observed with NBI at a moderate magnification, pitlike structure is recognized at the right upper position with a yellow arrow. Small and round pits are regularly aligned, and the lesion is diagnosed as a non-tumorous area. Meanwhile, a mixture of structures of pits and villi is observed at the site with a red arrow. The shape of villi is irregular and heterogeneous in size and the density is high. Taken together, the lesion is diagnosed as WDA (tub1) (Fig. 9.2a).

9.1.6 Let's Observe the Anal Side

- Pitlike structure is observed at the site with a yellow arrow. Small and round pits are aligned regularly, and the area is diagnosed as non-tumorous. Villi-like structure is observed at the site with a red arrow. The shape of villi is irregular and heterogeneous in size and the density is high. Taken together, the lesion is also diagnosed as tub1. The part shown with a blue arrow is a biopsy scar (Fig. 9.2b).

9.1.7 Let's Perform ESD

- The lesion is marked under NBI magnifying observation and performed en block resection by ESD (Fig. 9.2c).

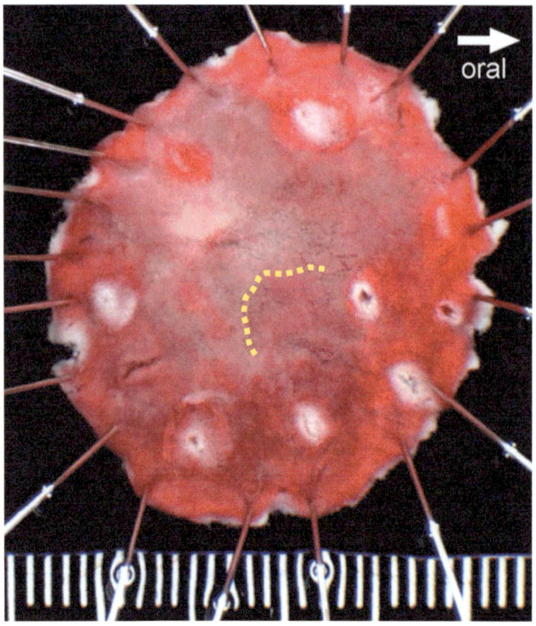

Fig. 9.3 Freshly resected specimen

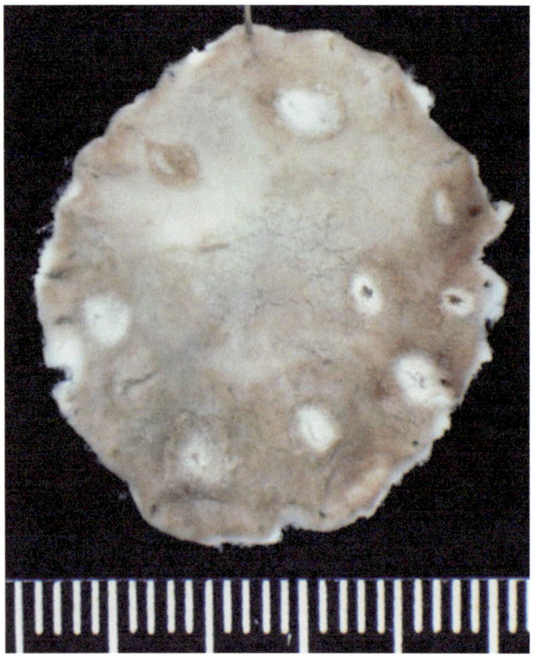

Fig. 9.4 Fixed specimen

9.2 From ESD to the Final Diagnosis

9.2.1 Let's Look at Fresh Resected Specimens

- The oral side is on the right.
- The inside of the lesion is a mixture of a faded color and redness.

  The surface is irregular compared with the adjacent mucosa, and fine gutter-like structure is recognized.
- It is possible to recognize the boundary of the lesion as the difference in color and structure.
- The reddish area on the right side of the dotted yellow line corresponds with the mildly reddish area by routine observation (Fig. 9.3).

9.2.2 Let's Observe Fixed Specimens

- When the specimen is fixed, surface structure is visualized more clearly.
- The surface is irregular with fine gutters, and it is possible to recognize the boundary from the adjacent mucosa (Fig. 9.4).

9.2.3 Let's Stain Specimens with Crystal Violet

- When the specimen is stained, the surface structure is visualized more clearly. The lesion shows villi-like structure heterogeneous in size with partial pitlike structure, and it is possible to recognize the boundary as the area shown in the black dotted line.
- The left side of the yellow dotted line shows fine villi-like structure heterogeneous in size, and the right side shows more coarse villi mixed with pitlike structure (Fig. 9.5a).

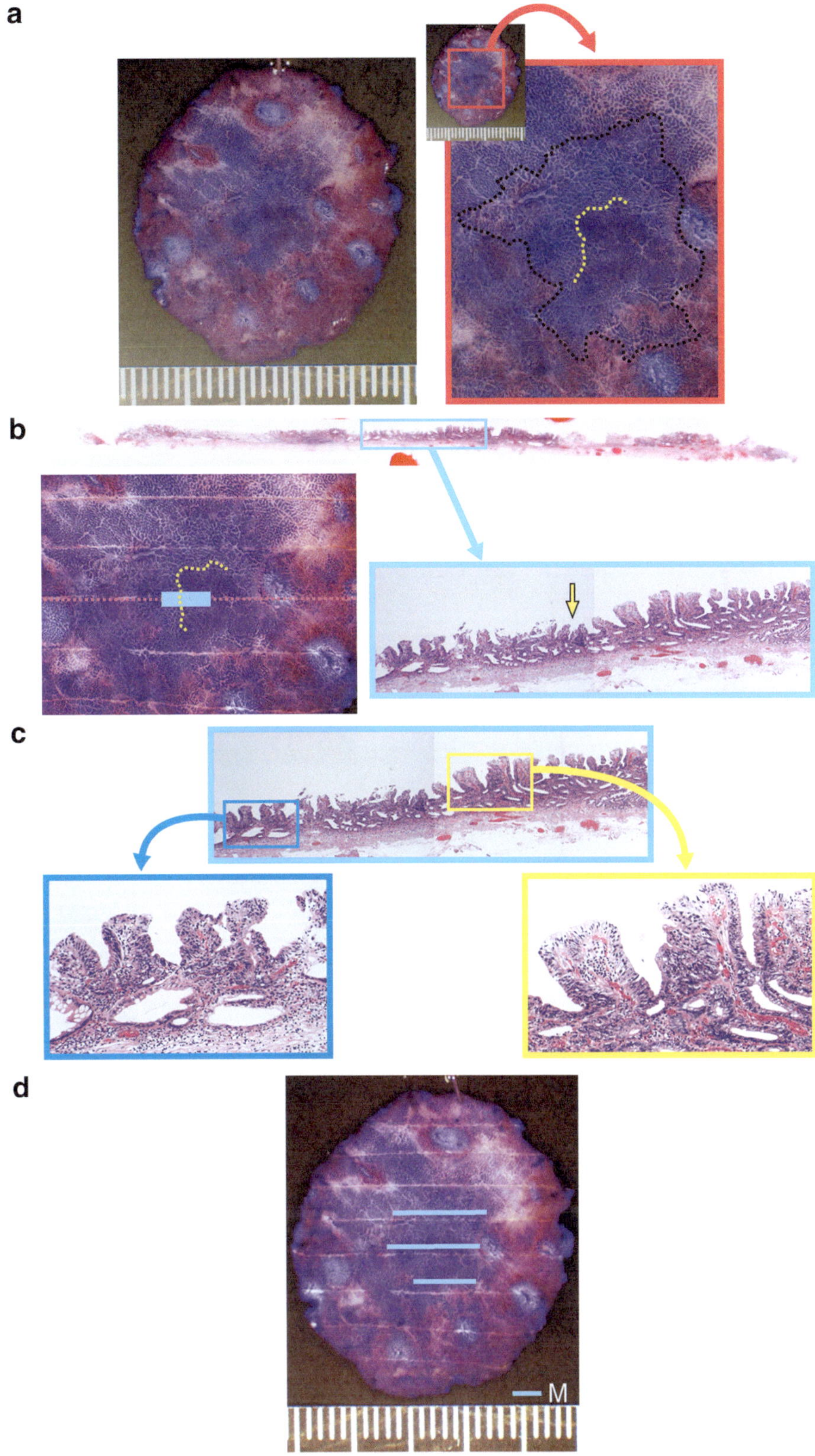

Fig. 9.5 Specimens stained with crystal violet. (**a**) Vill like structure (**b**, **c**) Histology image of the center of the lesion (**d**) Mapping of cancer distribution on the specimen

The lesion is recognized at the center with almost no difference in height compared with the adjacent mucosa (Fig. 9.5b). This is the histpathology of the center of the lesion (HE stained). Swollen nuclei and pseudostratification are recognized, but glandular structure is maintained. Therefore, tub1 is diagnosed. The yellow dotted line in the left panel of Fig. 9.5b corresponds with the site with a yellow arrow in the right panel, and there is a slight difference in height of tumor glands between the right and left sides.

The magnified view on the left of Fig. 9.5c exhibits swollen nuclei and the stroma of the glands is narrow in width. On the other hand, the magnified view on the right of Fig. 9.5c exhibits wide stroma with a number of blood vessels visible. It is presumed that the difference in these structures causes the color difference. The muscularis mucosae is maintained, and WDA with invasion depth of M is diagnosed.

Conslusive Diagnosis (Fig. 9.5d)
Gastric adenocarcinoma, Tub1, T1(M), ly0, v0, LM(−), VM(−), pType 0-IIb, 10 × 9 mm, L, Post.

Summary
The lesion on the posterior wall of the lesser curvature of the gastric antrum is diagnosed as 0-IIb with a mixture of a faded color and redness. The lesion is well-delineated by WL imaging, but since it is a 0-IIb lesion with little difference in height, it unexpectedly becomes unclear by indigo carmine spraying. The lesion is more clearly recognized by NBI magnifying observation, and a dense mixture of irregular villi and pitlike structure is recognized inside the lesion, which leads to the diagnosis of WDA (tub1).

Type 0-IIc Gastric Cancer

10

Akiko Takahashi

A. Takahashi (✉)
Division of Endoscopy, Saku Central Hospital, 197 Usuda, Saku,
Nagano 384-0301, Japan
e-mail: aurevoireurope@yahoo.co.jp

T. Oyama (ed.), *Endoscopic Diagnosis of Superficial Gastric Cancer for ESD*, DOI 10.1007/978-4-431-54469-2_10

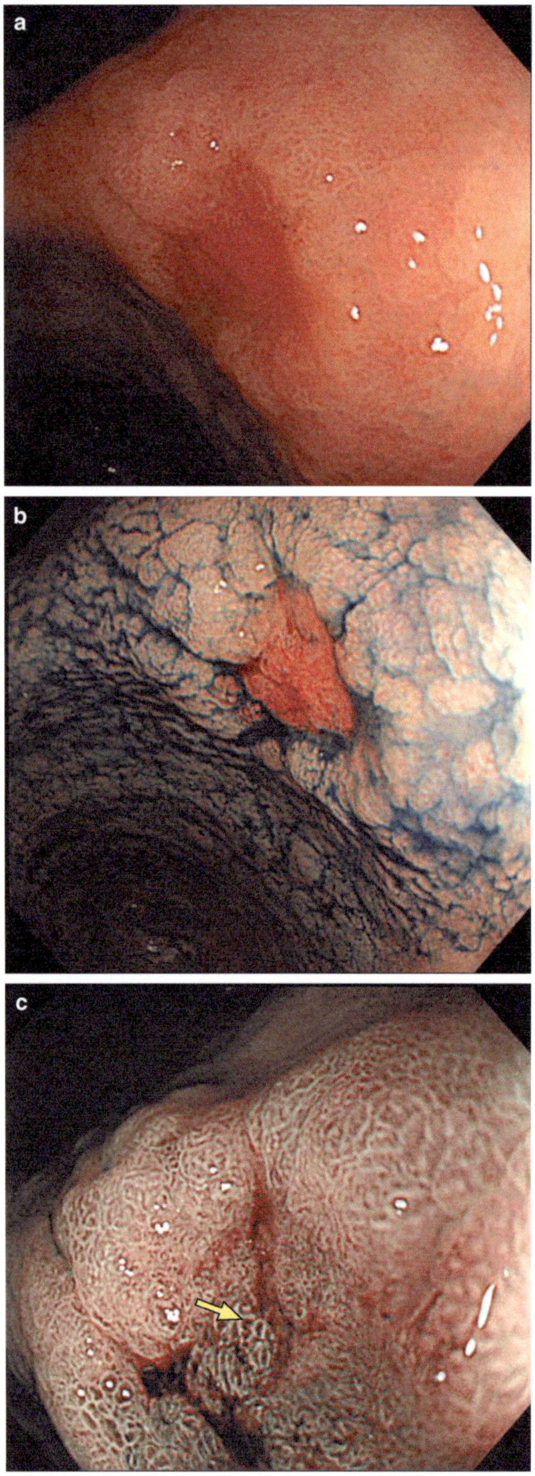

Fig. 10.1 (**a**) WL endoscopic image (**b**) Indigo carmine stained image (**c**) NBI endoscopic image

10.1 Let's Try to Diagnose This Lesion

10.1.1 Let's Look at a Reddish Depression

- WL endoscopy shows a reddish, irregular, and depressed lesion with surrounding protuberance on the posterior wall of the gastric angle.
- The margin of the lesion is unclear. Therefore, the lesion must be distinguished between cancer and noncancer (inflammation) (Fig. 10.1a).

10.1.2 Let's Spray Indigo Carmine

- The surface pattern can be analyzed in detail after indigo carmine spraying.
- Chromoendoscopy using indigo carmine shows a regular areal pattern in the background mucosa. However, it doesn't show areal patterns inside of the depression. In addition, the margin of the depression appears clear (Fig. 10.1b).

10.1.3 Let's Magnify with NBI

- To distinguish between cancer and noncancer by WL endoscopy and chromoendoscopy using indigo carmine is difficult. Therefore, NBI magnified endoscopy is used next.
- NBI magnified endoscopy of the oral side of the lesion shows regular pitlike and villous patterns in the background mucosa.
- The yellow arrow in this NBI magnified endoscopic image shows an irregular villous pattern with variable size and of high density in the depression. However, vascular patterns cannot be recognized (Fig. 10.1c).

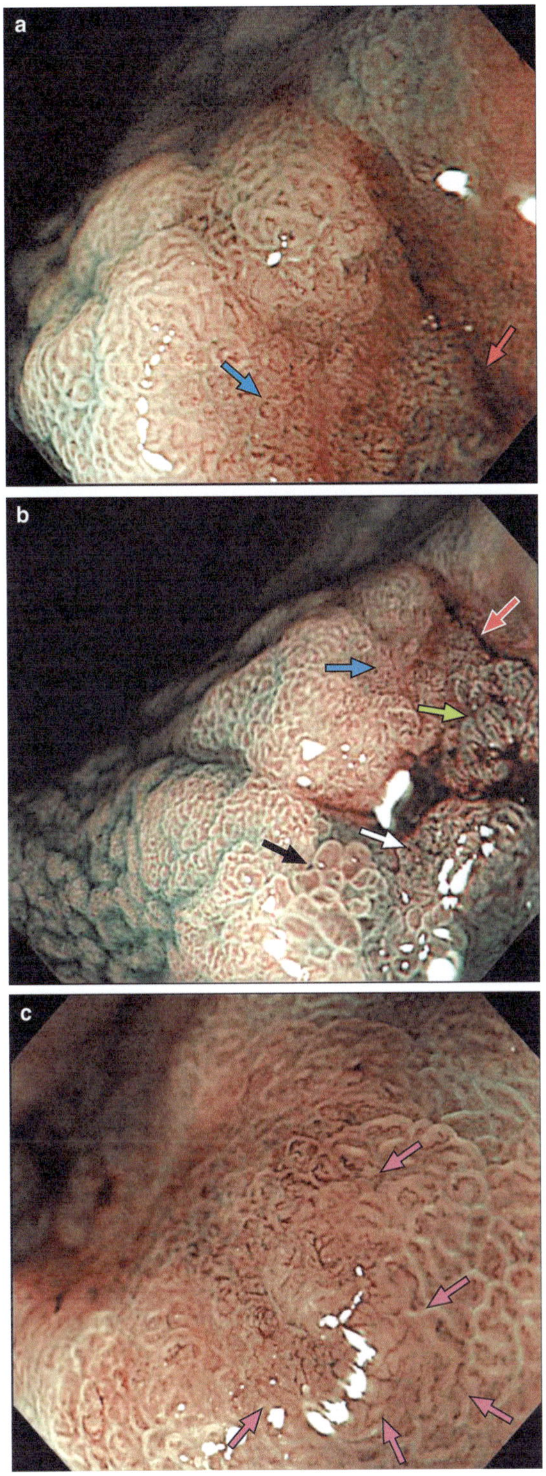

Fig. 10.2 (**a**) Magnified image of the oral side of the lesion (**b**) Magnified image of the anterior wall of the lesion (**c**) Magnified image of the anal side of the lesion

10.1.4 Let's Magnify the Oral Side of the Lesion More

- The pink arrow in this NBI magnified endoscopic image shows irregular villous patterns (pink arrow) (Fig. 10.2a).
- On the other hand, the blue arrow shows an area with villous patterns of variable size and mild irregularity.
- Network patterns are noted partially.

10.1.5 Let's Magnify the Anterior Wall of the Lesion

- The pink and the blue arrows are the same as in the previous NBI magnified image (Fig. 10.2b).
- The light-green arrow shows irregular villous patterns of variable size. Vascular pattern cannot be recognized.
- The black arrow shows irregular villous patterns with variable size. Vascular pattern cannot be recognized.
- The white arrow shows highly dense small villous patterns. NBI magnified endoscopy shows abnormal vessels with caliber changes and partial running irregularity.

10.1.6 Let's Magnify the Anal Side of the Lesion

- NBI magnified endoscopy shows villous patterns of variable size. The surface pattern is unclear partially. NBI magnified endoscopy shows abnormal vessels with caliber changes and running irregularity (Fig. 10.2c).
- The background mucosa shows a regular villous pattern. The area indicated by the pink arrows is diagnosed as the margin of the lesion by difference of surface patterns.
- The lesion is diagnosed endoscopically as gastric adenocarcinoma, well-differentiated type, T1a-M. The lesion was marked circumferentially and was resected en bloc by ESD.

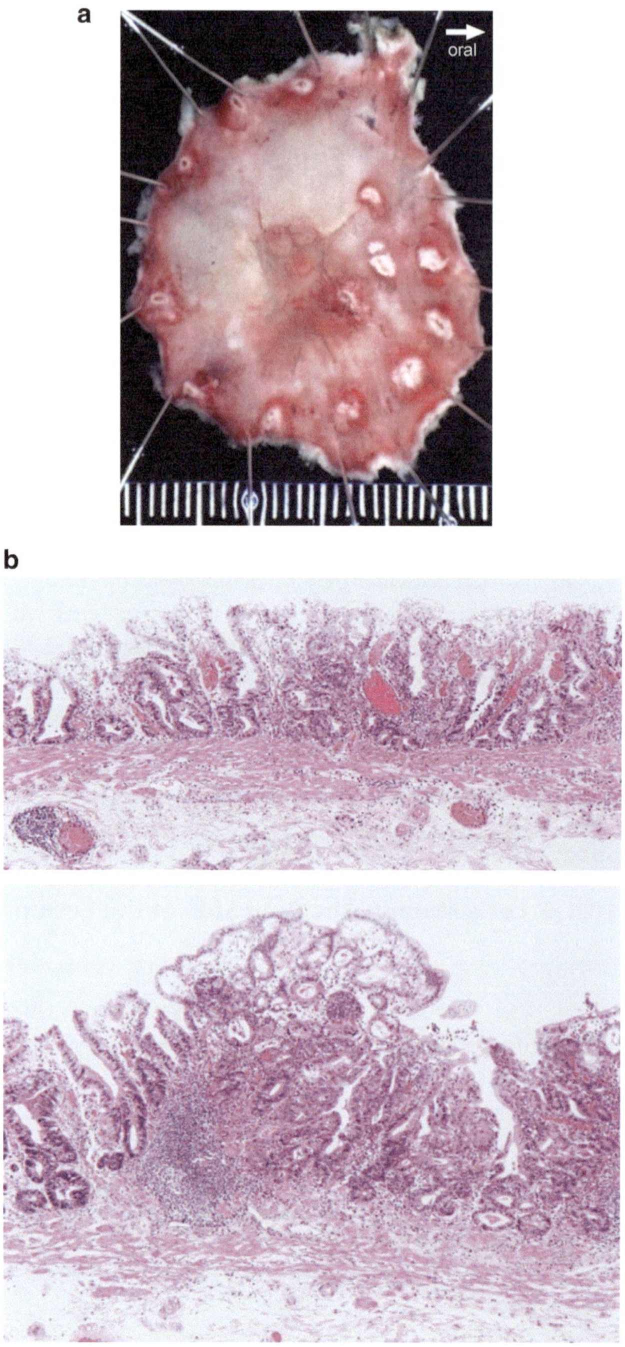

Fig. 10.3 (a) Freshly resected specimen (b) Histology image of the lesion

10.2 From ESD to the Final Diagnosis

10.2.1 Let's Look at the Freshly Resected Specimen

- The right side of the image is the oral side (Fig. 10.3a).
- The irregular and reddish depression with a clear margin is observed in the center of the specimen. The small protuberance is shown inside of the lesion partially.
- The margin of the lesion can be clearly traced by difference in coloration and depression.

10.2.2 Let's Look at Pathological Findings

- This image shows the pathological finding (HE stained) of a representative section.
- The tumor cells with nuclear swelling made tubular formation.
- The lesion was diagnosed as WDA, T1a-M, because of mild structural atypia.
- The protuberant part in the oral side of the lesion was diagnosed as WDA, because of mild structural atypia (Fig. 10.3b).
- Comparison between the depressed part and the surrounding protuberant part is shown. (The white dotted line: the line of section imposed on the endoscopic picture. The yellow line: the part shown by the pathological finding. The light blue line: the extent of mucosal cancer.) (Fig. 10.4)
- The pathological image is viewed from the direction of the red arrow.
- The pathological finding shows WDA extending from the depressed part to the periphery of the surrounding protuberance. (Fig. 10.4)

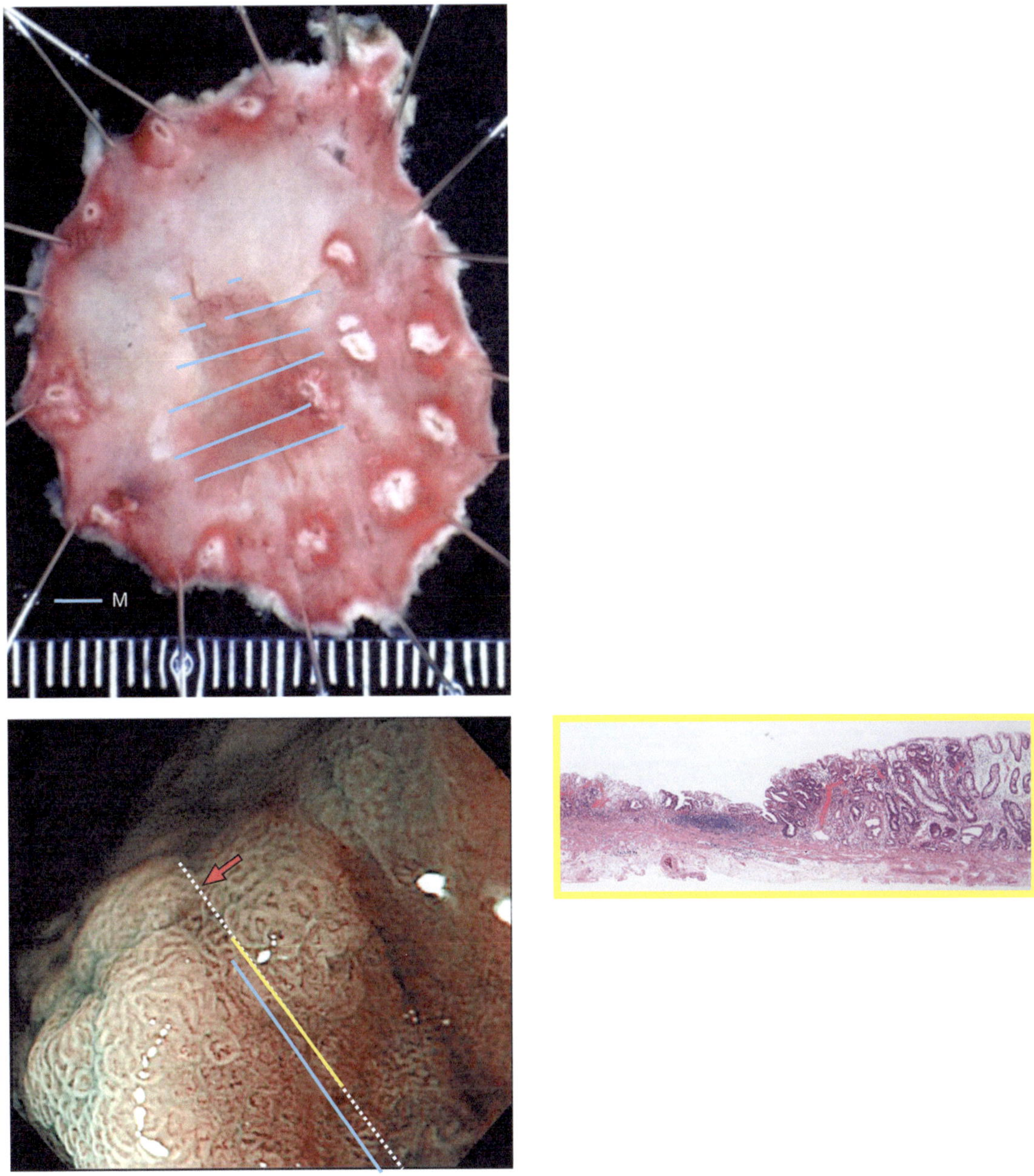

Fig. 10.4 Mapping of the cancer distribution displayed on the fresh specimen and histology image of the lesion. Comparison between the depressed part and the surrounding protuberant part

Conclusive Diagnosis

Gastric adenocarcinoma, tub1, T1(M), ly0, v0, LM (−), VM(−), pType 0-IIc, 12 × 10 mm, M, Post.

Summary

The final diagnosis is gastric WDA, T1a-M, pType 0-IIc, 12 × 10 mm, M, Post. Lymph duct and venous invasions are absent. The lateral and the vertical margins are free of cancer.

This was a reddish, irregular, and depressed lesion with unclear margin on the posterior wall of the gastric angle. It was necessary to distinguish whether the lesion was cancer or noncancer (inflammatory change).

NBI magnified endoscopy revealed irregular villous structures and abnormal vessels with network formations.

These findings helped diagnose this lesion as WDA.

Gastric Cancer: SM1 Invasion

11

Akiko Takahashi

A. Takahashi (✉)
Division of Endoscopy, Saku Central Hospital, 197 Usuda, Saku,
Nagano 384-0301, Japan
e-mail: aurevoireurope@yahoo.co.jp

T. Oyama (ed.), *Endoscopic Diagnosis of Superficial Gastric Cancer for ESD*, DOI 10.1007/978-4-431-54469-2_11

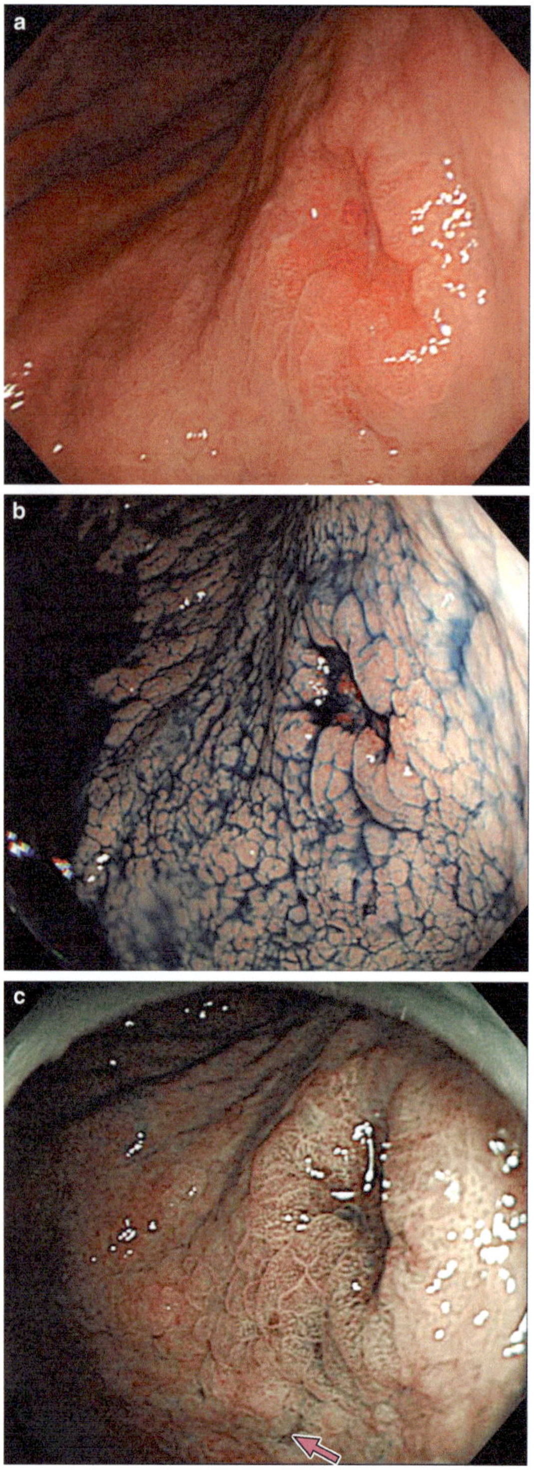

Fig. 11.1 (a) WL endoscopic image (b) Indigo carmine stained image (c) NBI endoscopic image

11.1 Let's Try to Diagnose This Lesion

11.1.1 Let's Look at the Reddish Part

- WL endoscopy shows a reddish, irregular, and depressed lesion with a clear margin on the posterior wall of the gastric upper body.
- WL endoscopy reveals an even more reddish part within the depression.
- The depressed area is surrounded by a circumferential protuberance (Fig. 11.1a).

11.1.2 Let's Spray Indigo Carmine

- Chromoendoscopy using indigo carmine shows more clearly the margin of the depressed lesion as compared with WL endoscopy. It also shows irregular edges referred as "worm-eaten appearance."
- Chromoendoscopy using indigo carmine shows slightly rough and large areal patterns in the surrounding protuberance as compared with the areal patterns of the background mucosa (Fig. 11.1b).

11.1.3 Let's Magnify with NBI

- NBI shows an irregular brownish area.
- The pink arrow in this NBI shows a small depression on the greater curvature. This part is examined further with NBI magnified endoscopy (Fig. 11.1c).

11.1.4 Let's Examine More with Magnified NBI

- The central part of the main lesion is evaluated with NBI magnified endoscopy at moderate magnification.
- The pink arrow in this NBI magnified endoscopy shows pitlike structures.
- NBI magnified endoscopy shows vascular pattern with caliber changes, running irregularities, and network formations (Fig. 11.2a).

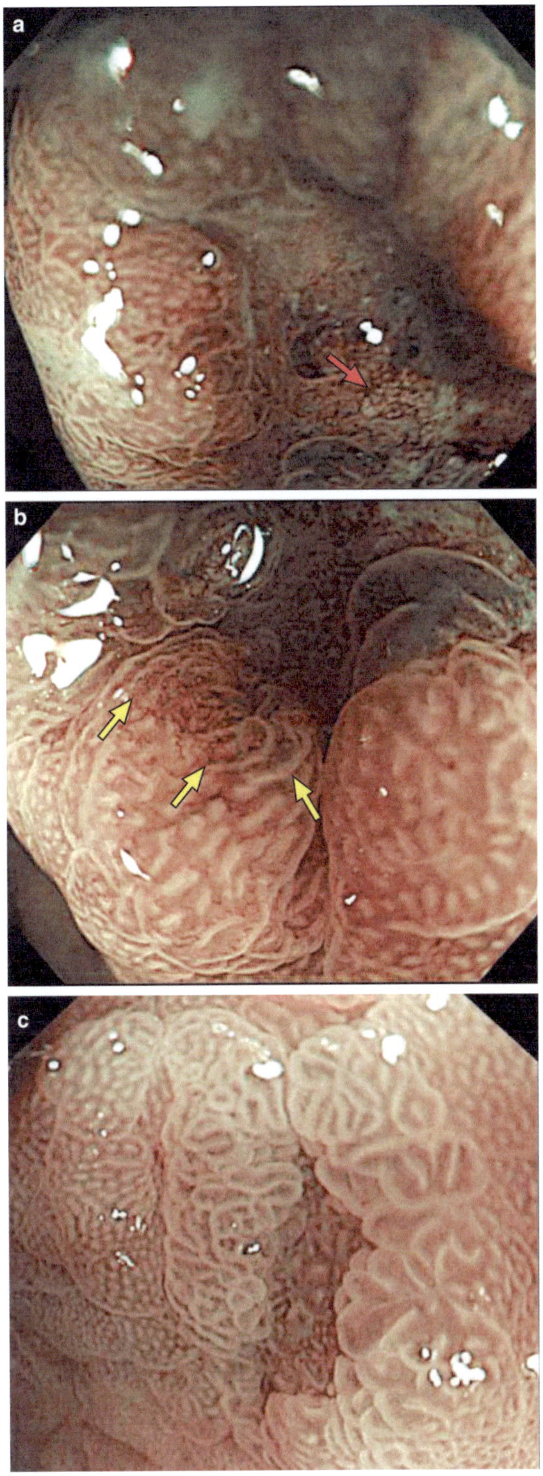

Fig. 11.2 (a) Moderate magnification NBI endoscopic image (b) Lateral margin in the greater curvature side of the lesion (c) Oral side of the lesion

11.1.5 Let's Magnify the Lateral Margin in the Greater Curvature Side of the Lesion

- NBI magnified endoscopy shows a villous pattern consisting of villi of variable sizes extending from the depression up to about half the height of the surrounding protuberance. Vascular patterns with caliber changes and running irregularities are noted on the depression side.
- The background mucosa shows a regular villous pattern. The part designated by yellow arrows is diagnosed as the demarcation line of the lesion by differences in surface patterns.
- Therefore, this main lesion is diagnosed as gastric adenocarcinoma, well-differentiated type, T1a-M (Fig. 11.2b).

11.1.6 Let's Carefully Observe the Oral Side of the Lesion

- NBI magnified endoscopy shows a pitlike pattern with variable pit sizes in the depressed lesion extending toward the greater curvature side. (This small depression on the greater curve side of the main lesion is same as noted by the pink arrow in the first NBI image.)
  NBI magnified endoscopy shows abnormal vessels with caliber changes, running irregularities, and network formations.
- This depressed part is also diagnosed as WDA (tub1). The lesion is thought to be extending orally along a crease from the main lesion.
- Therefore, the lesion is diagnosed as gastric adenocarcinoma, well-differentiated type, 0-IIc, T1a-M. This lesion was resected enbloc by ESD after putting the markings around the lesion (Fig. 11.2c).

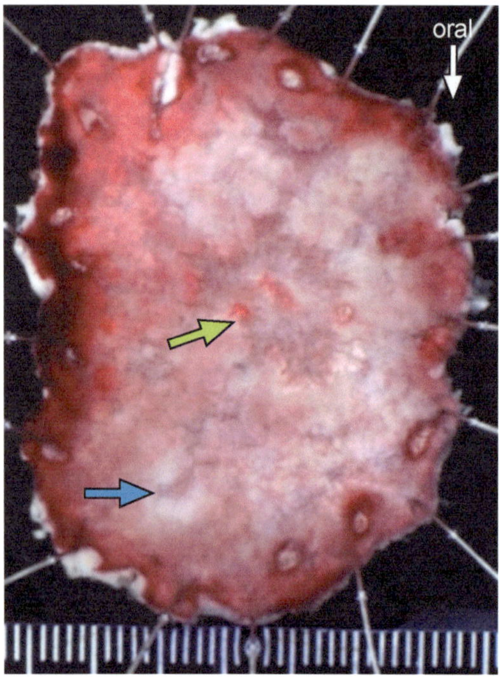

Fig. 11.3 Freshly resected specimen

11.2 From ESD to the Conclusive Diagnosis

11.2.1 Let's Examine the Freshly Resected Specimen

- The lower side of the image is the oral side (Fig. 11.3).
- The irregularly shaped, reddish depression is observed in the center of the specimen. A protuberance is noted within the depression as designated by a light green arrow. The demarcation of the lesion can be followed by differences in color and height of the lesion against its surrounding mucosa.
- The blue arrow in the fresh specimen denotes the smaller depression continuous with the central main depressed lesion via a narrow groove (Fig. 11.3).

11.2.2 Let's Compare the Fresh Specimen with the Endoscopic Image

- The reddishness in the center of the depression (light green arrow) and the depression extended to greater curvature side (blue arrow) correspond (Fig. 11.4a).
- This image shows a pathological finding (HE stained) of a representative section of the central part of the lesion (Fig. 11.4b).
- The tumor cells with swollen nuclei are noted to form irregular glandular tubules and can be diagnosed as WDA, T1-M (Fig. 11.4b).
- The pathological finding in the central part of the lesion shows an invasion of tumor into the submucosal layer, with the invasion depth of SM1 (400 μm) (Fig. 11.4c).

The depression marked by the green arrows in the oral side of the lesion extending like a groove was also a part of the lesion. In addition, MDA (tub2) was noted in part, and its surface was covered by nonneoplastic mucosa (Fig. 11.5).

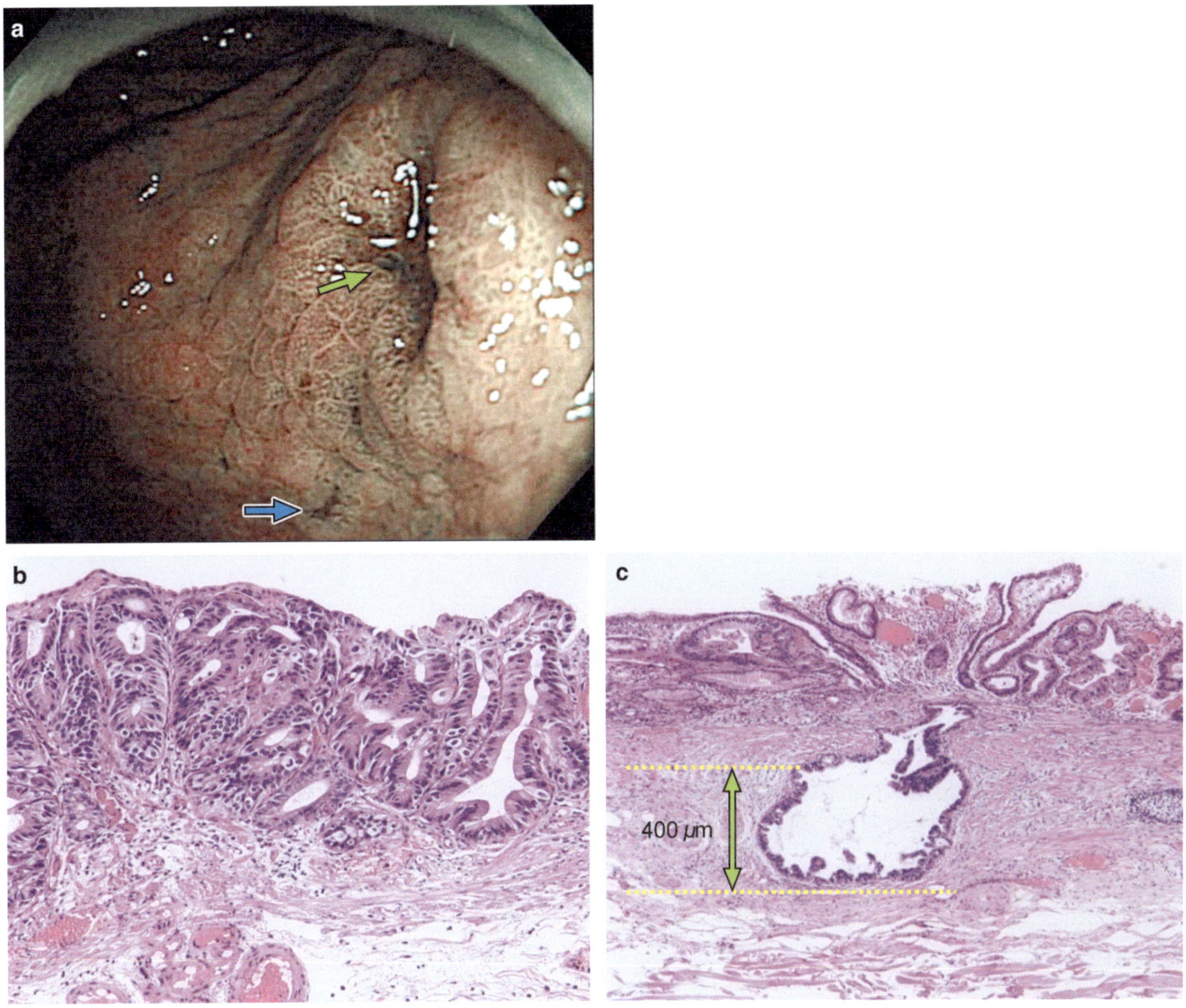

Fig. 11.4 NBI endoscopic image (**b**) Histological image of the lesion (**c**) Histological image of the central part of the lesion

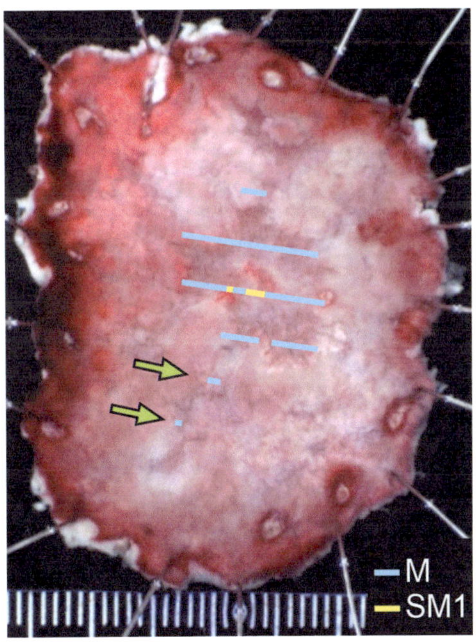

Fig. 11.5 Mapping of the cancer distribution projected on the freshly resected specimen

The protuberant part within the depression is shown in Fig. 11.6a. (The white dotted line represents the section line sliced on the resected specimen projected onto the endoscopic image on the left side. The yellow line represents the part shown by the microscopic image on the right side. The light blue line on the endoscopic image shows the extent of the intramucosal cancer.)

The microscopic image is shown by the direction of the red arrow (Fig. 11.6b).

The central part of the depression observed by NBI magnified endoscopy is WDA (tub1) (Fig. 11.7a).

The depression extending to the oral side is also well-differentiated adenocarcinoma (tub1) (Fig. 11.7b).

Conclusive Diagnosis

Gastric adenocarcinoma, tub1 >> tub2, T1 (SM1:400 μm), ly0, v0, LM(−), VM(−), pType 0-IIc, 19 × 12 mm, U, Post.

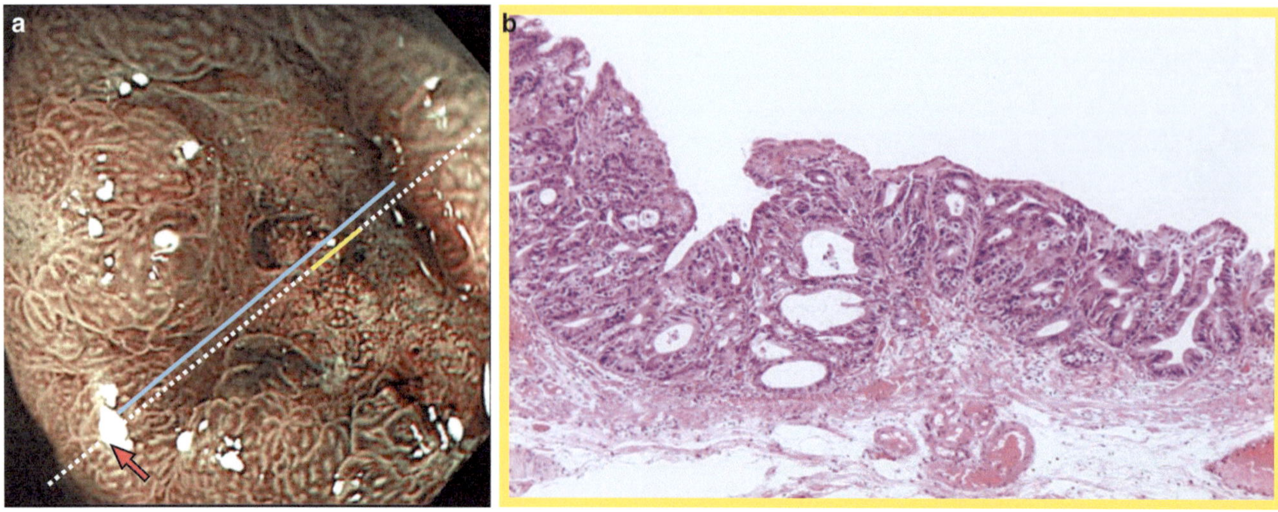

Fig. 11.6 (**a**) The endoscopic image of the protuberant part within the depression. (**b**) The microscopic image of the protuberant part within the depression

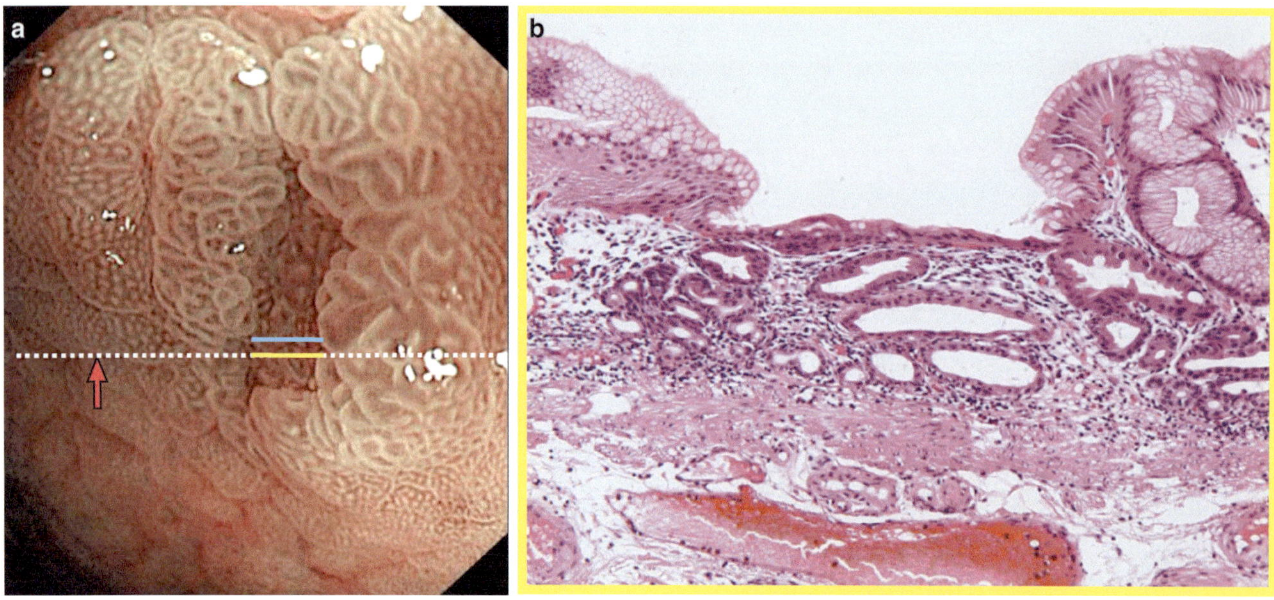

Fig. 11.7 (**a**) The endoscopic image of the central part of the depression. (**b**) The microscopic image of the central part of the depression

Summary

The conclusive diagnosis was gastric well- to MDA, T1b-SM1(:400 μm), pType 0-IIc, 19 × 12 mm, U, Post. Lymph duct and venous invasions were absent. Lateral and vertical margins were negative.

This case was a reddish and irregularly depressed lesion on the greater curvature of the gastric upper body. NBI magnified endoscopy revealed abnormal vessels with caliber changes and running irregularity within the lesion. It also revealed fine network patterns, making it possible to diagnose WDA (tub1). A portion of MDA (tub2), covered under nonneoplastic mucosal surface, could not be diagnosed by NBI magnified endoscopy. Since the depression was even without focal thickness, it was difficult to diagnose the lesion as SM invasive cancer. The depression extending to the oral side showed abnormal vessels, making it possible to diagnose this part as WDA (tub1).

12 Ulcerating Early Gastric Cancer

Shuko Morita

S. Morita (✉)
Department of Gastroenterology, Kobe City Medical Center General Hospital, 2-2-1, Minatojimaminamimachi, Chuo-ku, Kobe-city, Hyogo 650-0047, Japan
e-mail: shuko@crocus.ocn.ne.jp

T. Oyama (ed.), *Endoscopic Diagnosis of Superficial Gastric Cancer for ESD*, DOI 10.1007/978-4-431-54469-2_12

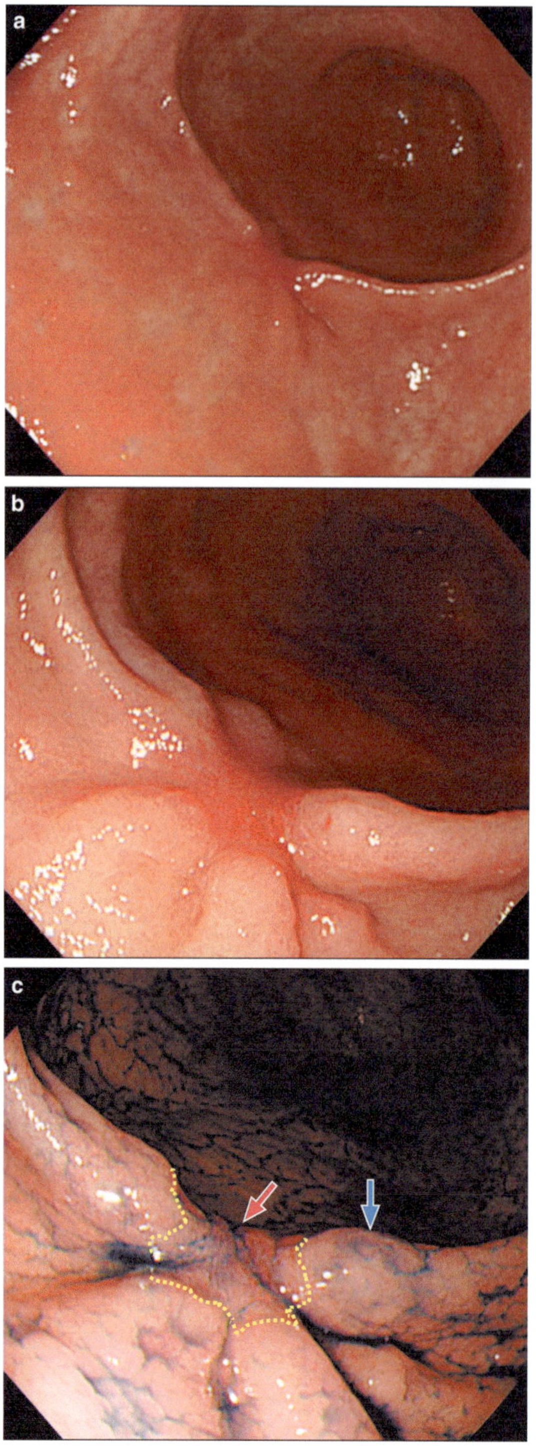

Fig. 12.1 (**a**) WL endoscopic image (**b**) Magnified image (**c**) Indigo carmine stained image

12.1 Let's Try to Diagnose This Lesion

12.1.1 Let's Pay Attention to the Surrounding Mucosa

- The background mucosa shows multiple small whitish depressed lesions and visible submucosal blood vessels, consistent with the presence of atrophic gastritis (Fig. 12.1a).

12.1.2 Let's Note the Gastric Folds

- Typically, the folds of the greater curvature course longitudinally. There are no folds in the antrum, but a pseudo-ring that runs circumferentially.
- In this case, a traversing fold is noted in the distal gastric body to the antrum. The fold is interrupted in the middle forming a shallow depressed area which is suspicious for cancer (Fig. 12.1a).

12.1.3 Let's Take a Closer Look

- The border of the lesion is unclear. Indigo carmine spraying may be helpful in enhancing the border and surface structure.
- Air volume changes the shape of the folds, making them appear rather soft. But the shape of the depressed lesion does not change, making this area to appear hard (Fig. 12.1b).

12.1.4 Let's Spray Indigo Carmine

- Though indigo carmine spraying may make the color of the lesion unclear, it enhances the surface structure (Fig. 12.1b).

12.1.5 Let's Note the Surface Structure of the Border and the Depressed Lesion

- Although the border of the depressed lesion can be recognized as a slight height difference of the surface (yellow dotted line of Fig. 12.1c), it is unclear.
- Compared with the background mucosa, the surface structure of the depressed lesion noted by pooling of indigo carmine is small and dense.
- The depressed area with a border and dense surface structures inside suggests this lesion to be a tumor. Further observation with magnifying endoscope is necessary to get more detailed information (Fig. 12.1c).

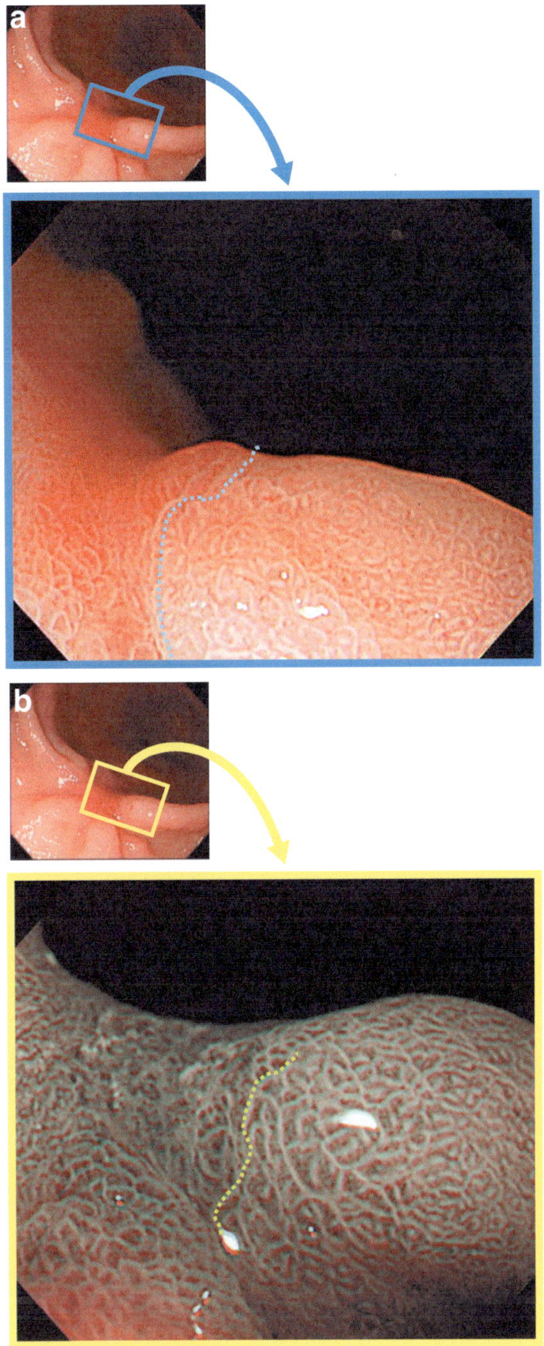

Fig. 12.2 (a) Magnified image of the lesion (b) NBI magnified endoscopic image of the lesion

12.1.6 Let's Focus on the Fold

- Though a blue arrow points to a slightly enlarged fold, the fold is not fused with adjacent folds. This finding suggests that this lesion does not invade the submucosal layer.
- Gathering of folds to a red arrow suggests the presence of an ulcer scar, which makes the depressed lesion appear stiff (Fig. 12.1c).

12.1.7 Let's Magnify

- When examined with a magnifying endoscope, the surface pattern consists of small and round shapes with regularity to the right side of the blue dotted line.
- The surface pattern consists of irregularly shaped villi to the left side of the blue dotted line.
- There is a clear border between these two different surface patterns indicated by the blue dotted line. Therefore, the left side of the blue dotted line is diagnosed as carcinoma.
- NBI is easier to evaluate for close-up view of the surface structures on magnification than WL imaging (Fig. 12.2a).

12.1.8 Let's Use NBI

- Magnification with NBI makes it easy to see the surface structures and vessels.
- Surface structure: The surface structure to the right side of the yellow dotted line appears to be regularly shaped pits, while the left side appears irregularly shaped villi. The border is clear.
- Vessels: The vessels are not examined enough in this case. But the surface structure is useful to diagnose this lesion.
- Based on these findings, the diagnosis of the lesion to the left side of the yellow dotted line is WDA (Fig. 12.2b).

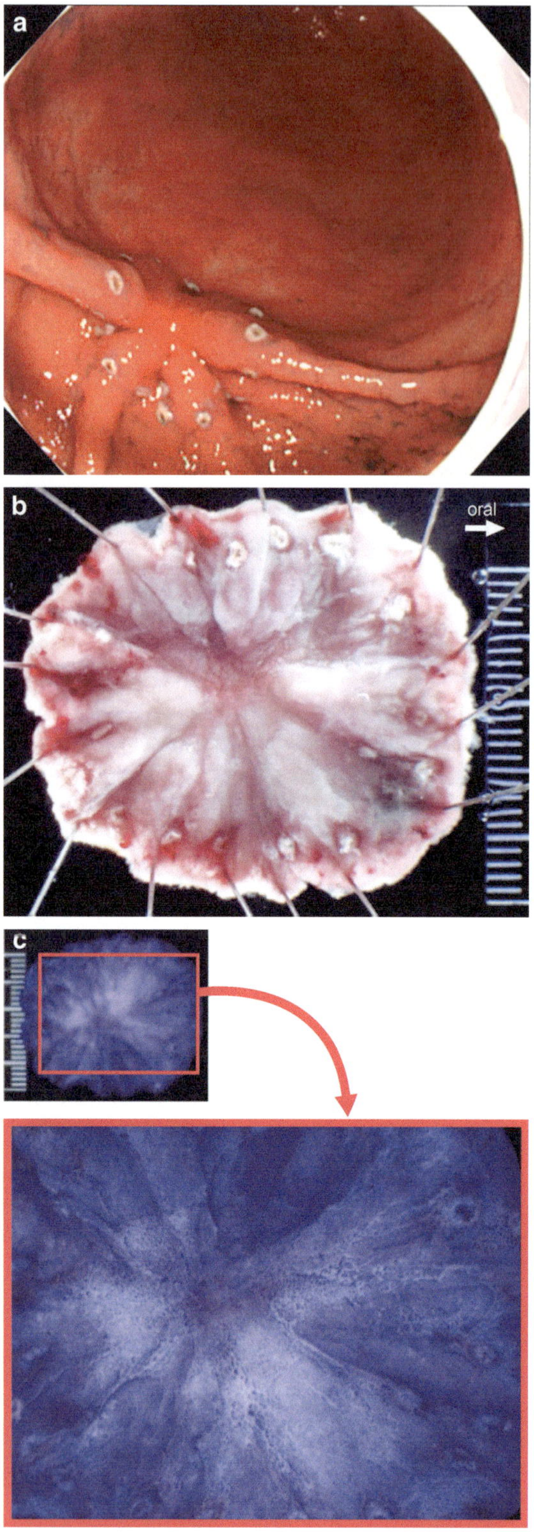

Fig. 12.3 (a) Endoscopic image of marking before ESD (b) Resected specimen (c) The specimen stained with crystal violet

12.2 From ESD to the Final Diagnosis

12.2.1 Let's Perform ESD

- Diagnosis based on endoscopic findings: Adenocarcinoma with invasion depth of M, largest diameter about 15 mm, and ulcer scar (+). This meets an expanded indication for ESD.
- The border of this lesion was diagnosed and marked based on magnifying endoscope with NBI and magnifying endoscope after spraying indigo carmine. The lesion was resected en bloc by ESD (Fig. 12.3a).

12.2.2 Let's Look at the Resected Specimen

- The right side of the specimen is the oral side.
- The red and depressed lesion is located in the middle of the specimen. The border is relatively clear (Fig. 12.3b).

12.2.3 Let's Stain the Specimen with Crystal Violet

- The surface structure becomes clear after staining with crystal violet.
- The surface pattern around the depressed lesion consists of small and round-shaped structures.
- The surface pattern of the depressed lesion itself appears to consist of irregularly shaped villi which are smaller and denser than the surrounding surface structures (Fig. 12.3c).

This is the histopathology of the depressed lesion with HE stained. Tumor cells with enlarged nuclei form highly dense ducts consistent with MDA (tub2) (Fig. 12.4).

There is intricately intertwined fibrosis at the submucosal layer, which makes this lesion to be diagnosed as UL (+). Histological invasion depth of the lesion is intramucosal (Fig. 12.5).

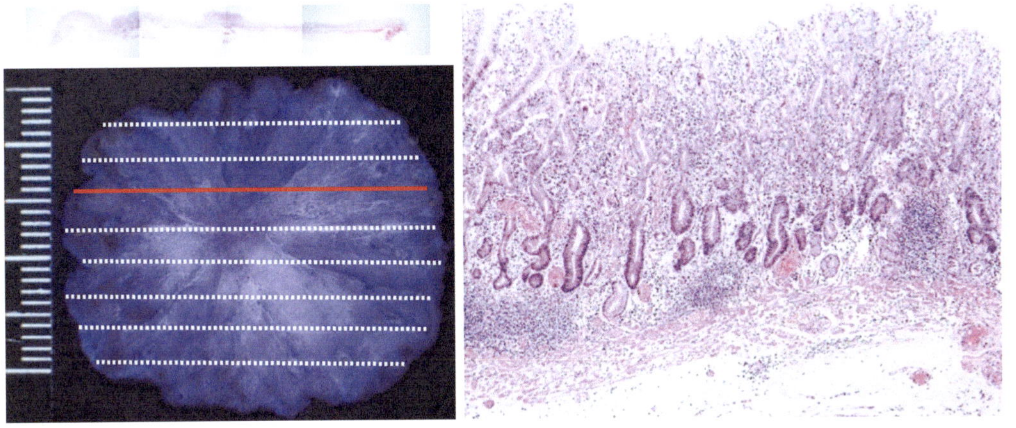

Fig. 12.4 Histology image of the depressed lesion (HE stained)

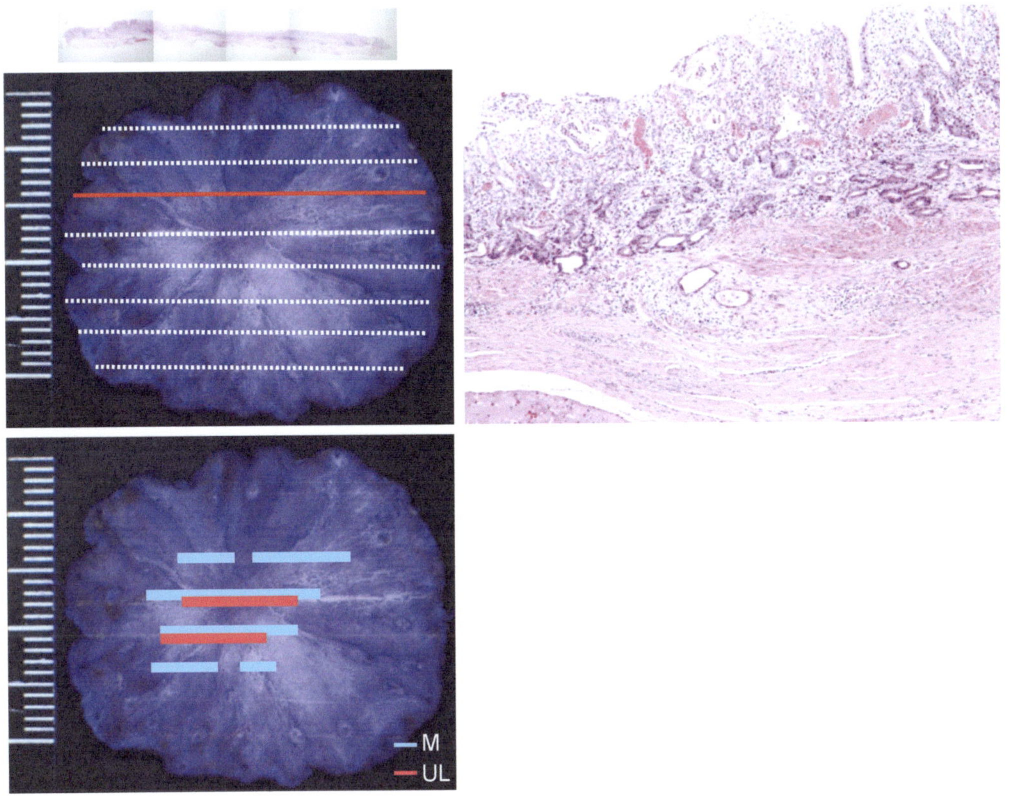

Fig. 12.5 Histology image and the mapping of the cancer distribution projected on the lesion (HE stained)

Conclusive Diagnosis

Gastric adenocarcinoma, tub2, T1(M), ly0, v0, UL(+), LM(−), VM(−), pType 0-IIc, 15 × 14 mm, L, Gre.

Summary

This case is a reddish depressed lesion with a UL scar at the greater curvature of the proximal antrum. The border of the lesion is unclear without magnifying NBI. But the border and irregular villous structures could be easily detected with magnifying NBI, leading to the diagnosis of MDA. The lesion did not appear to change shape by increasing or decreasing the air volume, and the apparent hardness of the lesion was felt to be because of ulcer scar formation (UL (+)) and not due to tumor invasion of the submucosal layer.

Signet Ring Cell Carcinoma

13

Masaki Tanaka

M. Tanaka (✉)
Division of Endoscopy, Shizuoka Cancer Center, 1007
Shimonagakubo, Nagaizumi-cho, Sunto-gun, Shizuoka 411-8777,
Japan
e-mail: ma.tanaka@scchr.jp

T. Oyama (ed.), *Endoscopic Diagnosis of Superficial Gastric Cancer for ESD*, DOI 10.1007/978-4-431-54469-2_13

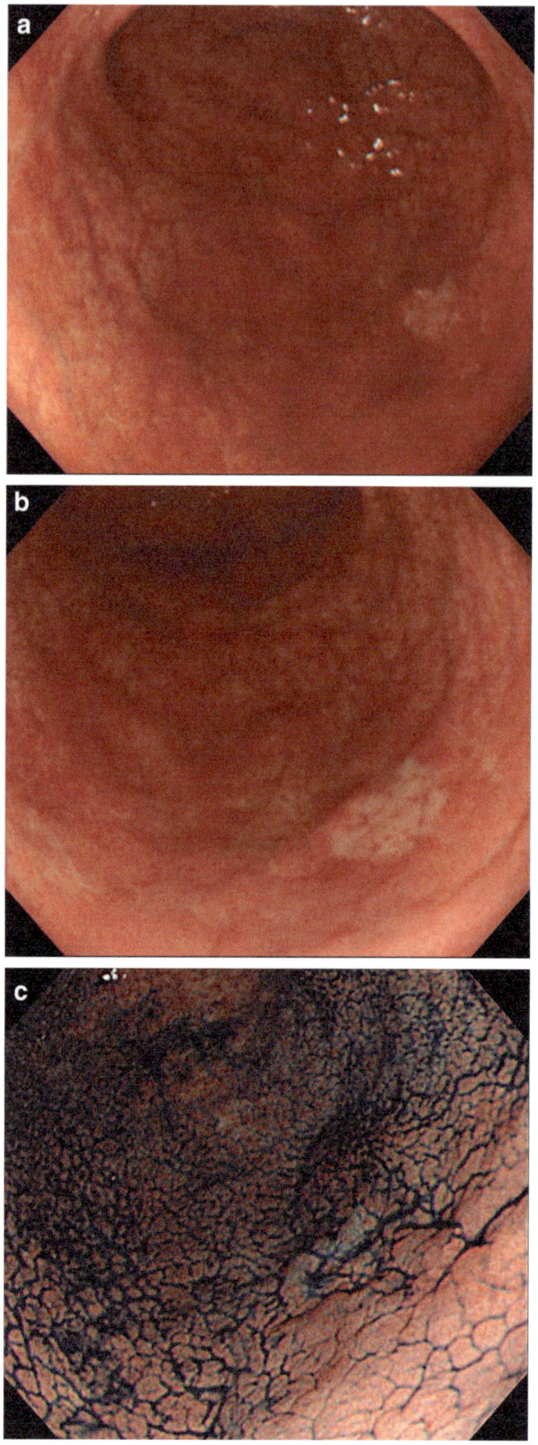

Fig. 13.1 (**a, b**) WL endoscopic image (**c**) Indigo carmine stained image

13.1 Let's Try to Diagnose This Lesion

13.1.1 Let's Take Notice of the Discoloration of Gastric Mucosa

- A small depressed lesion is located on the posterior side of greater curvature of the gastric body.
- Although gastric cancer is strongly suspected because of its clear margin and irregular shape, we have to make more detailed examination to differentiate it from other surrounding discolored lesions (Fig. 13.1a).

13.1.2 Let's Take Notice of the Background Mucosa

- We can see the atrophic changes of the mucosa, including visible submucosal vessels due to thinning of the gastric mucosa and mixed (red and white) color of the gastric mucosa, on the anal side of the lesion.
- On the other hand, there is no such finding in the oral side of the lesion.
- So we can conclude that the lesion is located around the border of the atrophic change (Fig. 13.1a).

13.1.3 Let's Take a Closer Look on the Lesion

- We can recognize the lesion by its distinct whitish depressed area compared to the surrounding atrophic mucosa.
- The surface structure of the depressed area is uniform, and there are no apparent irregularities.
- Gastric cancer is suspected because of a clearly demarcated irregular depressed lesion. However, we cannot diagnose definitely (Fig. 13.1b).

13.1.4 Let's Spray Indigo Carmine

- Although we cannot evaluate the color of the lesion after spraying indigo carmine, we can easily observe the surface structure and difference in height of the lesion against the background mucosa (Fig. 13.1c).

13.1.5 Let's Pay Attention to the Depressed Area

- The surface pattern of the surrounding mucosa is regular. However, the surface pattern of the depressed area is unclear.

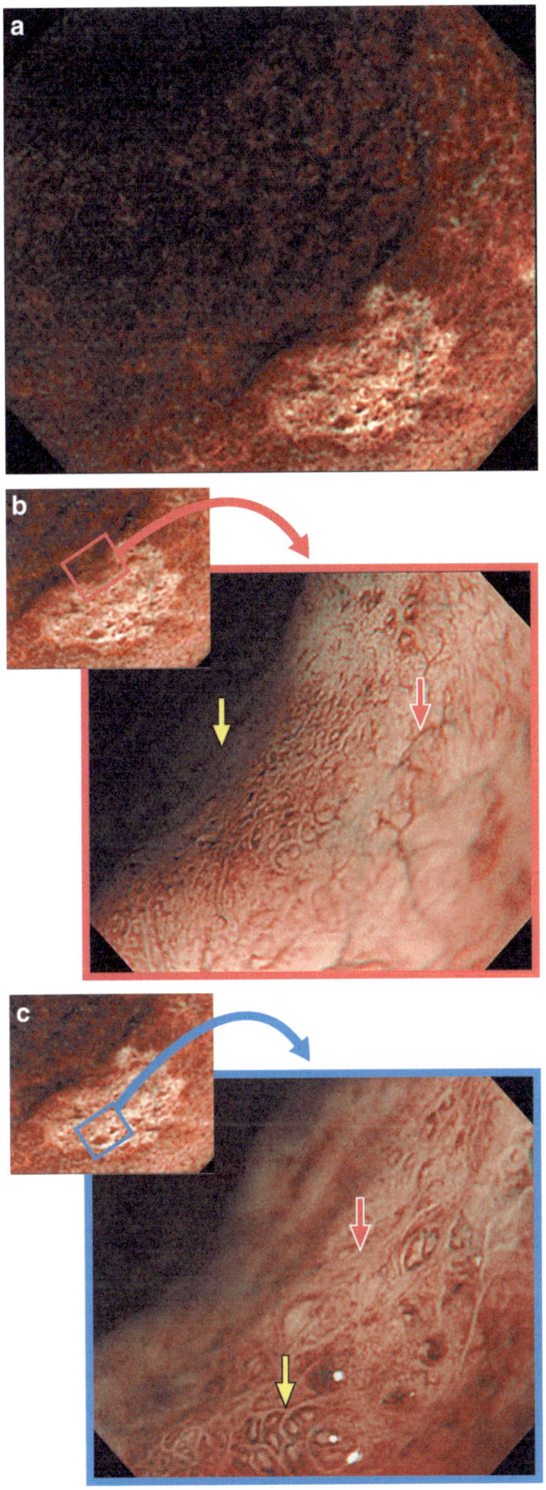

Fig. 13.2 (a) NBI endoscopic image (b) Magnified image of the anal side of the lesion (c) Magnified image of the oral side of the lesion

- Although the shape of the depressed lesion is irregular, the surface of the lesion is not so irregular. Gastric cancer is strongly suspected. But we cannot make a definite diagnosis (Fig. 13.1c).

13.1.6 Let's Use NBI

- With NBI, we can clearly see the margin of the discolored lesion as a whitish irregularly shaped depressed lesion.
- Although the irregularity of the surface is not so distinct by WL, we can see some island-shaped brownish areas within the depressed lesion by NBI.
- No further information is available without magnification (Fig. 13.2a).

13.1.7 Let's Observe with Magnification the Anal Side of the Lesion

- With NBI magnified endoscopy, a regularly arranged tubelike surface pattern and regular vessels are observed near the anal side of the depressed lesion as indicated by the yellow arrow on the left side. Microvascular pattern and its distribution are also regular. So we diagnosed the area as nonneoplastic.
- On the other hand, we cannot see glandular surface patterns on the right side indicated by the red arrow. And the surface structure of this area is also irregular.
- Although we can only see sparse vessels in the area, caliber change and tortuous running are seen in each vessel, and they make up nonnetwork pattern of the vessels. So we diagnosed the lesion as PDA (Fig. 13.2b).

13.1.8 Let's Observe with Magnification the Oral Side of the Lesion

- NBI magnified endoscopy of the oral side of the depressed area is shown.
- The yellow arrow indicates an area with a pitlike surface pattern. As each pit is round and uniformly sized, this area is diagnosed as nonneoplastic.
- On the other hand, another area indicated by the red arrow shows unclear surface pattern.
- And the vessels are irregular with caliber changes and tortuous running without forming network patterns, leading to diagnosis of a PDA (Fig. 13.2c).

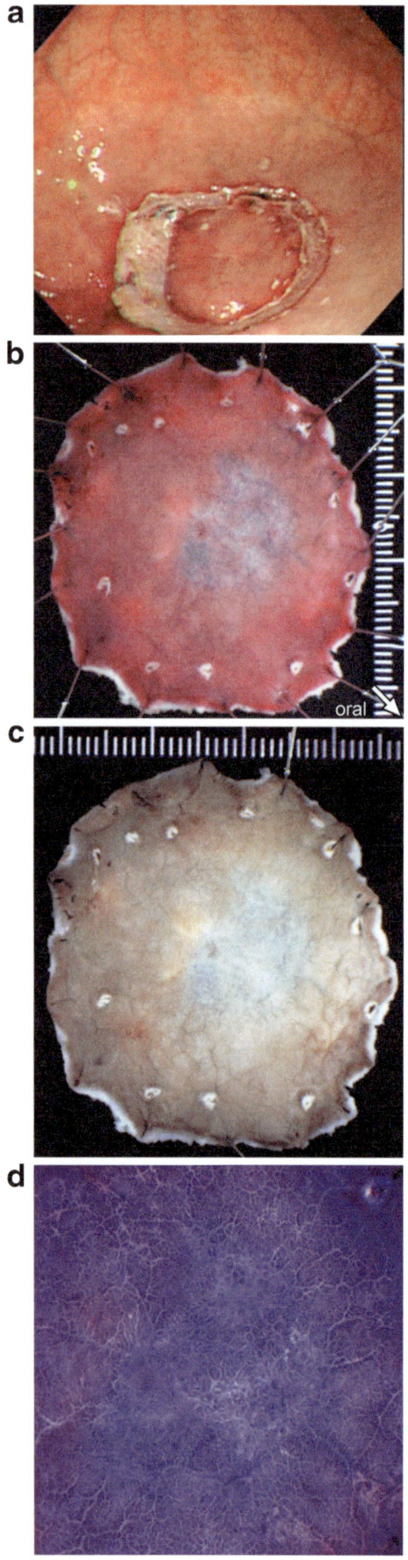

Fig. 13.3 (**a**) Endoscopic image of marking before ESD (**b**) The freshly resected specimen (**c**) Fixed specimen (**d**) The specimen stained with crystal violet

13.2 Making the Final Diagnosis from the ESD Specimen

13.2.1 Let's Perform ESD

- Because the histology of this lesion showed PDA, we confirmed the tumor extent by taking four-point negative biopsies around the lesion with 1 cm margin.
- We used magnification endoscopy with NBI to identify biopsy scars and placed markings outside these biopsy scars. ESD with en bloc resection was performed without any complications (Fig. 13.3a).

13.2.2 Let's Observe the Freshly Resected Specimen

- The lower right side of the figure is the oral side.
- The surrounding mucosa of the depressed area appears uniform with minimal atrophy consistent with fundic gland gastric mucosa.
- There is an irregular whitish depressed lesion in the center of the resected specimen, but its border is partially unclear (Fig. 13.3b).

13.2.3 Let's Observe the Formalin-Fixed Specimen

- After formalin fixation, we can see the surface structure more clearly.
- The surface of the depressed area is mostly unclear with some scattered tubular gland-like structures, which are larger than of the surrounding mucosa.
- The boundary with the surrounding mucosa is mostly clear (Fig. 13.3c).

13.2.4 Let's Stain with Crystal Violet and Observe with Magnification Using a Stereoscopic Microscope

- More detailed examination of the surface pattern can be made after crystal violet stain. The surface pattern of the surrounding mucosa appears to have regularly arranged glandular structures.
- On the other hand, the depressed lesion has larger irregularly shaped villi in part as well as parts which have no clear surface patterns with glandular structures obscured (Fig. 13.3d).

This figure shows the histopathology of the depressed area (HE stained) (Fig. 13.4a). Although there is a layer of regular foveolar epithelium on the surface of the mucosal layer, many mucus-filled eosinophilic cells with peripherally displaced nuclei are noted near the mucous neck region in the lamina propria. The lesion is diagnosed as a signet ring cell carcinoma.

As there were no findings of submucosal invasion, we diagnosed this lesion as a mucosal signet ring cell carcinoma. The lateral extent of the tumor conformed closely to the depressed area without any submucosal extension. There was no finding of ulcer scar or another lesion within the resected specimen (Fig. 13.4b).

We made a mapping of the tumor extent on a fresh specimen. After that, we matched the mapping image with the endoscopic image by adjusting the oral side of the lesion in the same orientation (Fig. 13.5).

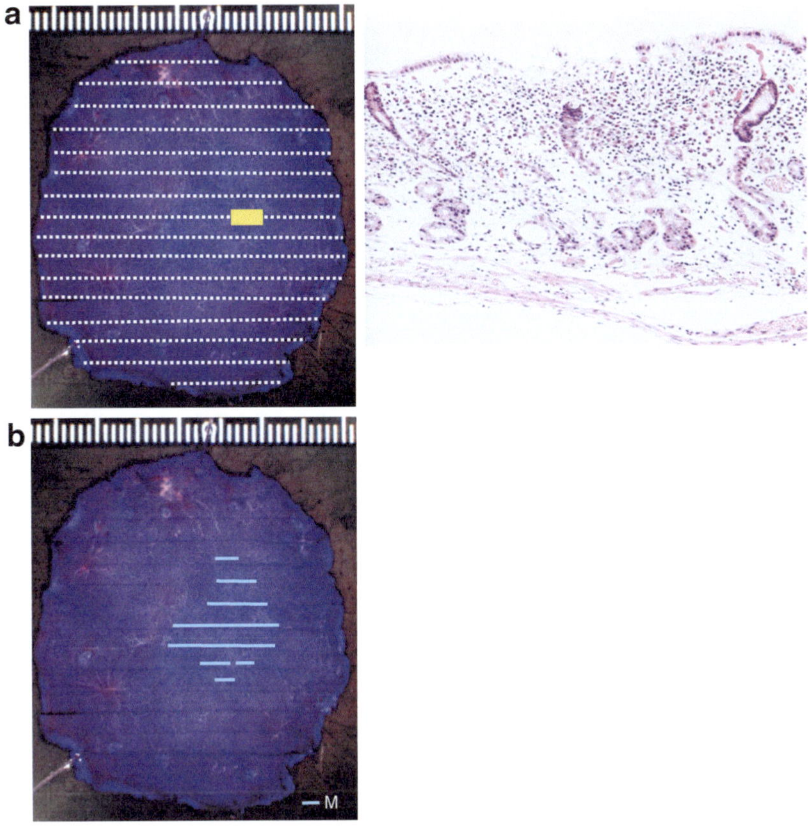

Fig. 13.4 Histology image of the depressed lesion (HE stained)

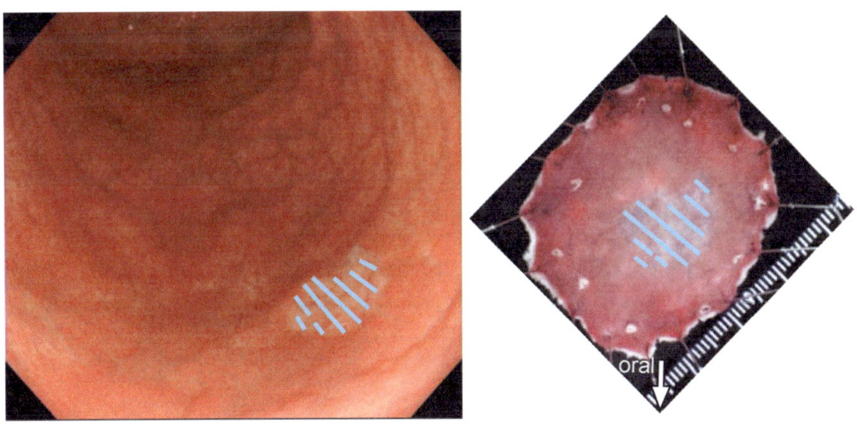

Fig. 13.5 Comparison between the endoscopic image and resected specimen. Mapping on cancer distribution on each image

Conclusive Diagnosis
Gastric adenocarcinoma, signet ring cell carcinoma, T1 (M), ly0, v0, Lateral margin (−), Vertical margin (−), pType 0 -IIc, 14 × 13 mm, M, Gre.

Summary
This tumor was a discolored depressed lesion located on the greater curvature of the gastric body. As it was located on the border between atrophic mucosa and normal mucosa, it was difficult to distinguish the tumor margin with WL imaging against the background discolored mucosa. With NBI magnification, we could see the change of surface structure and microvessels, such as loss of clear glandular structures and disappearance of vascular network. Furthermore, we could make a precise diagnosis not only about the lateral extent of the tumor but also about a prediction of its histological type.

(While arguments still remain as to including undifferentiated cancer for indication of ESD, we treated ESD for undifferentiated-type gastric cancer as an expanded indication in this section.)

14 Early Gastric Cancer with Large Size

Akiko Takahashi

A. Takahashi (✉)
Division of Endoscopy, Saku Central Hospital, 197 Usuda, Saku,
Nagano 384-0301, Japan
e-mail: aurevoireurope@yahoo.co.jp

T. Oyama (ed.), *Endoscopic Diagnosis of Superficial Gastric Cancer for ESD*, DOI 10.1007/978-4-431-54469-2_14

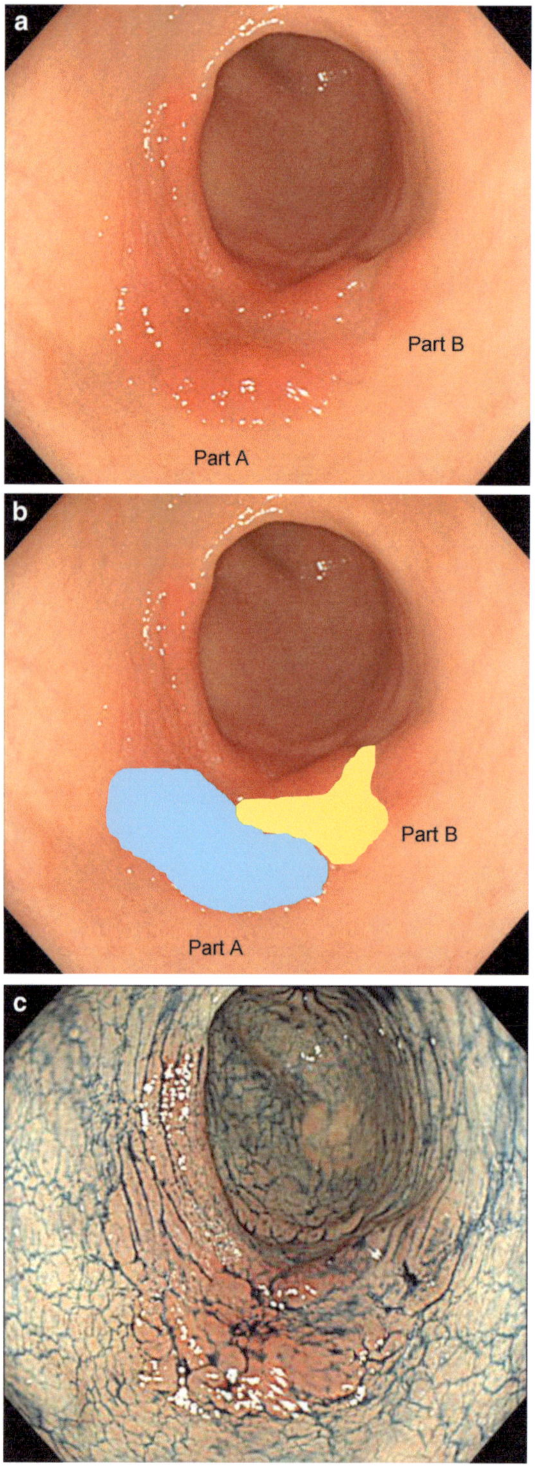

Fig. 14.1 (**a**) WL endoscopic image (**b**) WL endoscopic image with indicated the oral part and the posterior part (**c**) Indigo carmine stained image

14.1 Let's Try to Diagnose This Lesion

14.1.1 Let's Notice the Coloration of the Lesion

- WL endoscopy shows a reddish, flat, and protuberant lesion with a clear margin on the greater curvature of the gastric antrum.
- The surface is relatively smooth.
- The coloration is uneven. The oral part (Part A) and the central part of the lesion show more redness than other parts. In contrast, the posterior part (Part B) shows an irregularly shaped depression with some discoloration.
- Since larger gastric cancers tend to be of mixed pathological types, it is necessary to consider pathological types based on endoscopic findings (Fig. 14.1a).
- Parts A and B described above are colored by light blue for Part A and yellow for Part B (Fig. 14.1b).

14.1.2 Let's Spray Indigo Carmine

- Immediately following indigo carmine spraying, the surface pattern and protuberance can be observed in detail.
- The surface pattern of the lesion is irregular, particularly in the oral part where it is coarsely irregular.
- On the other hand, the discolored part on the posterior wall (Part B) shows slight depression with an irregular surface pattern.
- The margin of the lesion can be clearly recognized against regular areal surface pattern of the background mucosa (Fig. 14.1c).

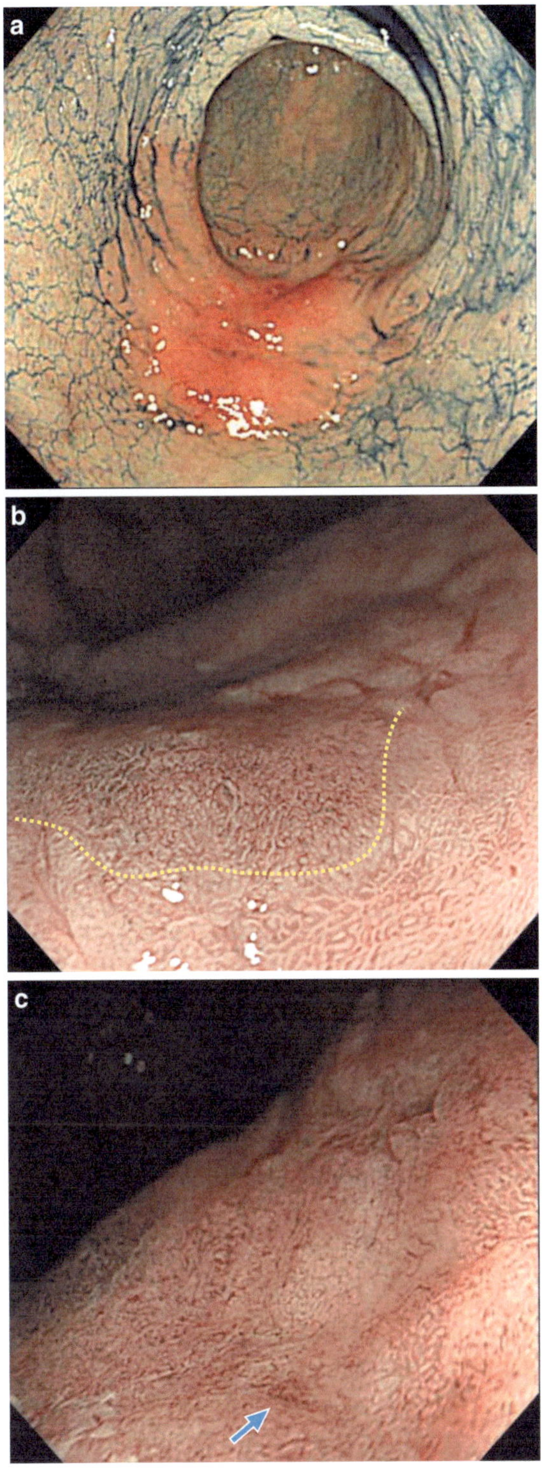

Fig. 14.2 (**a**) Indigo carmine stained image (**b**) NBI magnified endoscopic image of the oral side (**c**) NBI magnified endoscopic image of the posterior wall of the lesion

14.1.3 Let's Wait for a While, After Spraying Indigo Carmine

- It becomes easy to diagnose the margin of the lesion, 2–3 min after spraying indigo carmine because the lesion repels indigo carmine.
- The depressed part (Part B) of the posterior wall can be recognized as a part of the lesion (Fig. 14.2a).

14.1.4 Let's Magnify the Oral Side of the Lesion by NBI

- Next, we observe the lesion by NBI magnified endoscopy for pathological diagnosis.
- NBI magnified endoscopy with intermediate magnification of the oral side (Part A) of the lesion shows pitlike pattern with high density. Vascular pattern shows caliber changes and running irregularity and are highly dense. The oral side of the lesion is diagnosed as WDA (tub1).
- In addition, the background mucosa shows a mixture of regular pitlike pattern and villous pattern, making the margin of the lesion traceable by noticing the difference in surface pattern as indicated by the yellow dotted line (Fig. 14.2b).

14.1.5 Let's Magnify the Posterior Wall of the Lesion by NBI Magnified Endoscopy

- We observed the posterior wall (Part B) with intermediate magnification NBI.
- The surface pattern is villous and unclear partially. The vascular pattern shows caliber changes and running irregularity; however, network pattern could not be observed clearly (blue arrow). The vascular density is less compared with the reddish part. Therefore, the posterior part of the lesion is diagnosed as WDA (tub1).
- Therefore, the lesion was diagnosed as WDA, T1a-M, 0-IIa + IIc. After placing markings around, the lesion was resected en bloc by ESD (Fig. 14.2c).

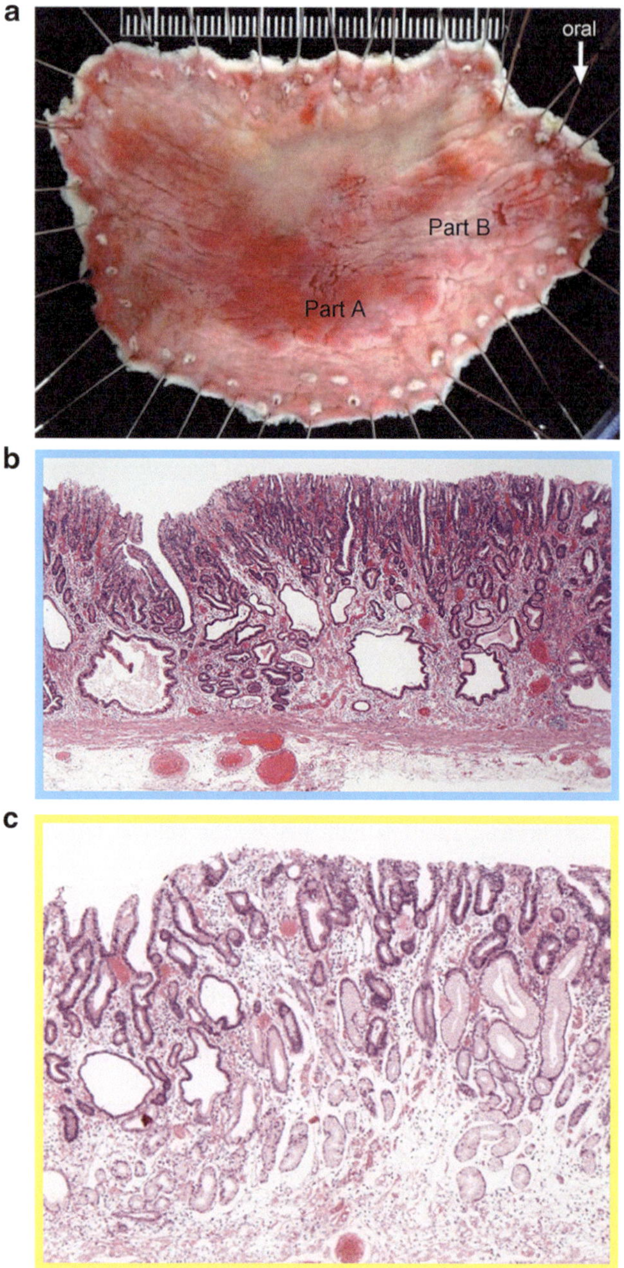

Fig. 14.3 (a) Freshly resected specimen (b) Histology image of the oral side of the lesion (c) Histology image of the posterior wall side of the lesion

14.2 From ESD to the Conclusive Diagnosis

14.2.1 Let's Observe the Freshly Resected Specimen

- The lower side of the image is the oral side.
- The fresh specimen shows strong reddish flat protuberance in the oral side (lower side) of the lesion. On the anal side, a discolored depressed lesion is noted. Because of its location, the lesion was not easily seen by endoscopy.
- On the other hand, the freshly resected specimen shows a slightly reddish depressed lesion on the posterior side (right side). It could be pointed out by endoscopy.
- The margin can be traced clearly and totally based on coloration and unevenness of the surface (Fig. 14.3a).

14.2.2 Let's Observe Histopathology of the Oral Side of the Lesion

- Histopathology (HE stained) of the reddish flat raised part on the oral side of the lesion (Part A) is shown as a representative section.
- The tumor cells with swollen nuclei are forming dense tubular glands and are diagnosed as WDA, T1a M.
- There are a lot of vessels in the interstitial, which explain redness observed by WL endoscopy (Fig. 14.3b).

14.2.3 Let's Observe Histopathology of the Posterior Wall Side of the Lesion

- Histopathology of the slightly discolored depressed part (Part B) of the posterior wall side is shown.
- The tumor cells with swollen nuclei are forming tubular glands in two layers with very little structural atypia, consistent with WDA (tub1).
- There are very few interstitial vessels accounting for discoloration noted by WL endoscopy (Fig. 14.3c).
- The conclusive diagnosis is a gastric WDA, T1a-M, pType 0-IIa + IIc, 63 × 51 mm, L, Gre. Both lymph duct and venous invasions are negative, and lateral and vertical margins are free of cancer.
- A comparison of the reddish flat raised part on the oral side of the lesion is shown (Fig. 14.4a). The white dotted line is an imaginary line of resection of the resected specimen imposed on an endoscopic image. The yellow line shows where the corresponding histopathological

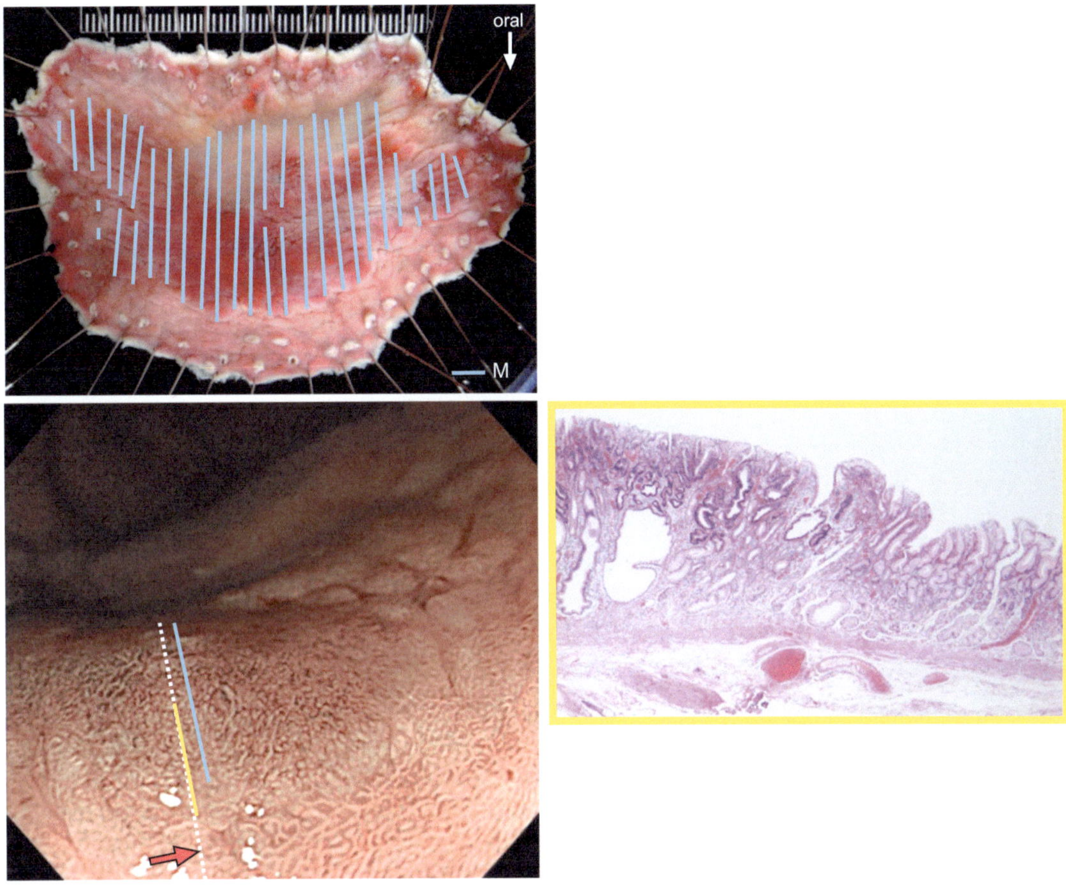

Fig. 14.4 (**a**) Mapping of the cancer distribution on the fresh specimen (**b**) Mapping on the NBI magnified endoscopic image (**c**) The histology image : seen from the direction of the *red arrow* of (**b**)

image (in the yellow frame) is. The light blue line shows the extent of the mucosal cancer (Fig. 14.4b).

- The histopathology image is seen from the direction of the red arrow (Fig. 14.4c).
- The areas observed with high vascular density by magnified NBI are WDA containing rich interstitial vascularity accounting for red coloration.

Conclusive Diagnosis

Gastric adenocarcinoma, tub1, T1(M), ly0, v0, LM (−), VM(−), 0-IIa + IIc, 63 × 31 mm, L, Gre.

Summary

The lesion is 0-IIa + IIc noted on the greater curvature of the gastric antrum.

By WL endoscopy, gastric cancer of mixed pathological types was suspected because of color differences. However, NBI magnified endoscopy revealed findings of WDA (tub1) by surface pattern and vascular pattern. The color difference was thought to reflect the difference in densities of abnormal vessels.

Histopathology showed WDA (tub1) with increased interstitial vascularity accounting for its reddish coloration.

Part III

Practices

Question 1: What Is the Invasion Depth? 15

Koichi Okamoto

K. Okamoto (✉)
Department of Gastroenterology and Oncology, University of Tokushima, 2-24, Shinkura-cho, Tokushima 770-8501, Japan
e-mail: tagayasu33jp@yahoo.co.jp

T. Oyama (ed.), *Endoscopic Diagnosis of Superficial Gastric Cancer for ESD*, DOI 10.1007/978-4-431-54469-2_15

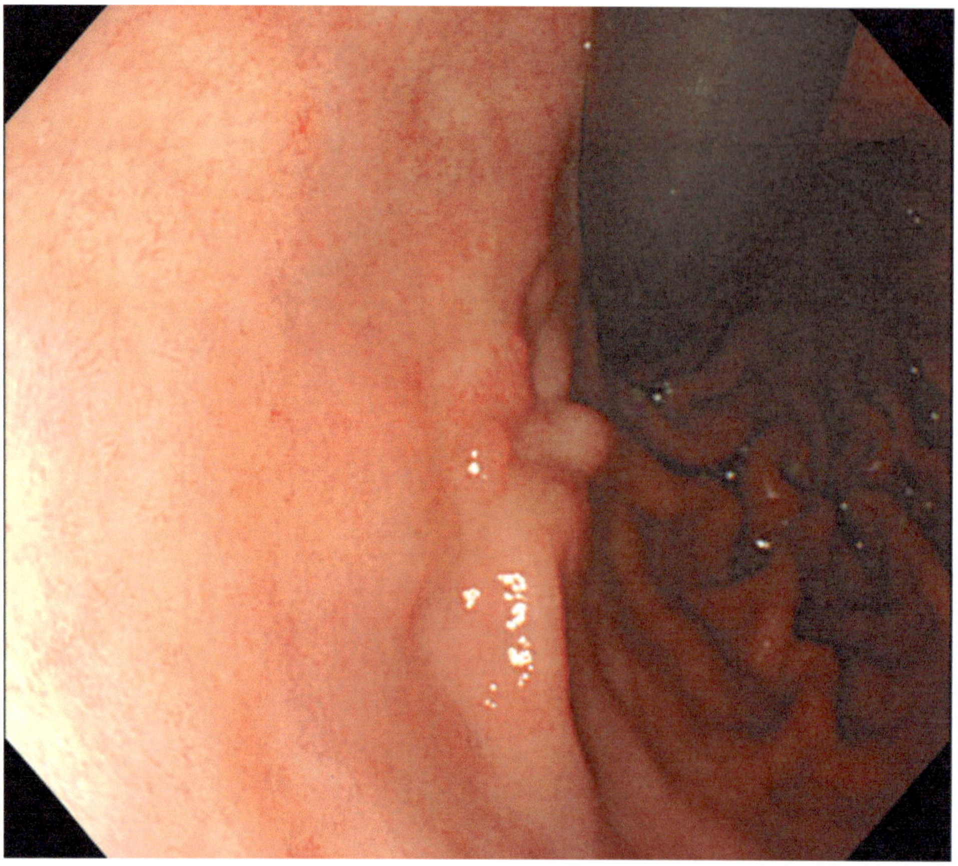

Fig. 15.1 What is the invasion depth?

Question: Which of the following answers is correct? (Fig. 15.1)

(1) M
(2) SM
(3) MP

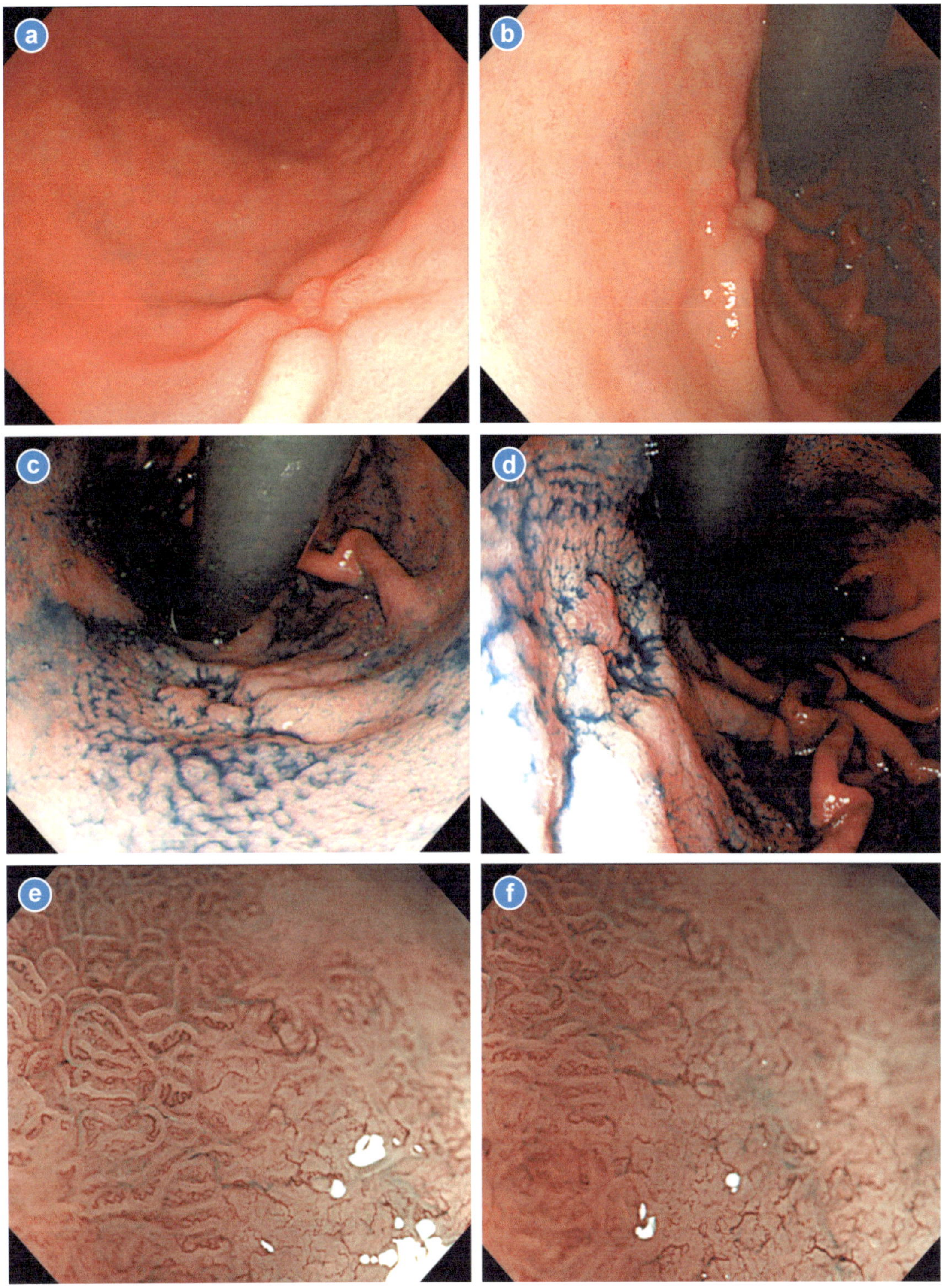

Fig. 15.2 Let's diagnose by observing these six images

15.1 Focus on These Points

15.1.1 Let's Focus on Fold Convergence

- There is a reddish depressed lesion with fold convergence at the posterior wall of the greater curvature of the gastric upper body. It is possible to follow the depressed boundary on the oral side, but the anal side is in the tangential direction and hard to see. Small nodules are recognized inside the depression.
- The fold convergence is focused on not one point but the depressed area. The tips of the folds are interrupted at the reddish part, but the folds show no thickening or fusion (Fig. 15.3a).

15.1.2 Let's Also Focus on the Background Mucosa

- No vascular image is seen through the adjacent mucosa, and gastric fundic gland mucosa without atrophy is diagnosed (Fig. 15.3a).

15.1.3 Let's Observe with a Retroflexed Endoscope

- The anal side of the lesion, which is hard to see by a looking-down approach, is observed more clearly. The reddish area is just a part of the whole lesion, and the whole lesion is recognized as a depressed lesion with discoloration, but the boundary is obscure (Fig. 15.3b).

15.1.4 Let's Focus on the Inside of the Depression

- There are two small reddish nodules within the depression (Fig. 15.3b).

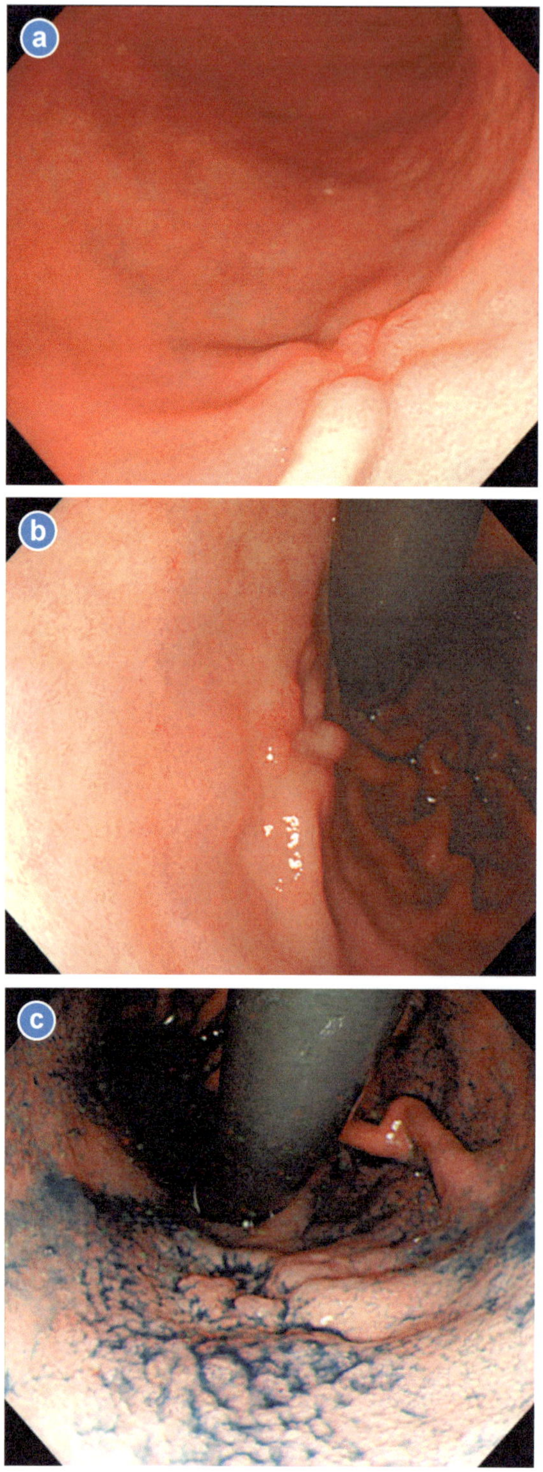

Fig. 15.3 Same images as Fig. 15.2

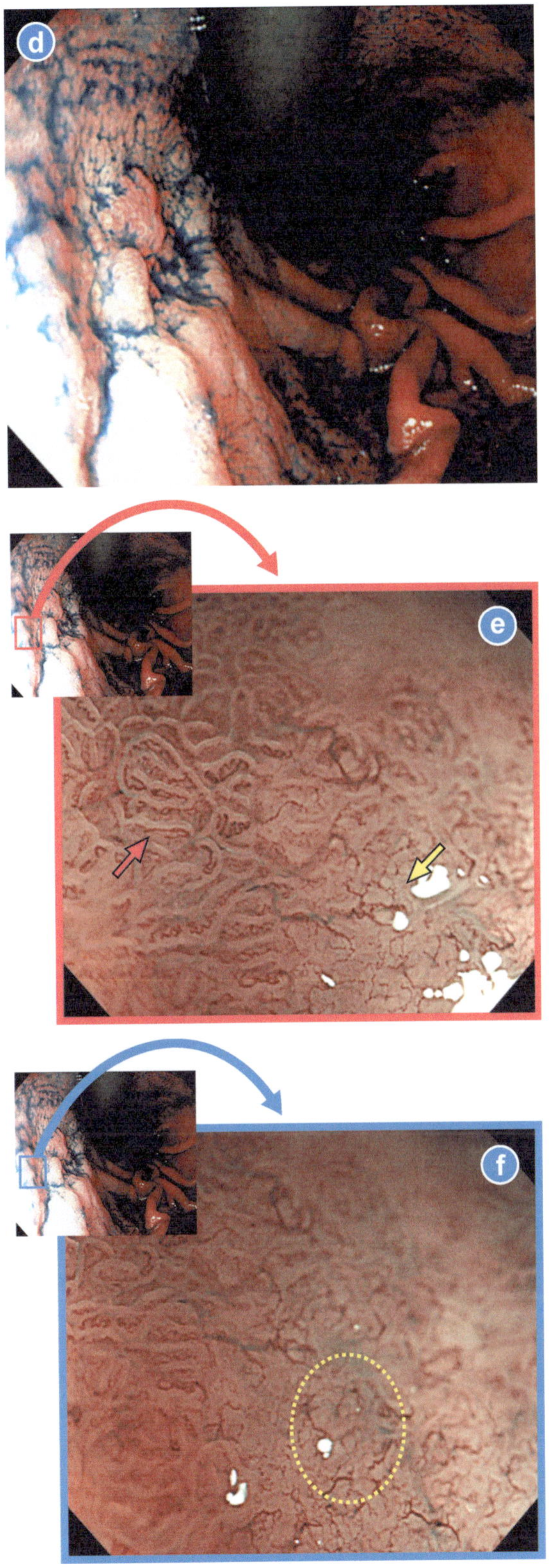

Fig. 15.3 (continued)

15.1.5 How Should We Interpret These Findings

- The cause of fold convergence is fibrosis in the submucosal layer, and the cause of fibrosis is either ulcer or submucosal invasion of cancer. In this case, there is no fold thickening or fusion suggesting submucosal invasion, and a change of peptic ulcer scar is diagnosed (Fig. 15.3b).

15.1.6 Let's Focus on the Boundary

- When indigo carmine is sprayed, the boundary of the depression is more clearly visible, and irregular dye pooling is recognized as the site almost corresponding with the depressed area with discoloration noted by WL imaging. The image of fold interruptions at the greater curvature is also recognized more clearly. The boundaries of two small nodules in the depression are visualized more clearly (Fig. 15.3c).

15.1.7 Let's Focus on Air Volume Changes

- Compared with the image by WL imaging, the status of the fold on the greater curvature suggests that the image is obtained with the stomach extended with air. The lesion is relatively well extended and invasion depth of M is diagnosed (Fig. 15.3c).

15.1.8 Let's Carry Out Close-Up Observation

- The inside of the depression is recognized as fine gutter-like structure, and the boundary is well delineated. The interrupted folds on the greater curvature are clearly recognized, but no fold thickening or fusion is observed (Fig. 15.3d).

15.1.9 Let's Focus on the Inside of the Depression

- Two small nodules are observed inside the depression. The surface of the nodules is smooth, and they are comparable in height with the adjacent non-tumorous mucosa. The mucosa shows a shape remaining like an island, and "Insel (island-like nodule)" is suspected.

- Taken together, the well-delineated depressed lesion mostly exhibits a white color and accompanies "Insel" or an island-like nodule in the depression. Since it can be extended well by air inflation, the lesion is diagnosed as 0-IIc PDA (por) with invasion depth of M and an ulcer scar (Fig. 15.3d).

15.1.10 Let's Carry Out NBI Magnified Endoscopy

- This is an NBI magnified view of the oral side of the lesion.
- The left side shown with a red arrow demonstrates villi-like structure, while the right side shown with a yellow arrow exhibits unclear surface structure and vascular structure with different diameters and irregular running.
- Vascular density is low, but a network is mildly developed. MDA (tub2) is diagnosed (Fig. 15.3e).

15.1.11 Let's Observe Vascular Structure More

- This is an NBI magnified endoscopic view of almost the same area. The vascular structure in the area surrounded with a yellow dotted line shows different diameters and irregular running with mild network development, and MDA (tub2) is diagnosed.
- Taken together, the lesion is diagnosed as 0-IIc tub2 about 15 mm in size with invasion depth of M and an ulcer scar. The lesion met extended indications for ESD, and ESD was carried out (Fig. 15.3f).

15.2 Let's Compare Fixed Specimens with Resected Specimens

"Fresh specimen, left panel": The oral side is on the right. There is a depressed lesion with a white color, and two small nodules with redness are observed in the depression (Fig. 15.4).

"Fixed specimen, right panel": When the specimen is fixed, the boundary of the lesion is more clearly visible (Fig. 15.4).

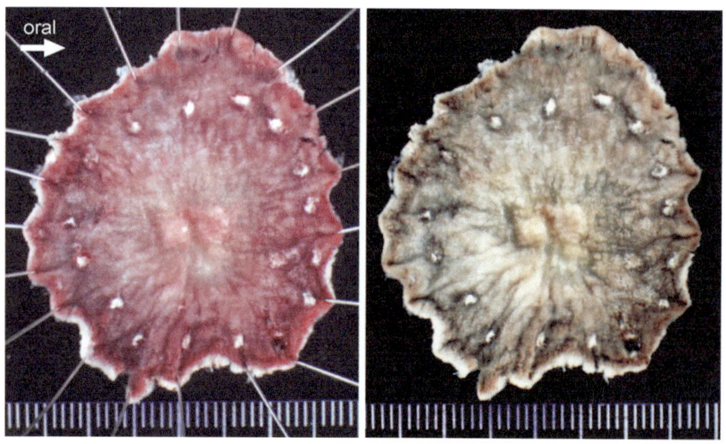

Fig. 15.4 *left* Fresh specimen, *right* Fixed specimen

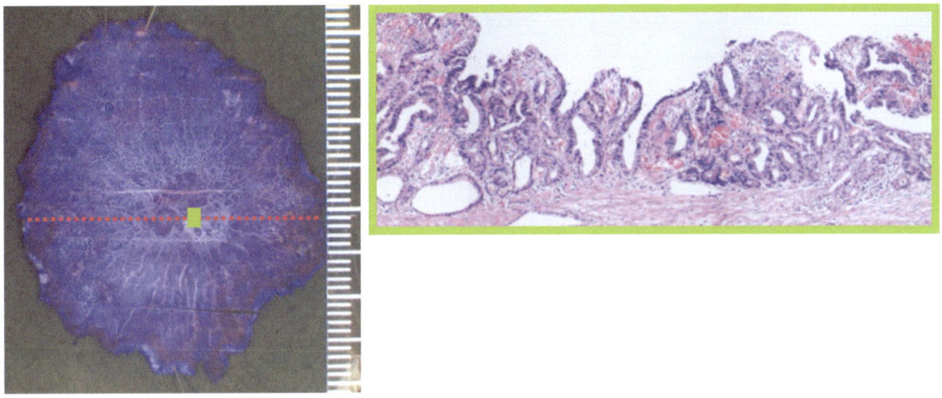

Fig. 15.5 Histopathology of the center of the lesion (HE stained)

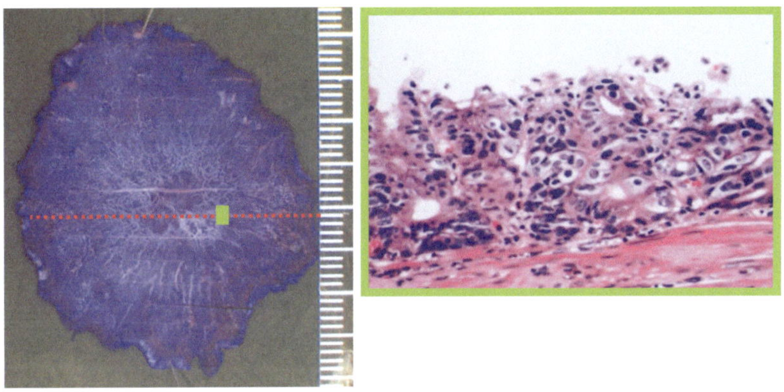

Fig. 15.6 Histopathology of the oral side of the lesion (HE stained)

Figure 15.5 shows histopathology of the center of the lesion (HE stained). Thickening of the muscularis mucosae and severe fibrosis in the submucosal layer are observed. MDA (tub2) with small glands is diagnosed.

Figure 15.6 is histopathology of the oral side of the lesion (HE stained). No glandular structure is observed and PDA (por) is diagnosed.

Figure 15.7 is histopathology of the center of the lesion (HE stained). A minute cancer invasion to the submucosal layer is recognized. The cancer with invasion maintains glandular structure, and WDA (tub1) is diagnosed. The depth of SM invasion is 150 μm from the lower end of the muscularis mucosae.

Conclusive Diagnosis

Gastric adenocarcinoma, tub2 > tub1 > por, T1 (SM1)(150 μm, tub1), ly0, v0, LM(−), VM(−), pType 0-IIc + UL-s, 18 × 15 mm, U, post.

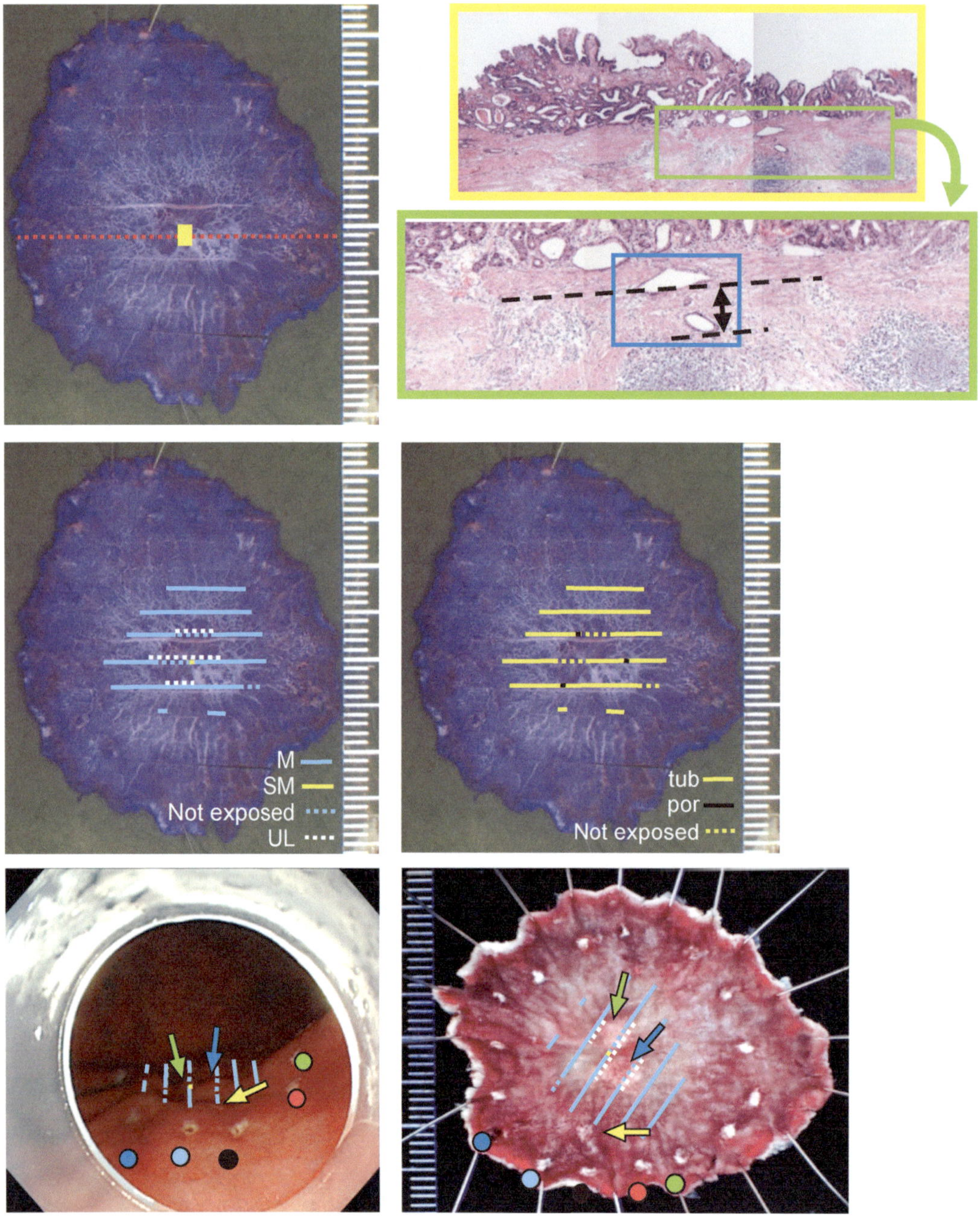

Fig. 15.7 Histopathology of the center of the lesion (HE stained)

Summary
This lesion on the posterior wall of the greater curvature of the gastric upper body is 0-IIc with fold convergence. It is often difficult to diagnose invasion depth of the lesion with fold convergence. The cause of fold convergence in this case is attributable to an ulcer scar, but minute cancer invasion to SM is recognized. However, SM invasion is not to the degree where it is reflected in macroscopic findings, and preoperative diagnosis of SM1 is considered difficult.

15.3 Answer

Invasion depth in this case is (1) M.

16 Question 2: Where Is the Lateral Boundary?

Koichi Okamoto

K. Okamoto (✉)
Department of Gastroenterology and Oncology, University of Tokushima, 2-24, Shinkura-cho, Tokushima 770-8501, Japan
e-mail: tagayasu33jp@yahoo.co.jp

T. Oyama (ed.), *Endoscopic Diagnosis of Superficial Gastric Cancer for ESD*, DOI 10.1007/978-4-431-54469-2_16

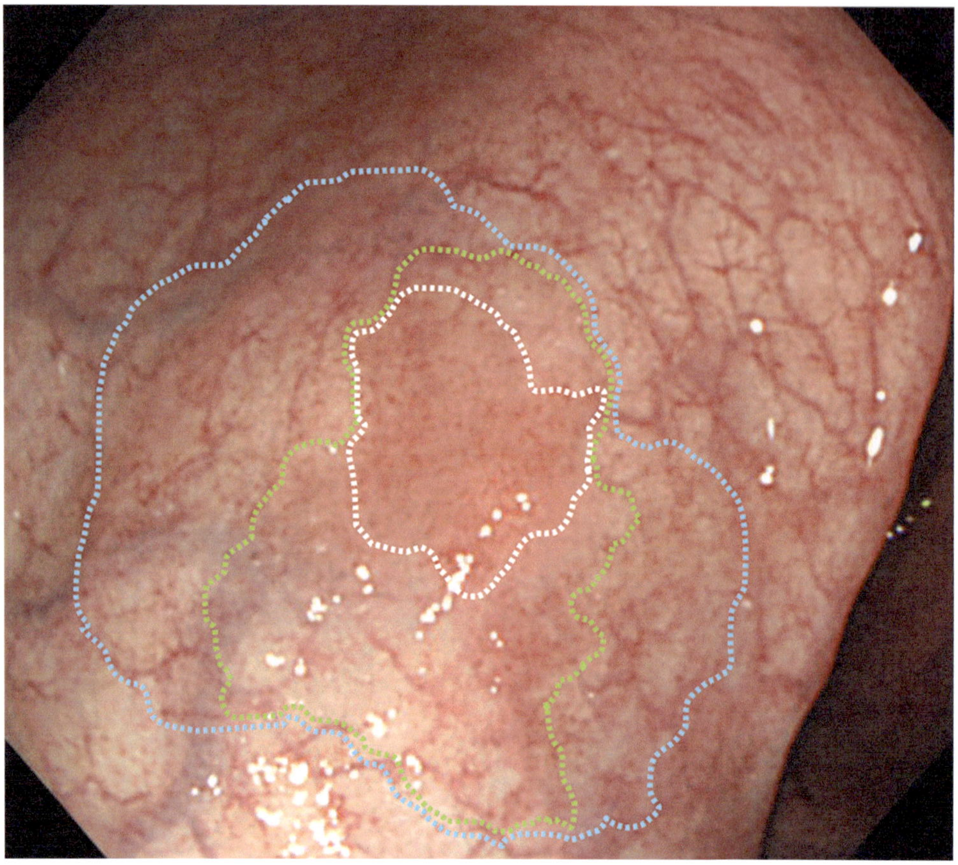

Fig. 16.1 Where is the lateral boundary

Where is the lateral boundary (Fig. 16.1)?
Choose your answer from 1 to 3.

(1) White dotted line
(2) Green dotted line
(3) Blue dotted line.

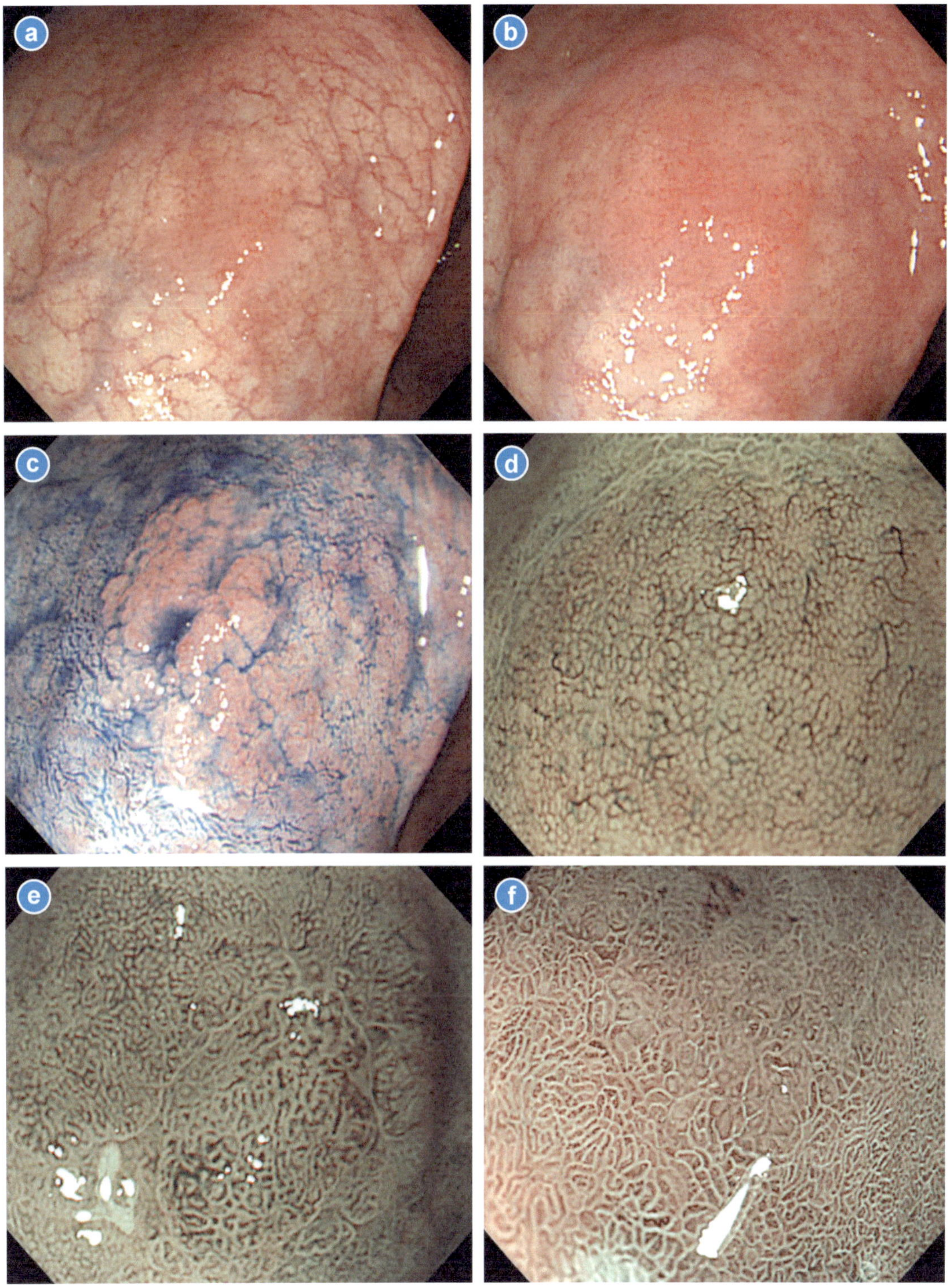

Fig. 16.2 Let's diagnose by observing these six images

16.1 Focus on These Points

16.1.1 Let's Focus on the Areas with Decreased Visibility of Blood Vessels

- There is a reddish elevated lesion at the lesser curvature of the gastric lower body, and the boundary is obscure.
- Careful examination reveals an area of decreased vascular visibility, and of partly white and partly reddish color, as indicated by the yellow arrows. But the boundary is still ill delineated (Fig. 16.3a).

16.1.2 Let's Focus on the Background Mucosa

- Blood vessels are clearly visible through the adjacent background mucosa, and atrophic gastritis is diagnosed (Fig. 16.3a).

16.1.3 Let's Make Close-Up Observation

- Relatively homogeneous redness is observed inside of the lesion, mixed with scattered spotty redness.
- An area with discoloration and reddish color and poorly visible blood vessels is observed at the anal and anterior sides of the reddish area as indicated by the yellow arrows, but the boundary is still obscure (Fig. 16.3b).

16.1.4 Let's Focus on Light Catching

- Light catching reflective of the irregular surface mucosa is recognized from the reddish area with an obscure boundary to the anterior wall (Fig. 16.3b).

16.1.5 Let's Focus on Surface Structure

- When indigo carmine is sprayed, the area with poor vascular visibility repels the dye and is recognized with rough areal patterns of variable sizes. The boundary is clearly visualized by dye spraying, but the boundary on the anal side of the lesion is still obscure.
- WL imaging and indigo carmine spraying reveal a relatively well-delineated reddish elevated lesion, leading to diagnosis of 0-IIa, WDA (tub1) with invasion depth of M. However, it is still difficult to tell which one is the true lateral boundary (Fig. 16.3c).

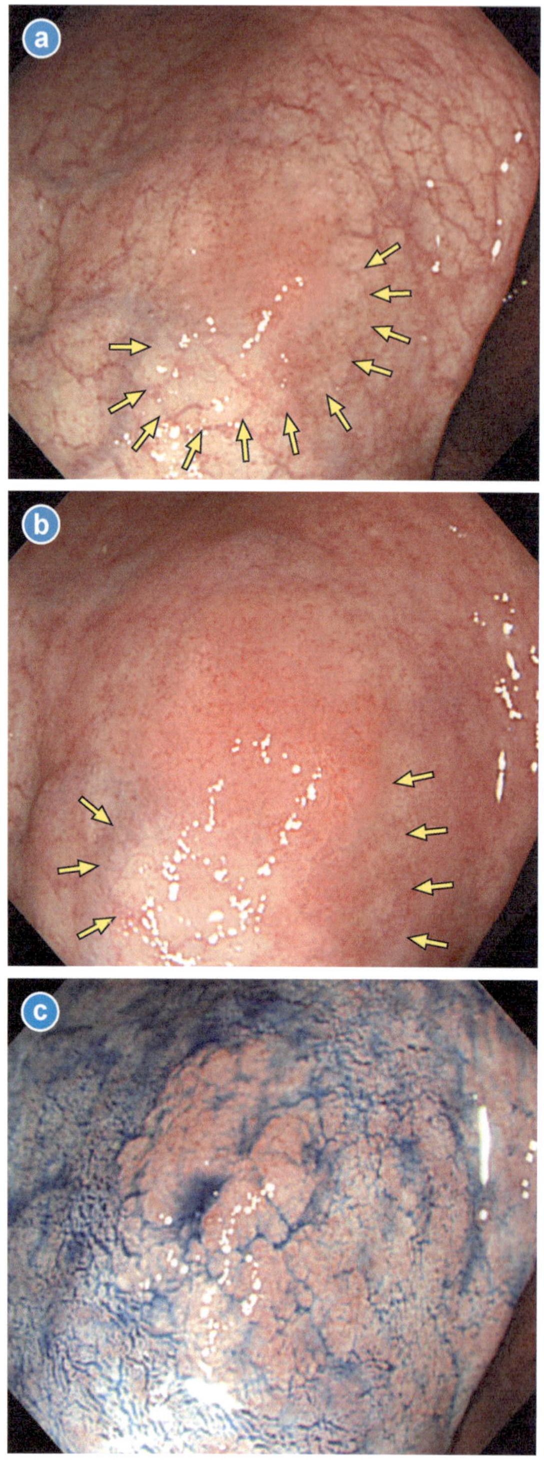

Fig. 16.3 Same images as Fig. 16.2

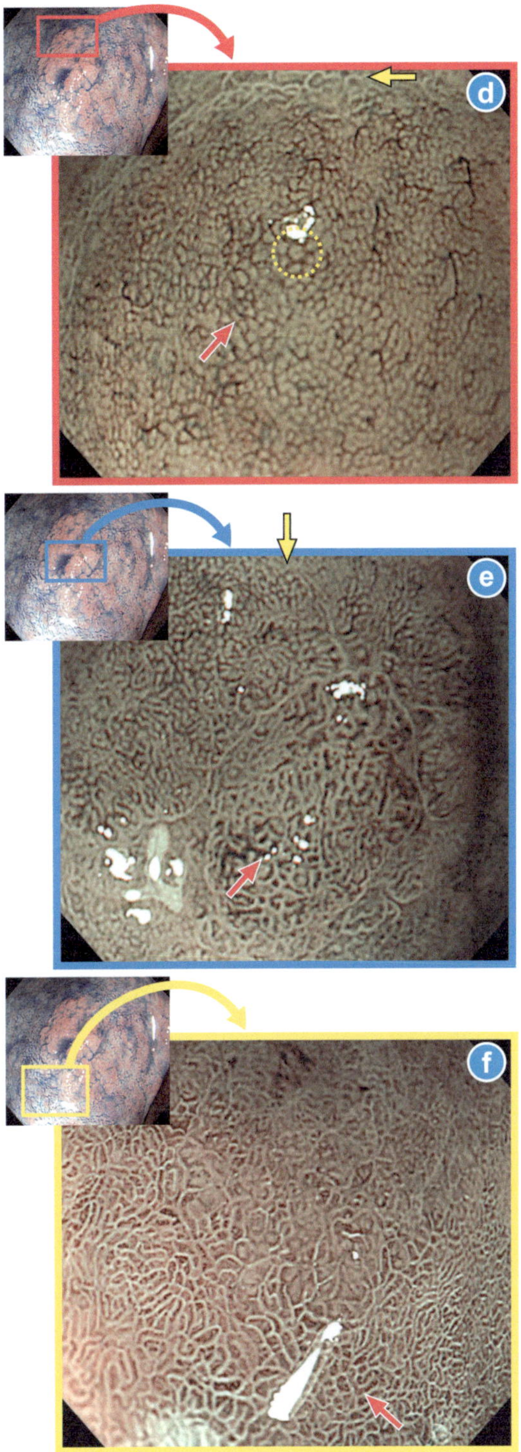

Fig. 16.3 (continued)

16.1.6 What Is the Next Step?

- The same area is examined by NBI magnified endoscopy for more detailed observation (Fig. 16.3c).

16.1.7 Let's Focus on Surface Structure

- An NBI magnified view of the oral side of the lesion is shown.
- Regular pits and villi-like structure are observed at the upper edge of the figure as indicated by the yellow arrow, whereas dense pitlike structure is recognized at the center of the figure as indicated by the red arrow, also showing vascular network formations. The boundary of the two areas is clearly visible, and WDA (tub1) is diagnosed (Fig. 16.3d).

16.1.8 Let's Focus on Pitlike Structure

- Pitlike structures consist of white areas surrounded with brown circles. Careful observation reveals a black spot in each of the white areas. This is how true pits should appear, as seen in the area circled with a yellow dotted line (Fig. 16.3d).

16.1.9 Let's Focus on the Center of the Lesion

- This is an NBI magnified view of the center of the lesion.
- Dense pitlike structures are observed at the upper side of the figure indicated by the yellow arrow, whereas villi structures are more predominantly observed in the center to the lower side marked by the red arrow.
- Villous structures of variable sizes are densely packed, confirming diagnosis of WDA (tub1) (Fig. 16.3e).

16.1.10 Let's Focus on the Anal and Anterior Sides of the Lesion

- This is an NBI magnified view of the anal and anterior sides of the lesion. Regular villi-like structures are observed at the lower side of the figure marked by the red arrow.

- However, villi-like structures at the center to the upper side of the figure marked with a yellow arrow are unclear, and this area can be diagnosed as cancer.
- Based on these, the lateral boundary of the lesion on the anal side is diagnosed as (2) (Fig. 16.3f).

16.2 Let's Compare Fixed Specimens with Resected Specimens

16.2.1 Let's Mark the Lesion

- The outside of the lateral boundary, diagnosed by NBI magnified observation, is marked. The left figure shows an endoscopic image after circumferential marking.
- The expansion of cancer diagnosed by NBI magnified endoscopy almost corresponds with the area that repels dye when indigo carmine is sprayed (Fig. 16.4).

(Fresh specimen: left figure) The oral side is on the right. An elevated lesion with a white color and redness is observed at the center. On its anal side, an area with a mixture of a white color and redness is observed, although the boundary is obscure (Fig. 16.5a).

(Fixed specimen: center figure) When the specimen is fixed, the boundary of the area shown with yellow arrows is more clearly visible (Fig. 16.5b).

(Crystal violet [Pyoktanin Blue®]-stained specimen: right figure) When the specimen is stained with crystal violet, it is possible to recognize surface structure more clearly (Fig. 16.5c).

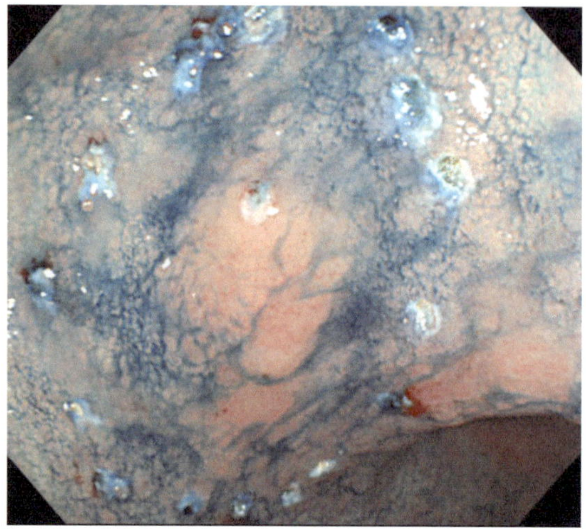

Fig. 16.4 Endscopic image after circumferencial marking

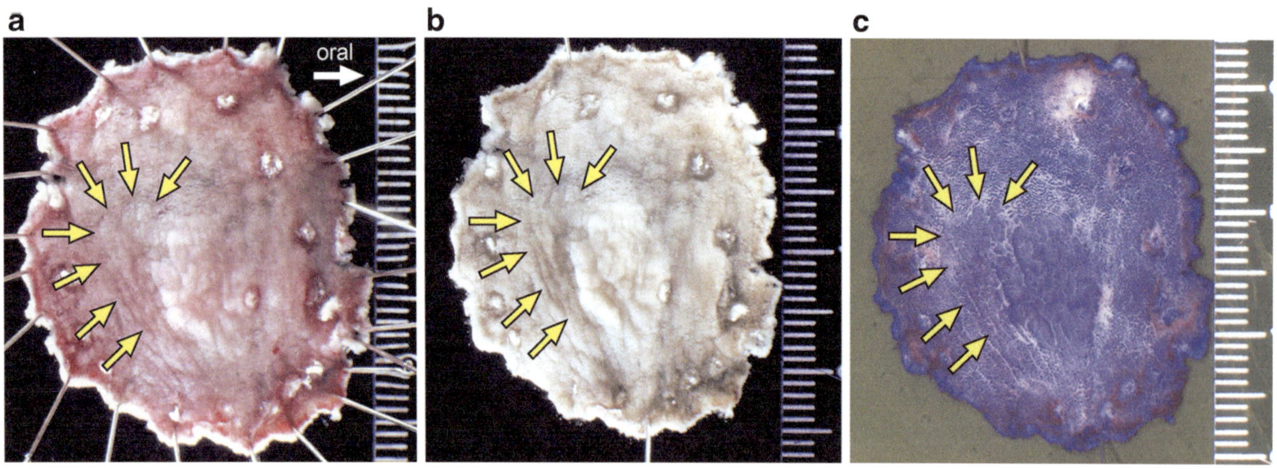

Fig. 16.5 (**a**) Fresh specimen. (**b**) Fixed specimen. (**c**) Crystal violet [Pyoktanin Blue®]-stained specimen

16.2.2 Images of Crystal Violet Staining (High Magnification) Are Comparable to NBI Images

- Regular villi-like structures are observed around the lesion, but each of the villi-like structures shown with yellow arrows is ill delineated and is noted to fuse one another.
- It is possible to recognize the same findings by NBI magnified observation (Fig. 16.6).

Histopathology of the center of the lesion is shown by HE stained. Swollen nuclei and pseudostratification are observed, but glandular structures are maintained. WDA (tub1) is diagnosed (Fig. 16.7).

Histopathology of the anal side of the lesion is shown. Swollen nuclei and pseudostratification are observed, but glandular structures are maintained, consistent with diagnosis of WDA (tub1) (Fig. 16.8).

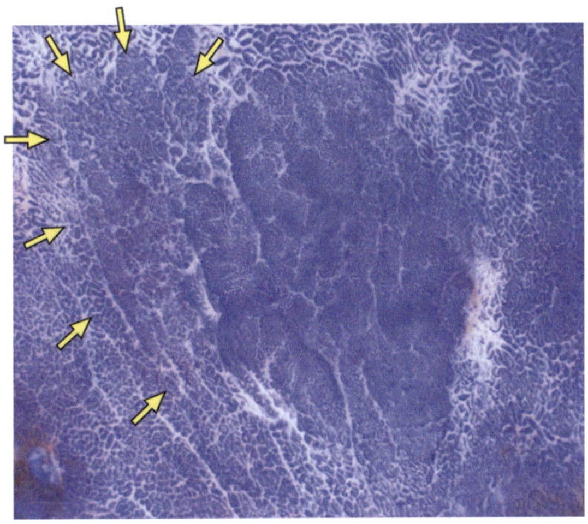

Fig. 16.6 The image of crystal violet stained

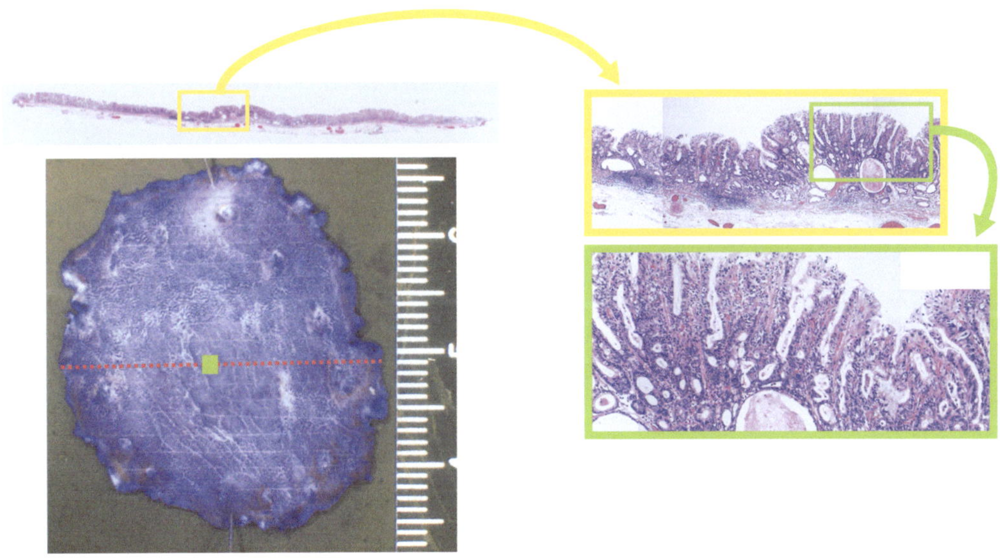

Fig. 16.7 Comparison with the resected specimen and the histological image of the center of the lesion

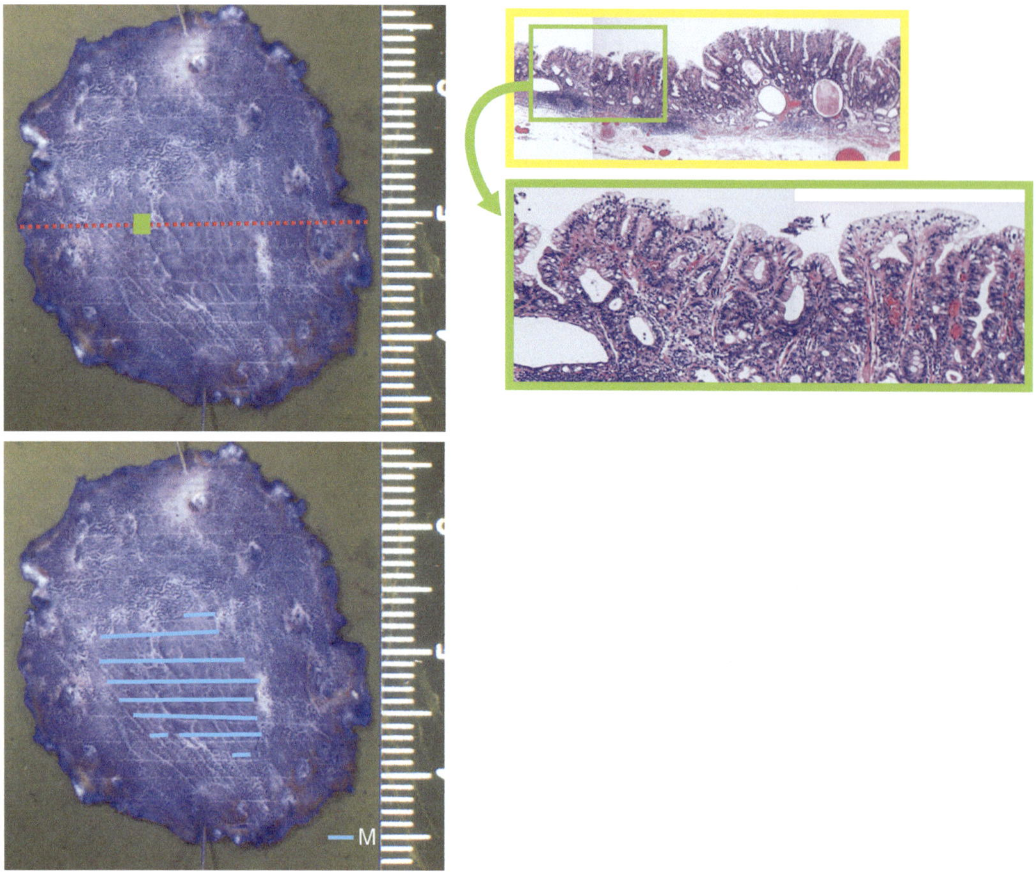

Fig. 16.8 Comparison with the resected specimen and the histological image of the anal side of the lesion

Conclusive Diagnosis
Gastric adenocarcinoma, tub1 > tub2, T1 (M), ly0, v0, LM (−), VM (−), pType 0-IIa, 15 × 9 mm, M, Ant.

Conclusions
It is an ill-delineated 0-IIa lesion with a mixture of redness and whitish color at the lesser curvature of the gastric lower body. Routine WL observation and chromoendoscopy with indigo carmine spraying could not tell the lateral boundary at the anal and anterior sides of the lesion. NBI magnified observation clearly visualized the boundary and fusion of villi-like structures at the anal and anterior sides of the lesion. These findings led to diagnosis of WDA (tub1).

16.3 Answer

Lateral boundary is (2) green dotted line.

Question 3: How Do You Diagnose Pathological Type?

17

Yoko Kitamura

Y. Kitamura (✉)
Department of Gastroenterology, Center for Digestive and Liver Diseases, Nara City Hospital, 1-50-1, Higashikidera-cho, Nara-Shi, Nara 630-8305, Japan
e-mail: humiokumiko@yahoo.co.jp

T. Oyama (ed.), *Endoscopic Diagnosis of Superficial Gastric Cancer for ESD*, DOI 10.1007/978-4-431-54469-2_17

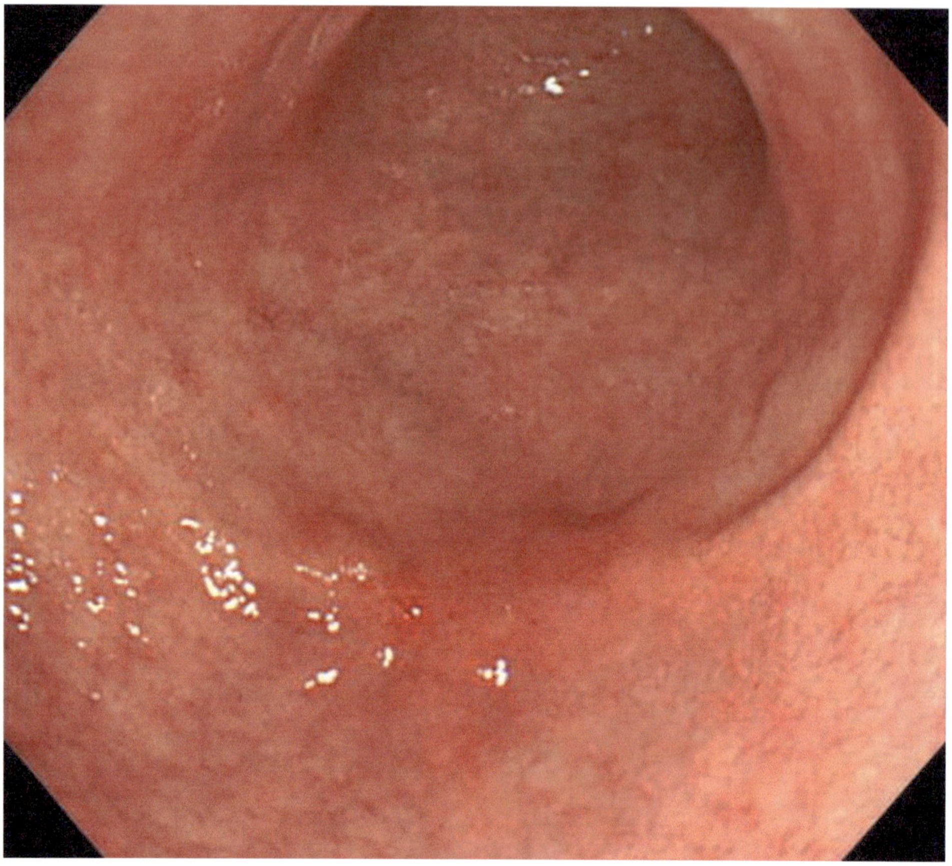

Fig. 17.1 How do you diagnose pathological type

How do you diagnose pathological type of the Fig. 17.1? Choose your answer from (1) to (3).

(1) WDA (tub1)
(2) MDA (tub2)
(3) PDA (por)

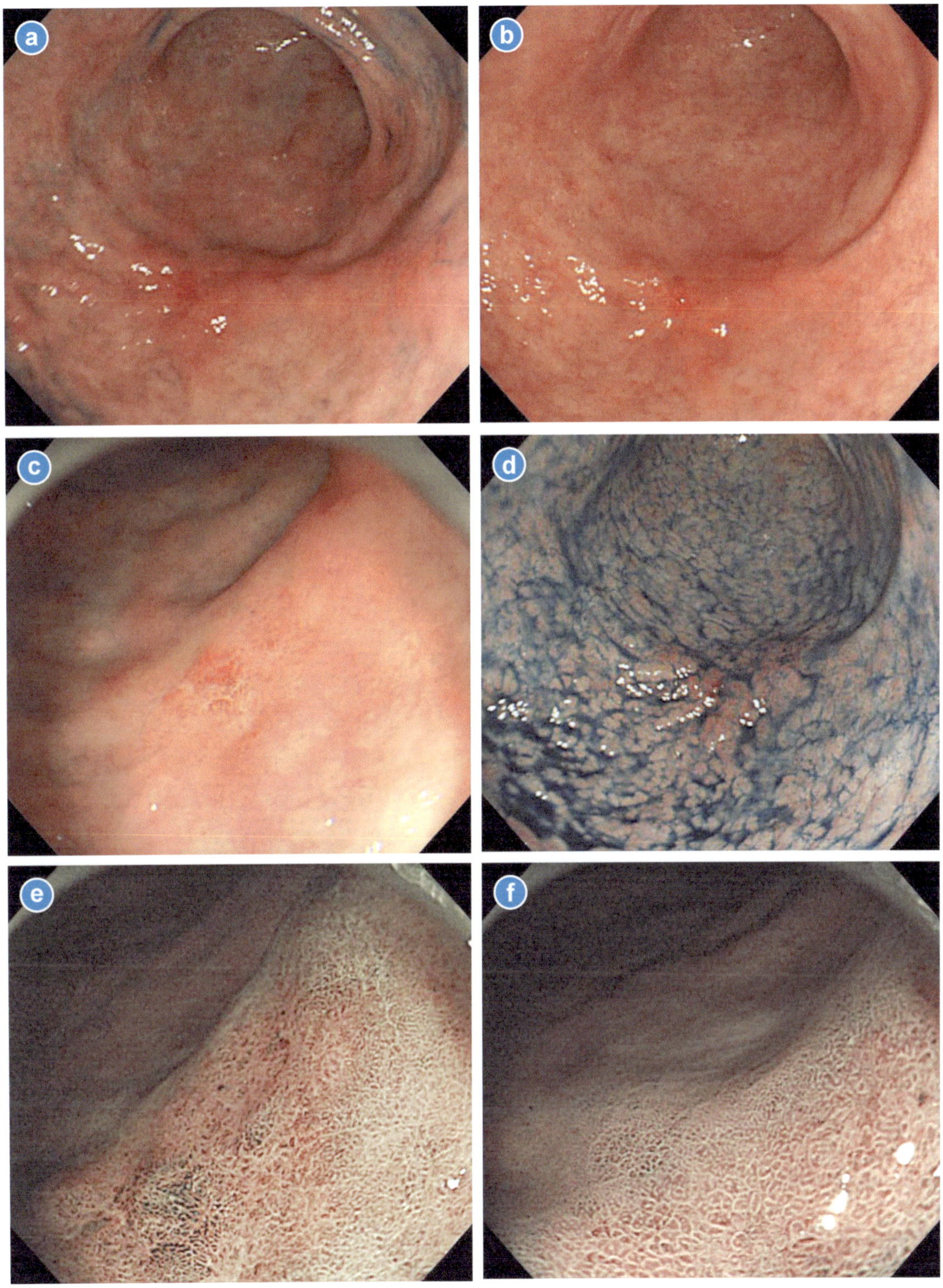

Fig. 17.2 Let's diagnose by observing these six images

17.1 Focus on These Points

17.1.1 Let's Notice the Reddish Part

- A reddish shallow depressed lesion is seen in the greater curvature of the antrum. The demarcation line of this lesion is unclear.
- The reddish part of the lesion appears slightly thick when inflated with small amount of air (Fig. 17.3a).

17.1.2 Let's Check if Fold Convergence Is Present

- Folds are noted to converge toward the slightly reddish elevation. However, converging folds are seen without clubbing or fusion of folds.
- Therefore, this lesion is noted to have a coexisting ulcer scar (Fig. 17.3a).

17.1.3 Let's Observe Under Inflation with Large Volume of Air

- When fully inflated with large volume of air, the background mucosa shows a mixture of spotty reddish and whitish mucosa consistent with atrophic gastritis.
- Under full inflation of air, the lesion does not appear to have much thickness and is seen as a slightly reddish depressed lesion.
- The center of the reddish part is noted with a small deeper red protuberance, and some mucosal convergence is seen toward the small reddish protuberance (Fig. 17.3b).

17.1.4 Let's Approach Closer

- When approaching closer to the lesion, the pale reddish lesion is found not to be homogenous in color, but as a mixture of reddish and whitish mucosa.
- The demarcation line of the lesion is unclear, making it necessary to include a differential diagnosis of PDA. NBI magnified endoscopy is useful for telling the lesion from PDA (Fig. 17.3c).

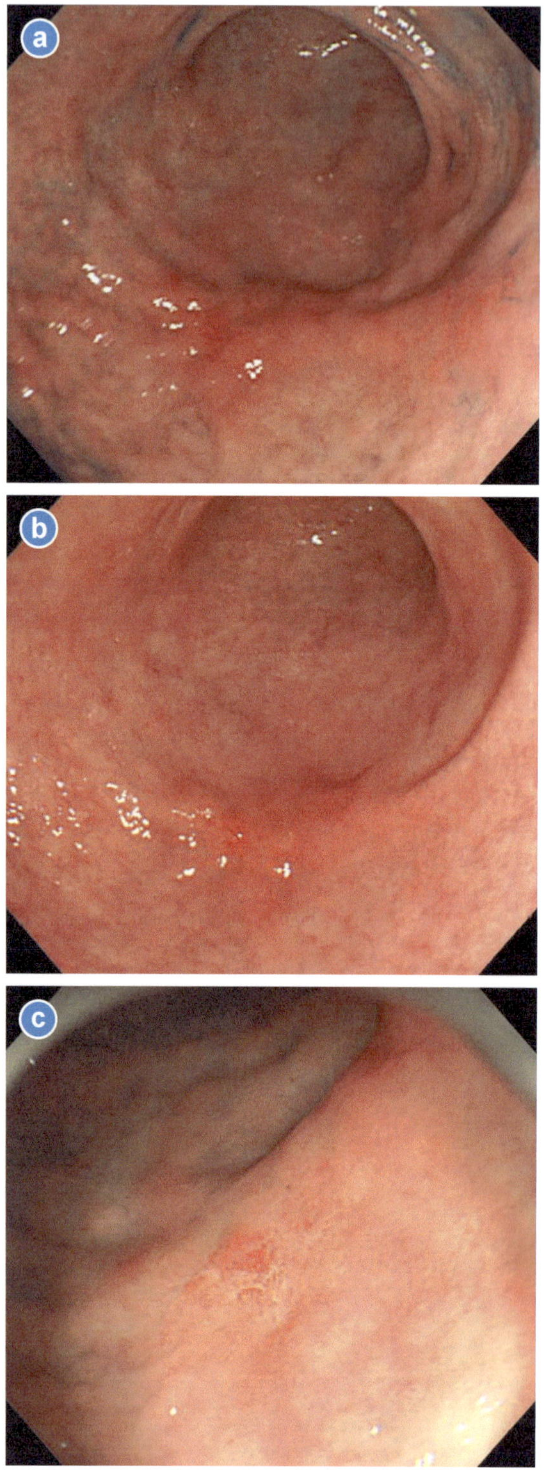

Fig. 17.3 Same images as Fig. 17.2

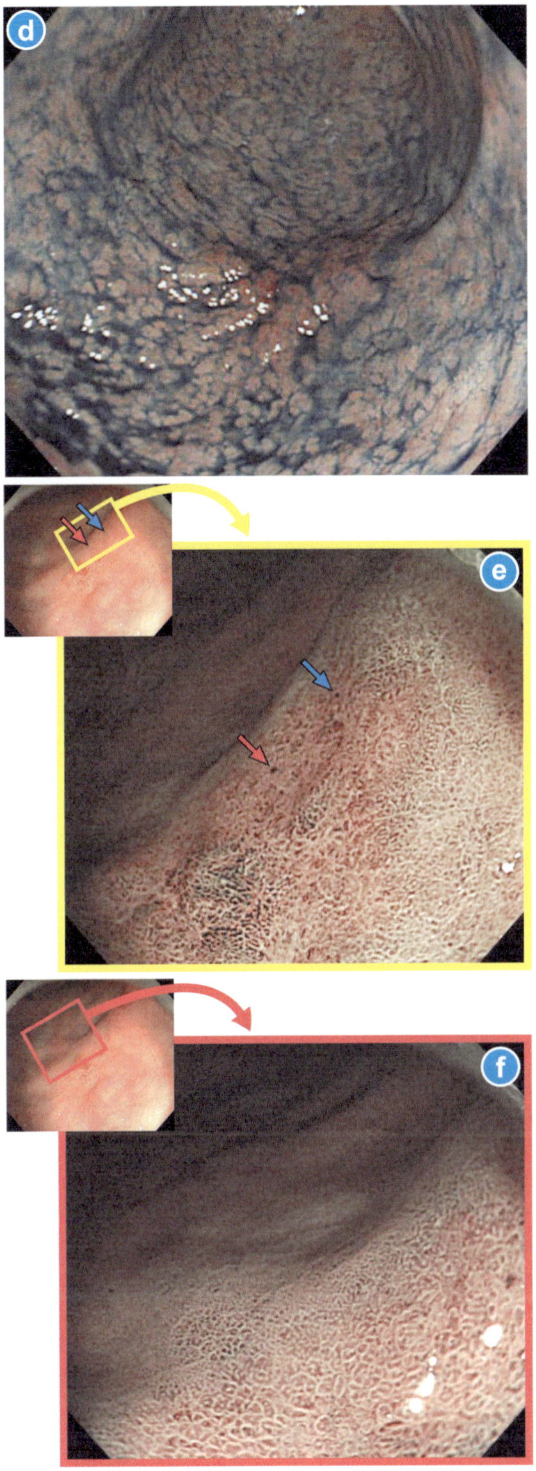

Fig. 17.3 (continued)

17.1.5 Let's Spray Indigo Carmine on the Lesion and the Surrounding Mucosa

- After indigo carmine spray, a lesion consisting of coarsely large and irregular gastric areas is noted, different from the areal patterns of the surrounding mucosa.
- But the border of the lesion is unclear, and the folds are noted to converge on one point (Fig. 17.3d).

17.1.6 Let's Observe the Lesion with Magnified NBI (1)

- The surrounding mucosa shows a mixture of regularly shaped villi and pit patterns. The red and blue arrows correspond with villous pattern and pit pattern within the lesion.
- While unmagnified WL endoscopy suggests a possibility of PDA, magnified NBI of the whitish area shows irregular villi consistent with WDA (Fig. 17.3e).

17.1.7 Let's Observe the Lesion with Magnified NBI (2)

- This view shows the anal part of the lesion.
- The background mucosa shows fine villi; however irregular villi of variable sizes and irregular pits are coexisting in the lesion. Therefore the demarcation of the lesion can be clearly recognized (Fig. 17.3f).

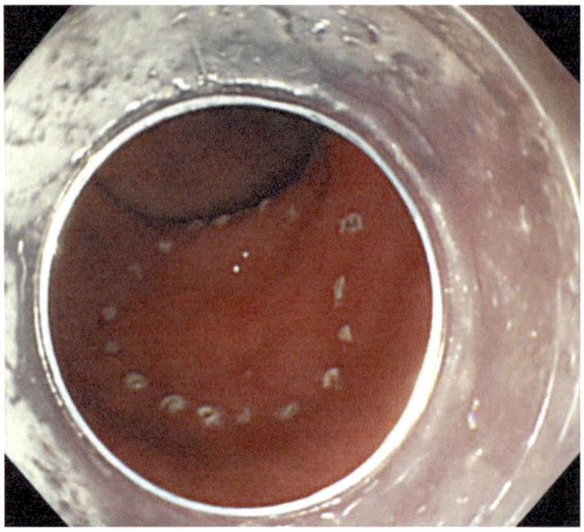

Fig. 17.4 Endscopic image after circumferencial marking

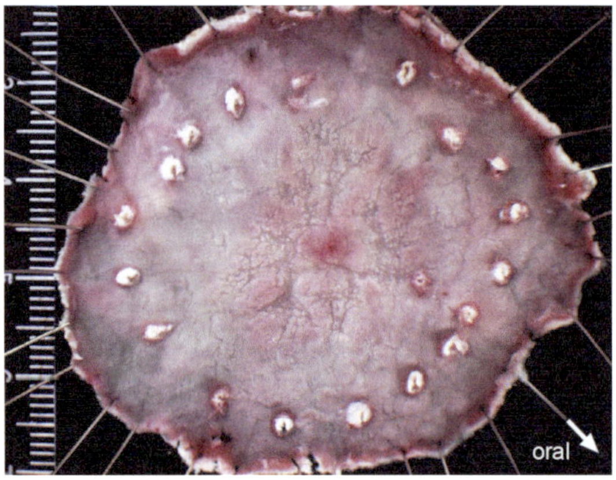

Fig. 17.5 Freshly resected specimen

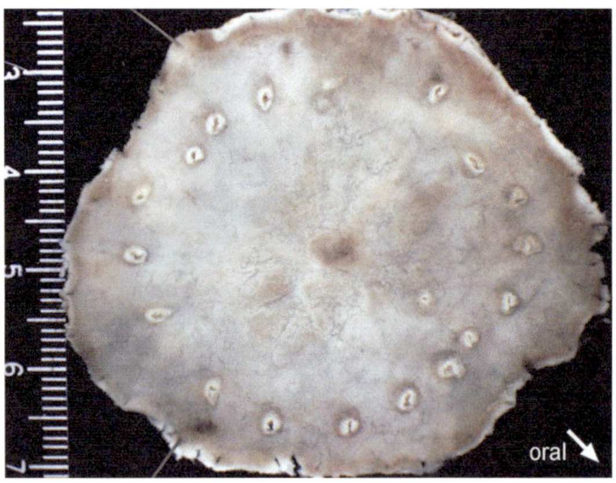

Fig. 17.6 Fixed specimen

17.2 Let's Compare the Endoscopic Picture with the Resected Specimen for the Conclusive Diagnosis

17.2.1 Let's Mark Surrounding the Lesion

- Multiple markings are placed 3 mm outside surrounding the lesion by applying coagulation current with back side of a hook knife under observation with NBI magnified endoscopy (Fig. 17.4).

17.2.2 Let's Pay Close Attention to the Color and the Surface Pattern

- This is the freshly resected specimen.
- A slightly depressed lesion is shown in the center of the specimen, and multiple flat reddish protuberances are shown within the depressed area. Also a small red nodule is shown in the center of the depressed area.
- The red nodule corresponds with the mucosal convergence noted by endoscopy. However, it is difficult to appreciate the presence of mucosal convergence in the resected specimen (Fig. 17.5).

17.2.3 Let's Examine the Surface Pattern in the Fixed Specimen

- This is the formalin-fixed specimen.
- The demarcation of the lesion after fixing with formalin remains unclear (Fig. 17.6).

This histopathological image is obtained of the red nodule in the center of the lesion as indicated by the yellow rectangle. The histological type of the area is diagnosed as WDA. The muscularis mucosa shows thickening with intricately overwrapping layers of multiple interrupted muscular fibers consistent with an ulcer scar (UL-IIs). On careful inspection, there is no submucosal invasion (Fig. 17.7a).

This histopathological image is of the whitish depressed area in conventional endoscopy. The histological type of the area is WDA (blue rectangle) (Fig. 17.7b).

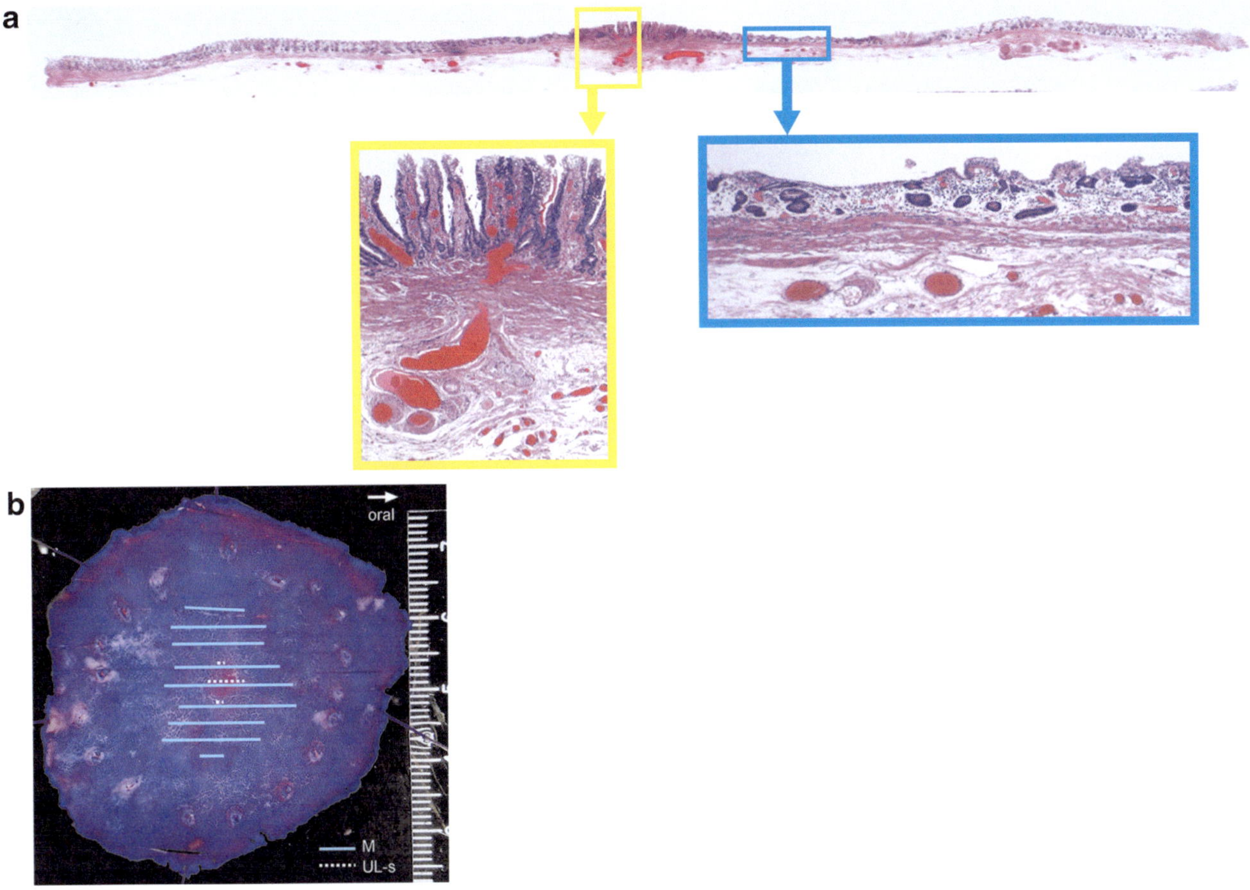

Fig. 17.7 Comparison with the histopathological image of the lesion (**a**) Resected specimen (**b**) Mapping of the cancer distribution

Conclusive Diagnosis

Gastric adenocarcinoma, tub1, T1 (M), ly0, v0, UL-IIs, LM (−), VM (−), pType0-IIc + IIa, 22 × 18mm, L, Gre.

Summary

In conventional endoscopy, the color of the lesion was heterogeneous; therefore we needed to tell the lesion from PDA. In NBI magnified endoscopy, the irregular villous pattern was shown in the lesion, supporting the diagnosis of the lesion as WDA.

The demarcation of the lesion was unclear because the lesion was flat and the surface pattern of the lesion was similar to the background mucosa, both being villous. Histologically speaking, the mucosal height of cancer was almost the same as of the surrounding noncancerous mucosa, making the demarcation of the lesion unclear.

The lesion was WDA with combined ulcer scar, M (depth), and 22 mm (tumor size); therefore the lesion was included in the expanded pathological criteria for curative endoscopic treatment, based on a retrospective analysis of a large series of surgical resection cases, determined to have a negligible risk of lymph node metastasis. Therefore, ESD was performed first.

17.3 Answer

The pathological type of the lesion is (1) WDA (tub1).

Question 4: Gastric Adenocarcinoma with Ulcer Scar – How Do You Diagnose the Depth of This Ulcer?

18

Yoko Kitamura

Y. Kitamura (✉)
Department of Gastroenterology, Center for Digestive and Liver Diseases, Nara City Hospital, 1-50-1, Higashikidera-cho, Nara-Shi, Nara 630-8305, Japan
e-mail: humiokumiko@yahoo.co.jp

T. Oyama (ed.), *Endoscopic Diagnosis of Superficial Gastric Cancer for ESD*, DOI 10.1007/978-4-431-54469-2_18

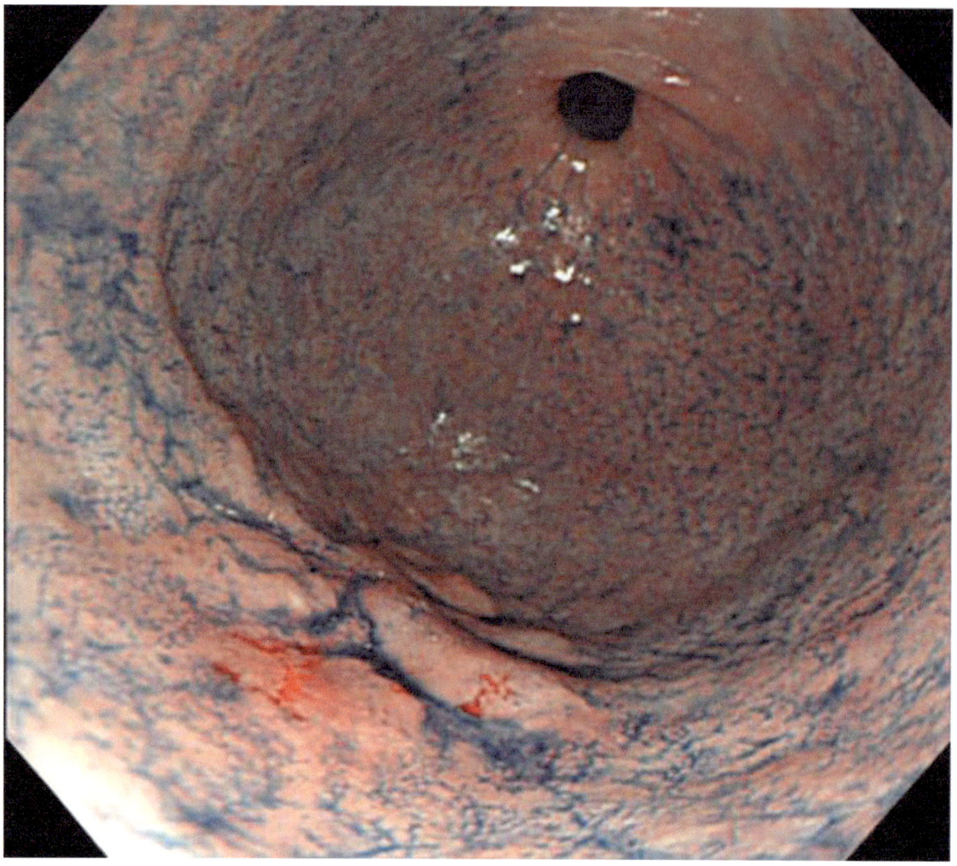

Fig. 18.1 How do you diagnose the depth of this ulcer

Gastric adenocarcinoma with ulcer scar (Fig. 18.1). How do you diagnose the depth of this ulcer? Choose your answer from 1 to 4.

(1) UL-Is
(2) UL-IIs
(3) UL-IIIs
(4) UL-IVs

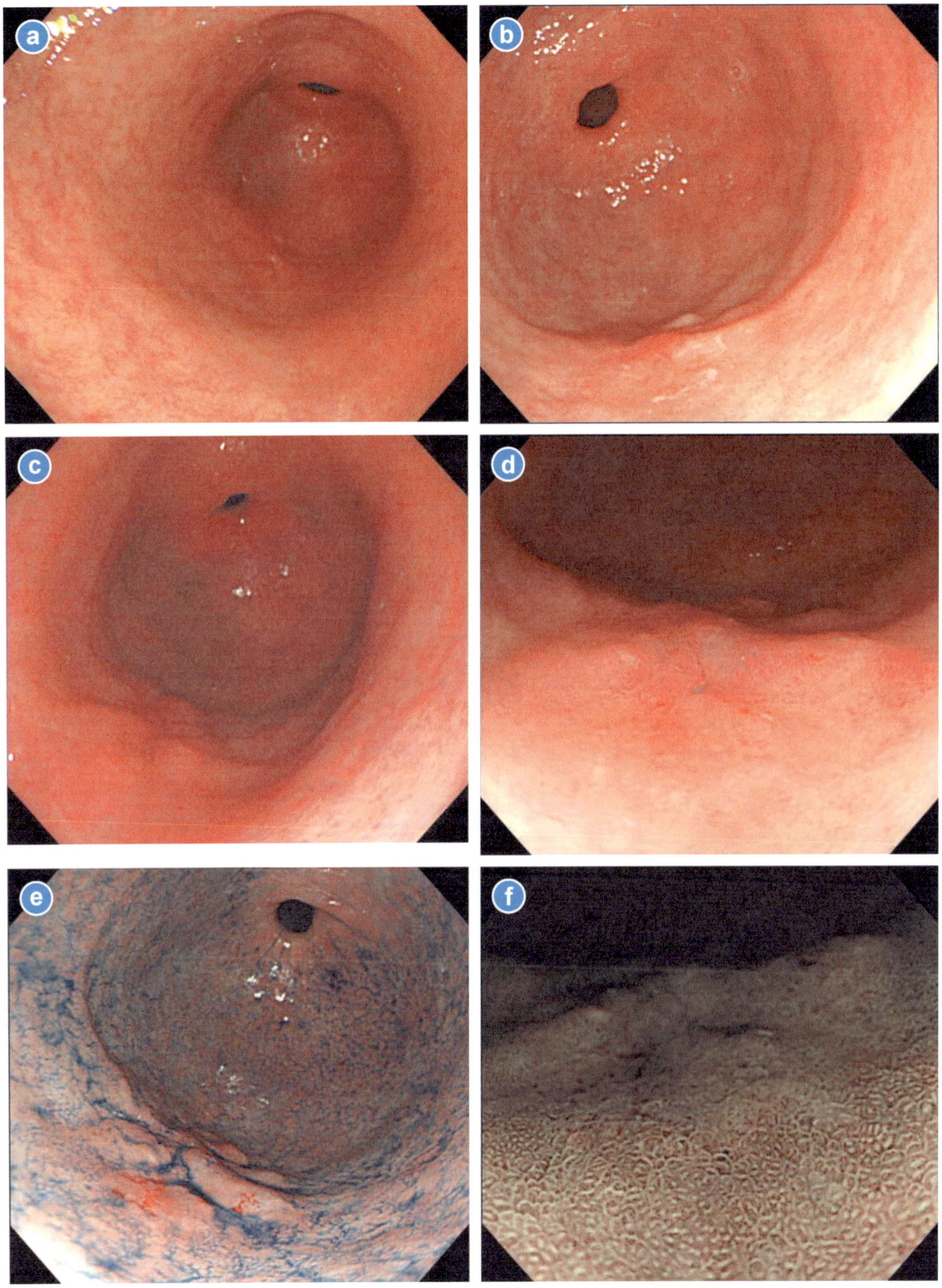

Fig. 18.2 Let's diagnose by observing these six images

18.1 Focus on These Points

18.1.1 Let's Notice the Slightly Reddish Part

- This image is obtained with full inflation of air.
- The background mucosa is a mixture of spotted reddish and whitish mucosa, consistent with a diagnosis of atrophic gastritis.
- There is a slightly reddish protrusion in the greater curvature of the antrum. However, the demarcation of the lesion is unclear. When evaluating a lesion with slight elevation, inflation with air stretches and changes its subtle difference in shape, making the demarcation unclear. Therefore, the next necessary step is to approach closer and reduce air volume (Fig. 18.3a).

18.1.2 Let's Approach Closer

- The reddish area with unclear demarcation is shown with smooth mucosal convergence surrounding the reddish part.
- No fusion or clubbing of converging folds suggestive of submucosal invasion is noted, leading to the diagnosis of combined ulcer scar (Fig. 18.3b).

18.1.3 Let's Deflate Air

- With small amount of air, mucosal convergence to one point is shown.
- Slightly reddish area is noted around the mucosal convergence. But the demarcation of the lesion is unclear with conventional endoscopy.
- Because of the fold convergence to one point, the depth of the ulceration is UL-IIs (Fig. 18.3c).

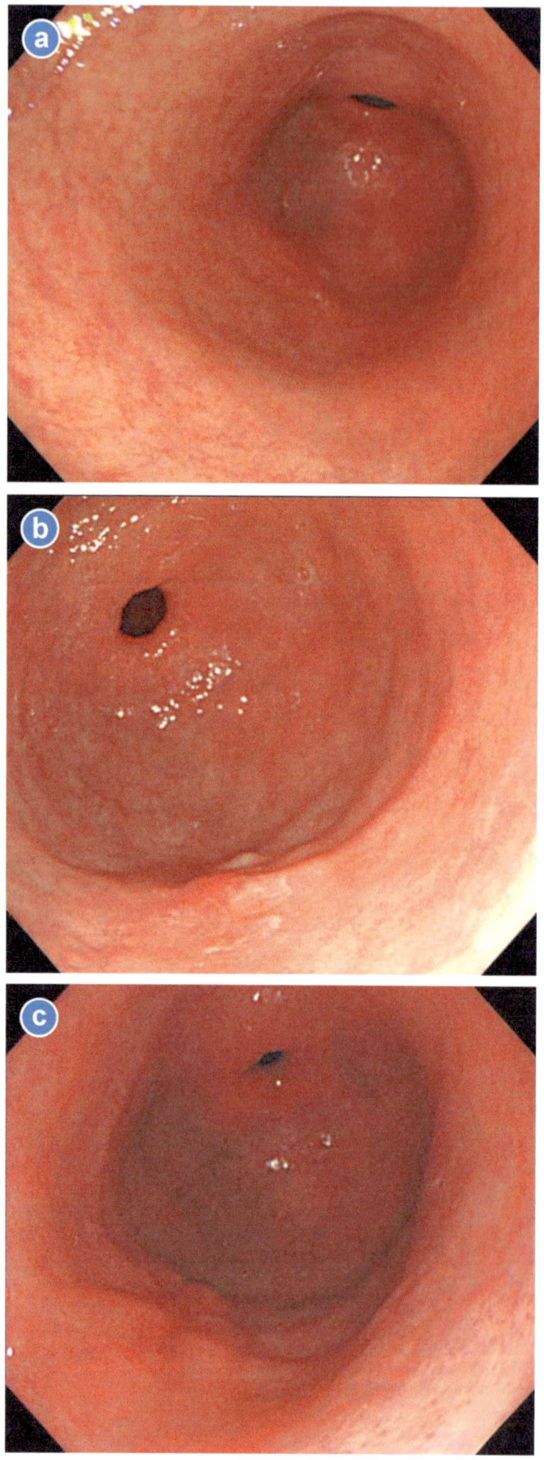

Fig. 18.3 Same images as Fig. 18.2

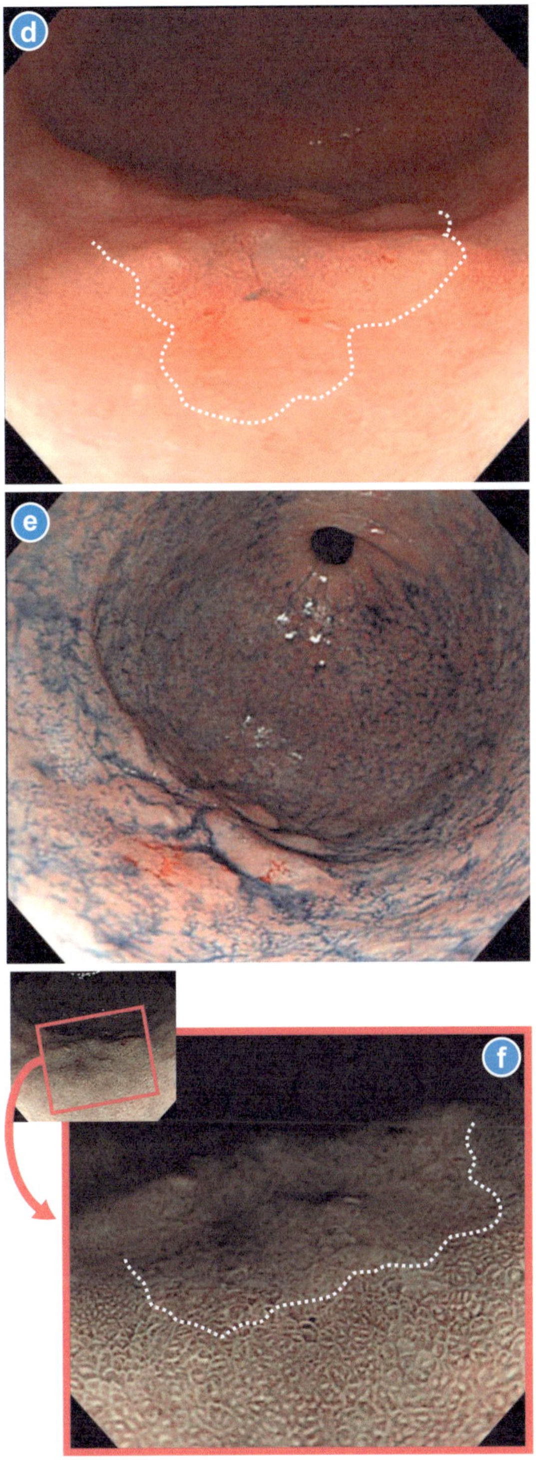

Fig. 18.3 (continued)

18.1.4 Let's Notice the Difference in Surface Pattern

- When carefully observing the surface pattern, the mucosal surface outside of the white-dotted line appears flat, while the mucosa inside of the white-dotted line shows irregular bumps and depressions (Fig. 18.3d).

18.1.5 Let's Spray Indigo Carmine for Observing the Surface Pattern Well

- Indigo carmine chromoendoscopy reveals multiple fine shallow streaks in the background mucosa pooling indigo carmine.
- The grooves between converging folds are noted to converge on one point.
- The lesion is shown as an elevated lesion repelling indigo carmine, and the demarcation of the lesion is mostly recognizable (Fig. 18.3e).

18.1.6 Let's Observe the Lesion Using Magnified NBI

- The oral side of the lesion is observed with low-power magnified NBI.
- The surface pattern of the background mucosa shows a mixture of regular small round pits and slightly irregular villi pattern. However, the surface pattern of the anal side of the dotted line shows a mixture of irregular pits and villi (Fig. 18.3f).

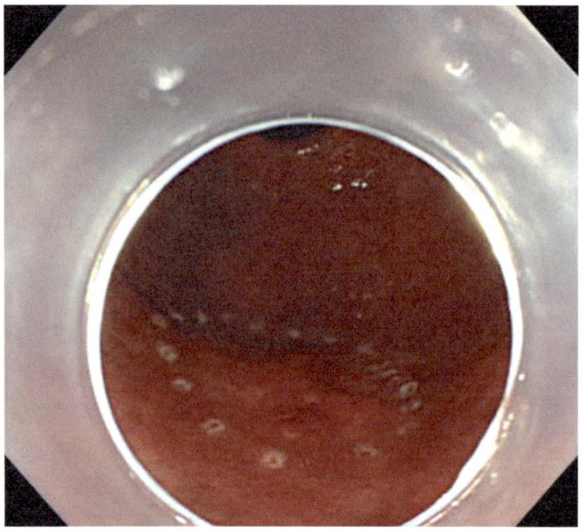

Fig. 18.4 Endscopic image after circumferencial marking

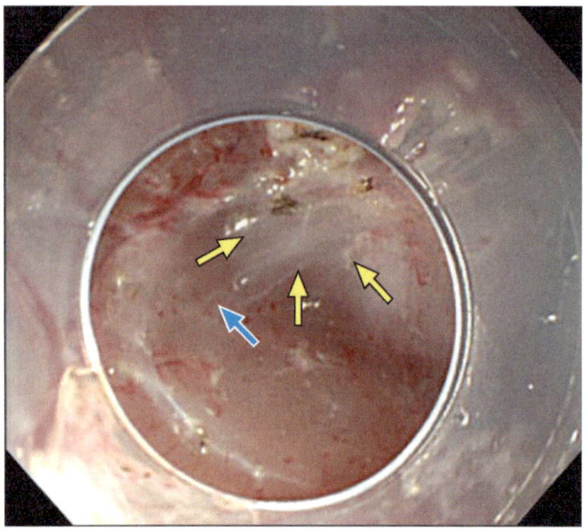

Fig. 18.5 Submucosal fibrosis

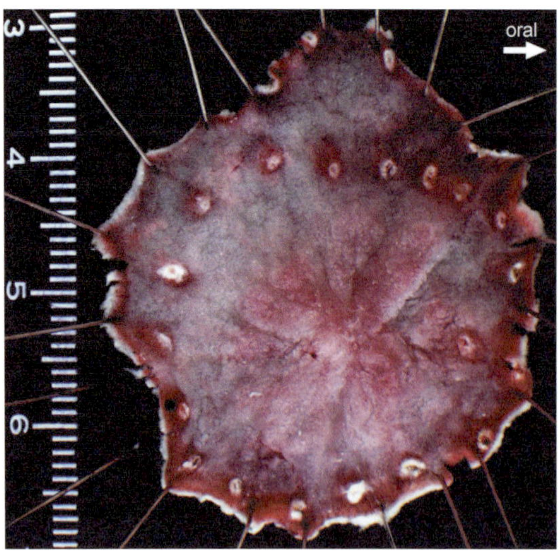

Fig. 18.6 Resected specimen

18.2 Let's Compare Fixed Specimens with Resected Specimens

18.2.1 Let's Mark Surrounding the Lesion

- Multiple markings are placed 3 mm outside surrounding the lesion by applying coagulation current with backside of a hook knife under observation with NBI magnified endoscopy. This conventional endoscopic image is obtained after marking.
- It is difficult to recognize the demarcation of the lesion by conventional endoscopy. However, it is possible to recognize the demarcation of the lesion and mark surrounding the lesion by NBI magnified endoscopy (Fig. 18.4).

18.2.2 Let's Check the Degree of Submucosal Fibrosis

- The opaque fibers are observed in the submucosa. And a small area of transparent submucosa is observed between the opaque fibers and the muscularis propria. Therefore, the depth of the ulcer scar can be diagnosed as UL-IIs.
- During submucosal dissection, we needed to dissect the tiny transparent layer to avoid cutting into the mucosal side (Fig. 18.5).

18.2.3 Let's Pay Attention to the Color

- The right side of the resected specimen is the oral side. The slightly reddish protuberant lesion is shown in the center of the resected specimen. The mucosal convergence is shown in the center of the reddish lesion.
- The lesion can be mostly identified as a slightly reddish area (Fig. 18.6).

18.2.4 The Surface Pattern Becomes Much Clearer on the Formalin-Fixed Specimen

- The surface pattern of the background mucosa shows regular small round pits and villi. However, the surface of the lesion shows a mixture of irregular pits and villi of variable sizes.
- The surface pattern of the formalin-fixed specimen shows surface patterns more clearly than the freshly resected specimen, making it easier to identify the demarcation of the lesion (Fig. 18.7).

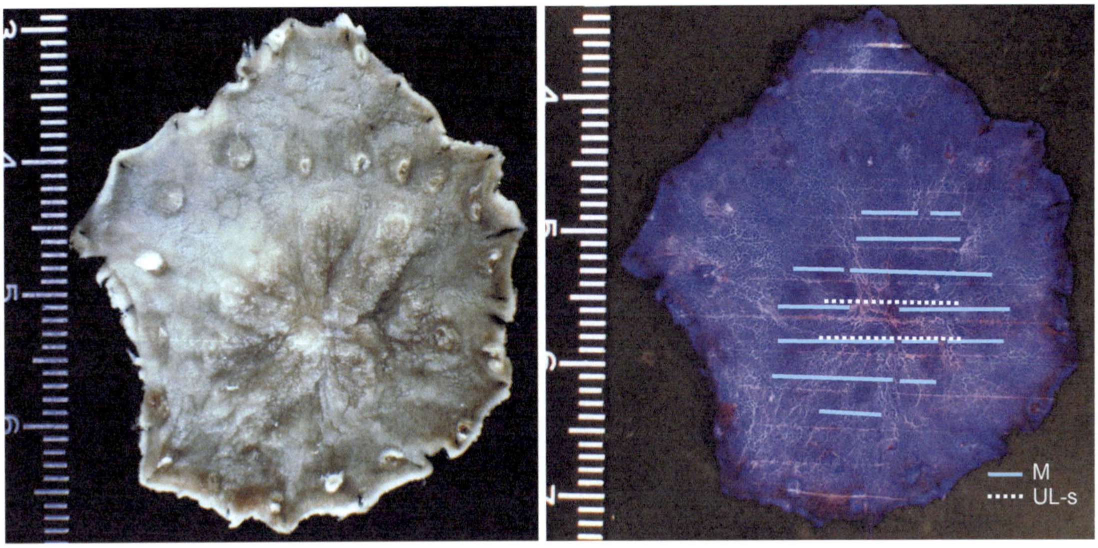

Fig. 18.7 The surface pattern on the formalin-fixed specimen and Mapping of the cancer distribution on the specimen

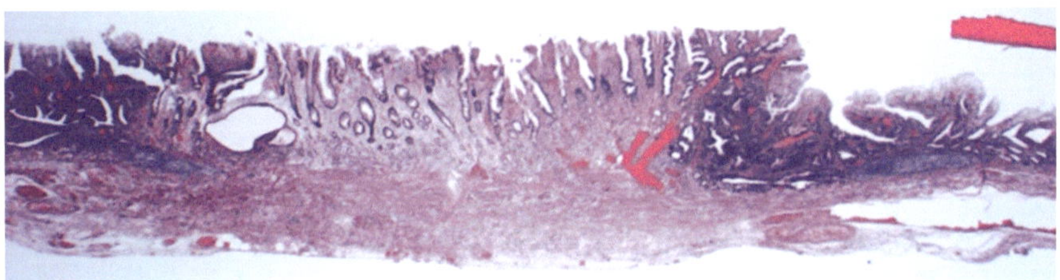

Fig. 18.8 Histopathological image taken from the center of the lesion with the ulcer scar

18.2.5 This Histopathological Image is Taken from the Center of the Lesion with the Ulcer Scar

- The submucosa under the center of the lesion show thickened and intricately woven muscularis mucosa confirming diagnosis of a combined ulcer scar (UL-IIs). However, submucosal invasion cannot be found in any of the sections.
- The histological type of the lesion is diagnosed as WDA (Fig. 18.8).

Conclusive Diagnosis
Gastric adenocarcinoma: tub1, T1(M), ly0, v0, UL-IIs, LM(−), VM(−), p-type 0-IIa, 19 × 19 mm, L, and Gre.

Summary
The conventional endoscopy and the chromoendoscopy revealed mucosal convergence. Mucosal convergence is found to be due to submucosal fibrosis. There are two possible explanations for submucosal fibrosis. First possible explanation is submucosal invasion of cancer. Second possible explanation is combined ulcer scar. Differentiating the two is very important for determining a treatment plan.

In this case, the mucosal convergence was to one point and smooth, with no fusion or clubbing. Therefore, we diagnosed the lesion as WDA with ulcer scar, which corresponded to the expanded pathological criteria for curative endoscopic treatment with a negligible risk of lymph node metastasis.

In case of UL-IIs, the mucosal convergence is shown toward one point. However in case of UL-IIIs, the mucosal convergence is shown toward a plane. This difference makes it possible to diagnose the depth of ulcer scars preoperatively.

18.3 Answer

The depth of the ulcer is (2) UL-IIs.

19 Question 5: How Far Is the Lateral Extension of This Lesion?

Yoko Kitamura

Y. Kitamura (✉)
Department of Gastroenterology, Center for Digestive and Liver Diseases, Nara City Hospital, 1-50-1, Higashikidera-cho, Nara-Shi, Nara 630-8305, Japan
e-mail: humiokumiko@yahoo.co.jp

T. Oyama (ed.), *Endoscopic Diagnosis of Superficial Gastric Cancer for ESD*, DOI 10.1007/978-4-431-54469-2_19

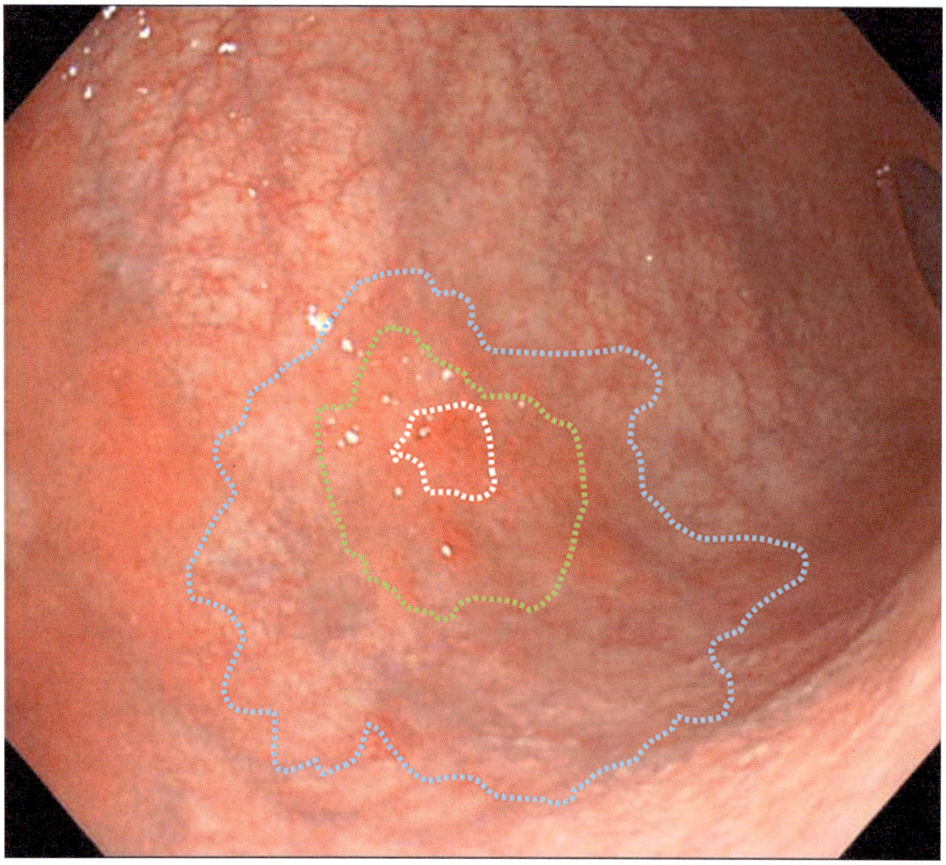

Fig. 19.1 How far is the lateral extension of this lesion?

How far is the lateral extension of this lesion (Fig. 19.1)? Choose your answer from 1 to 3.

(1) White dotted line
(2) Green dotted line
(3) Blue dotted line

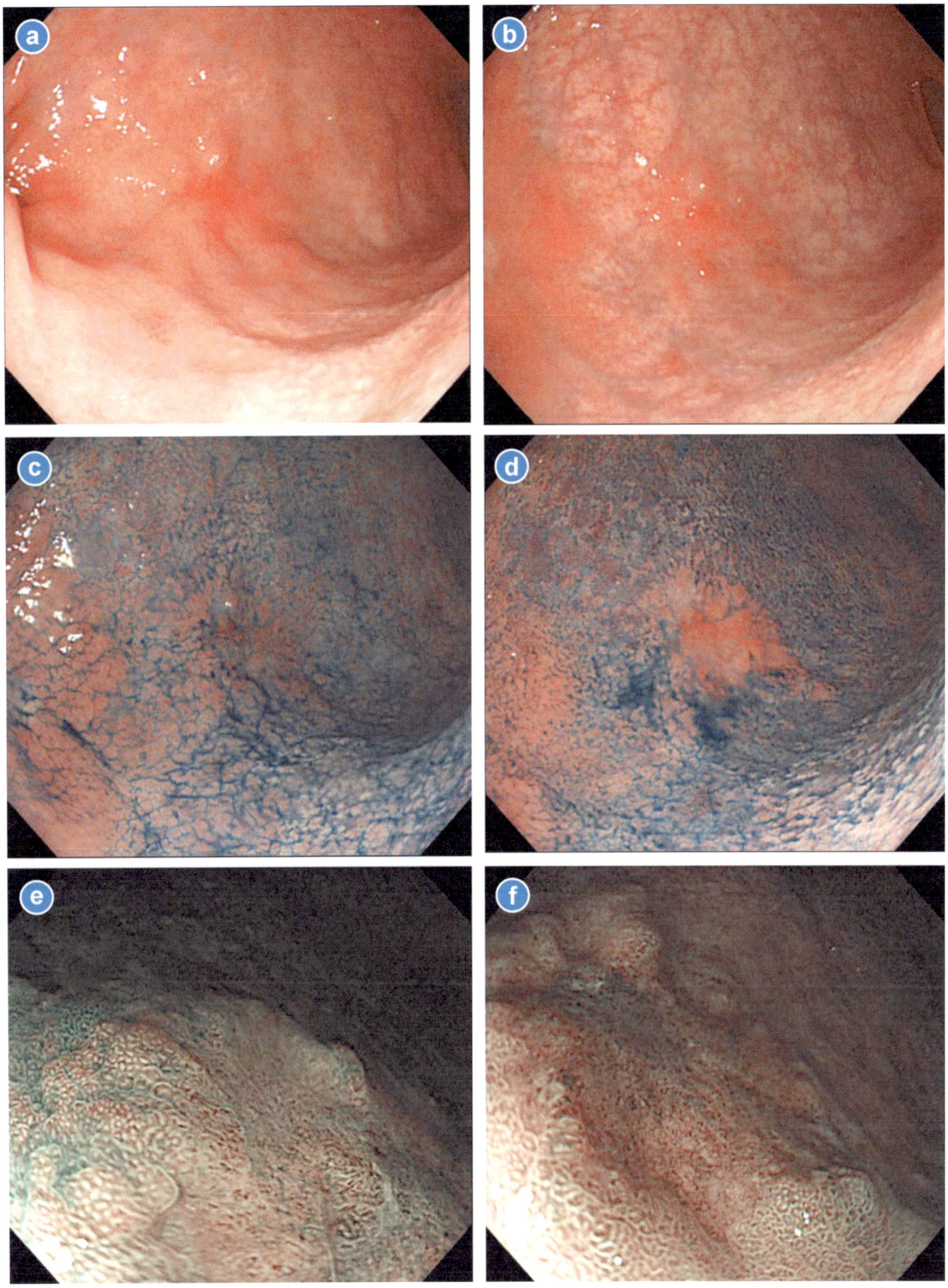

Fig. 19.2 Let's diagnose by observing these six images

19.1 Focus on These Points

19.1.1 Let's Notice the Reddish Part

- A reddish slightly protuberant lesion is shown in the greater curvature of the antrum. However, the demarcation line of the lesion is unclear (Fig. 19.3a).

19.1.2 Let's Check for Presence of Mucosal Convergence

- Converging folds are seen toward the slightly reddish elevated part, presenting this lesion as a combined ulcer scar.
- There are no clubbing or fusion of converging tips of folds (Fig. 19.3a).

19.1.3 Let's Observe with Full Inflation Air

- The stomach is fully inflated with air.
- **Background mucosa:** The background mucosa shows prominent visible blood vessels and loss of mucosal folds, consistent with atrophic gastritis.
- **The lesion:** The lesion is identified as the area of decreased vascular visibility. But its border is unclear, and the lesion itself is without much thickness. Since the mucosal convergence becomes rather indistinct with mass volume of air, the depth of the combined ulcer scar can be decided as UL-IIs (Fig. 19.3b).

19.1.4 Let's Spray Indigo Carmine

- Indigo carmine chromoendoscopy reveals shallow and irregularly shaped depressed lesion.
- The demarcation of the anal side of the lesion is unclear.
- No clear border is seen outside of the marginal swelling around the depression. Moreover, no difference is noted between the areal pattern of the marginal swelling and of the surrounding mucosa, concluding that the marginal swelling is caused by reactive inflammation (Fig. 19.3c).

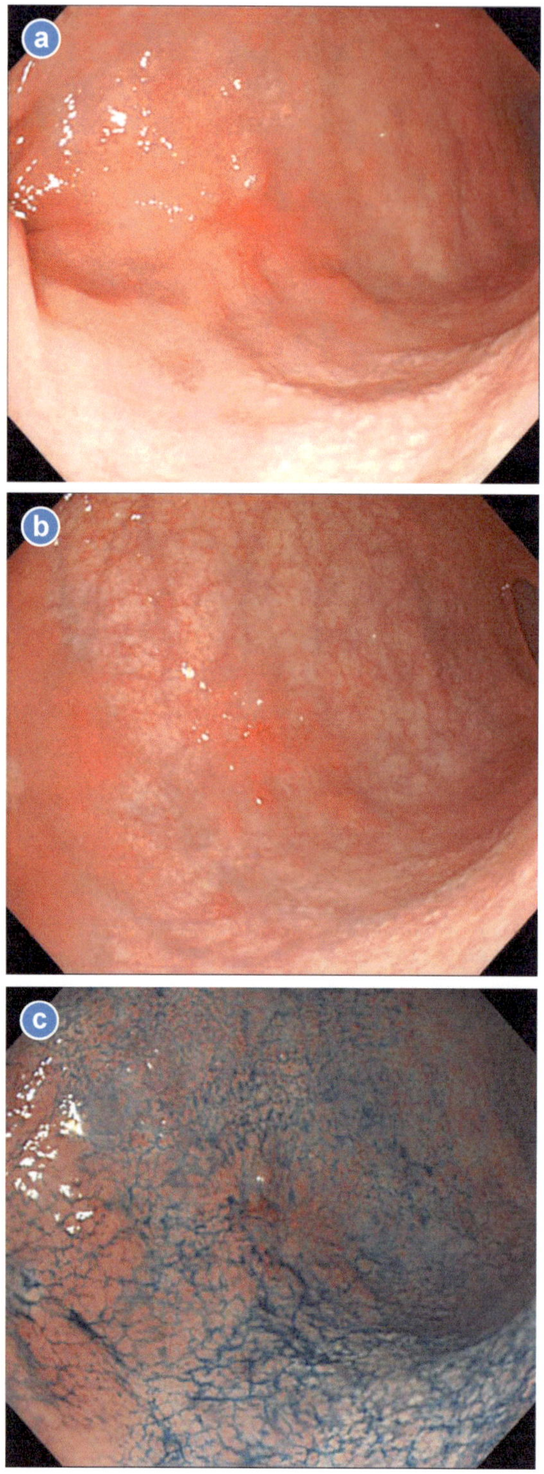

Fig. 19.3 Same images as Fig. 19.2

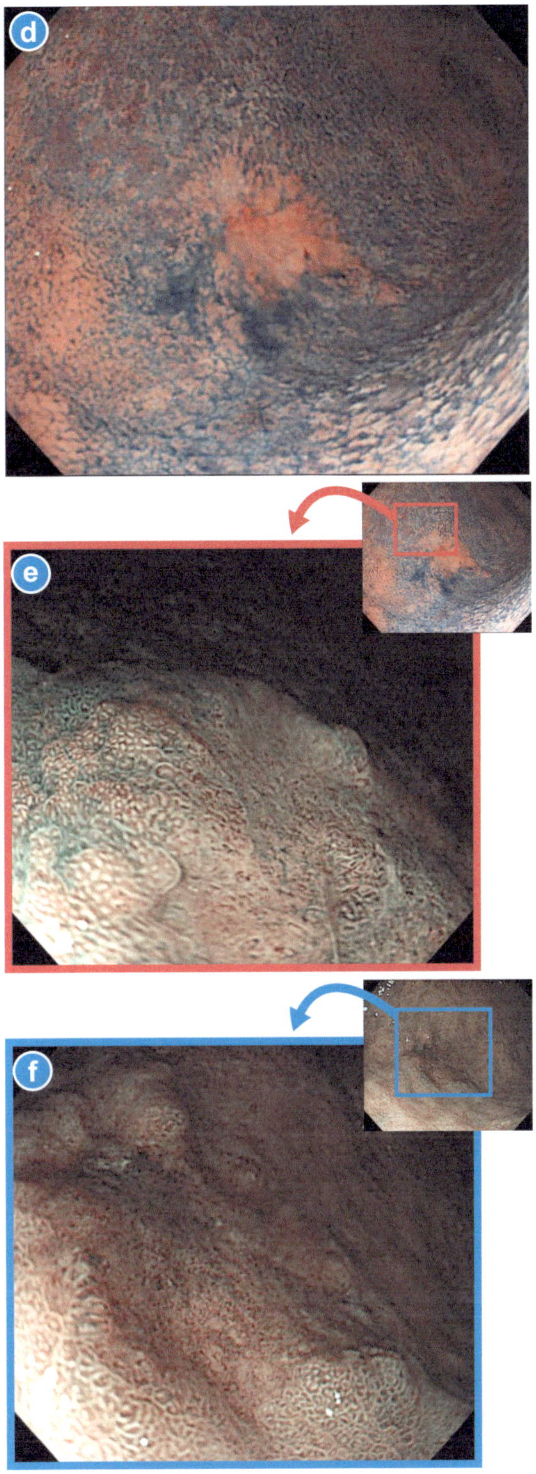

Fig. 19.3 (continued)

19.1.5 Let's Spray AIM

- This chromoendoscopic image is obtained a few minutes after spraying with 1.5 % acetic acid and indigocarmine mixture called AIM (acetic acid indigo carmine mixture).
- The depressed area diagnosed as the lesion strongly repels AIM, showing much more well-demarcated border than with indigo carmine (Fig. 19.3d).

19.1.6 Let's Observe the Lesion Using NBI Magnified Endoscopy (1)

- The background mucosa shows regular small round pits.
- The depressed area has irregular villi of variable sizes and parts with unclear structures.
- With use of NBI magnified endoscopy, the demarcation of the lesion has become clear by showing the surface pattern of the lesion against the background mucosa. With low power magnification, vascular patterns aren't seen. But the lesion may be diagnosed as WDA based on the irregular villous pattern (Fig. 19.3e).

19.1.7 Let's Observe the Lesion Using NBI Magnified Endoscopy (2)

- This NBI magnified endoscopic image shows the oral side of the lesion.
- The back ground mucosa shows a regular villi pattern, while the surface pattern of the depressed area is unclear (Fig. 19.3f).

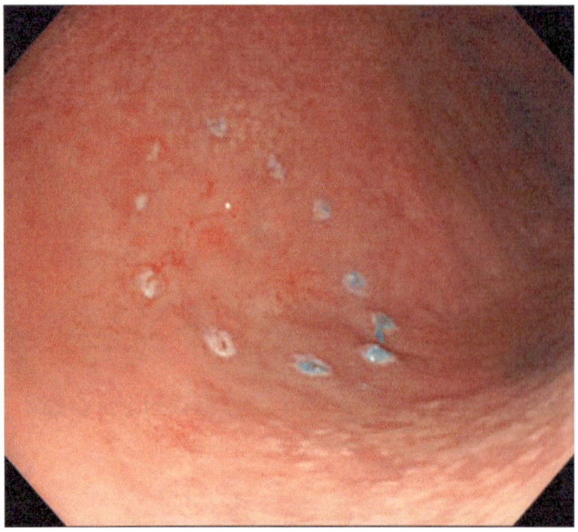

Fig. 19.4 Endscopic image after circumferencial marking

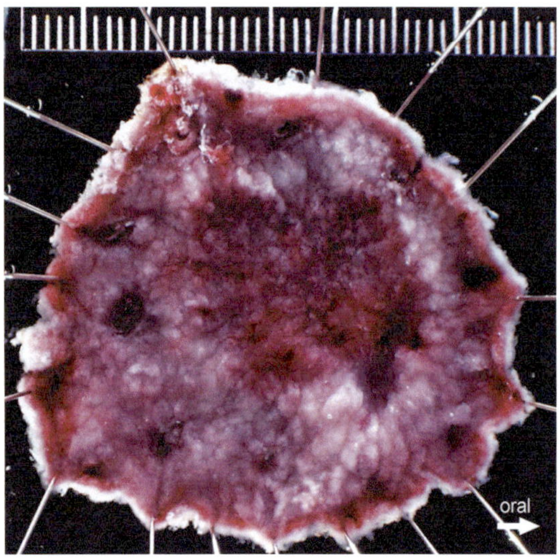

Fig. 19.5 Resected specimen

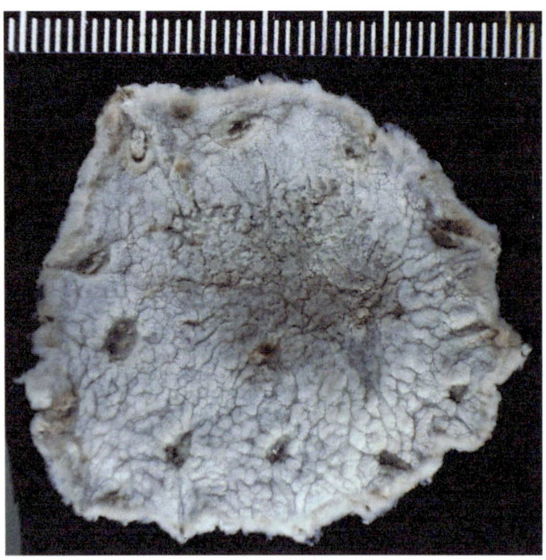

Fig. 19.6 Fixed specimen

19.2 Let's Compare Fixed Specimens with Resected Specimens

19.2.1 Let's Mark Surrounding the Lesion

- Markings are placed 3 mm outside surrounding the lesion by the back side of a hook knife under observation with NBI magnified endoscopy (Fig. 19.4).

19.2.2 Let's Pay Attention to Color and the Surface Pattern

- The right side of the resected specimen is the oral side.
- A slightly reddish depressed lesion is clearly seen in the center of the resected specimen.
- A small mucosal convergence is seen in the center of the reddish lesion (Fig. 19.5).

19.2.3 Let's Check the Surface Pattern of the Formalin-Fixed Specimen

- This image is of the formalin-fixed specimen.
- The lesion is recognized as an area of dense irregular surface pattern compared with the surrounding area (Fig. 19.6).

The lesion is diagnosed as WDA based on its structural atypia.

In conventional endoscopy, the demarcation of the lesion is unclear.

The black arrow indicates the demarcation of cancer and noncancer. The mucosal height of cancer and noncancer are almost the same, and this is why the demarcation is unclear by conventional endoscopy (Fig. 19.7a).

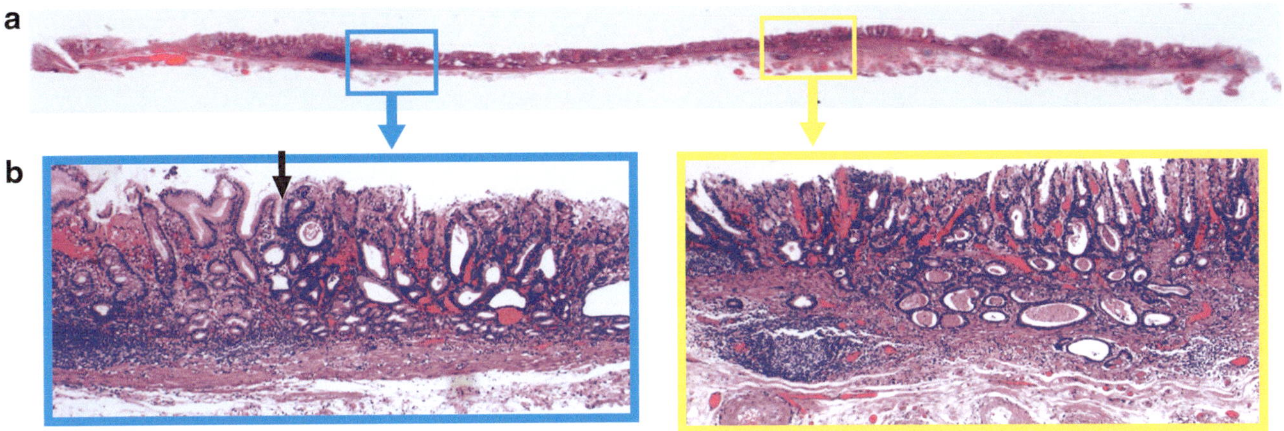

Fig. 19.7 Histological image of the specimen

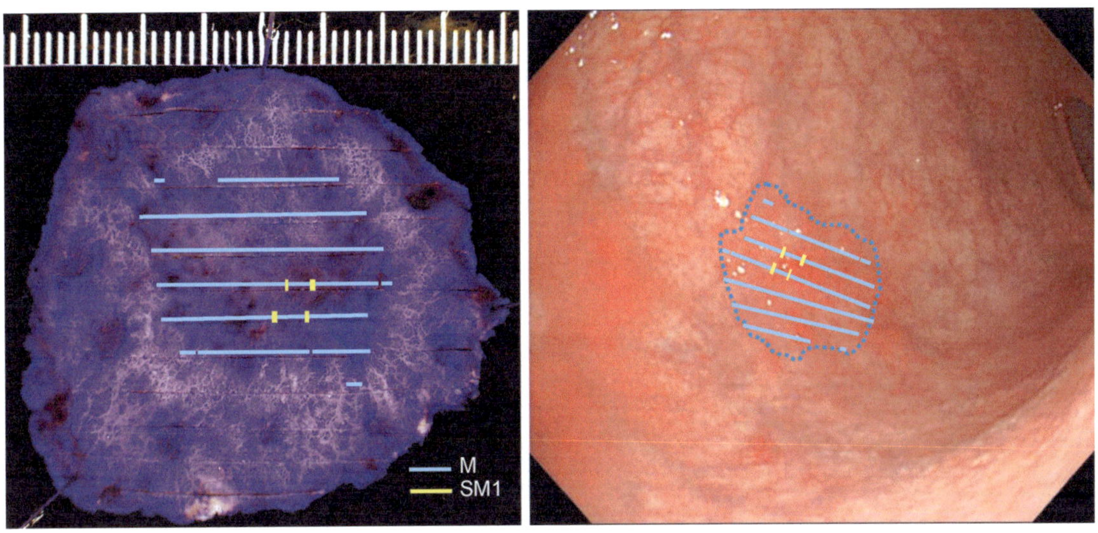

Fig. 19.8 Mapping of the cancer distribution projected on the specimen

This pathological image is of the small reddish protuberance noted by conventional endoscopy. The cancer glands are noted to invade into the muscularis mucosa and partially into the submucosa. The width of the invasion is very narrow, and it was not possible to diagnose submucosal invasion by endoscopic observation (Fig. 19.7b).

The mapping of the cancer is placed on the endoscopic image. The cancer matched with the area of decreased vascular visibility (Fig. 19.8).

Conclusive Diagnosis

Gastric adenocarcinoma, tub1, T1(SM1), ly0, v0, LM (−), VM(−), pType0-IIc, 24 × 20mm, L, Gre.

Conclusion

The reason why the demarcation was unclear was that the mucosal height of cancer and noncancer were almost the same. However the density of the cancer glands was higher than the surrounding mucosa, and it was possible to identify the demarcation of the lesion using NBI magnified endoscopy. The width of the invasion was so narrow that it was not possible to diagnose submucosal invasion in this case. The depth of the cancer was SM1 and tumor size was 24 mm. We diagnosed the lesion as was included expanded pathological criteria for curative endoscopic treatment based on a retrospective analysis of a large series of surgical resection cases in which patients suitable for such expanded criteria were determined to have a negligible risk of lymph node metastasis.

Based on these reasons, ESD was performed.

19.3 Answer

The lateral extension of the lesion is (2) green dotted line.

20 Question 6: Cancer or Adenoma?

Yoko Kitamura

Y. Kitamura (✉)
Department of Gastroenterology, Center for Digestive and Liver Diseases, Nara City Hospital, 1-50-1, Higashikidera-cho, Nara-Shi, Nara 630-8305, Japan
e-mail: humiokumiko@yahoo.co.jp

T. Oyama (ed.), *Endoscopic Diagnosis of Superficial Gastric Cancer for ESD*, DOI 10.1007/978-4-431-54469-2_20

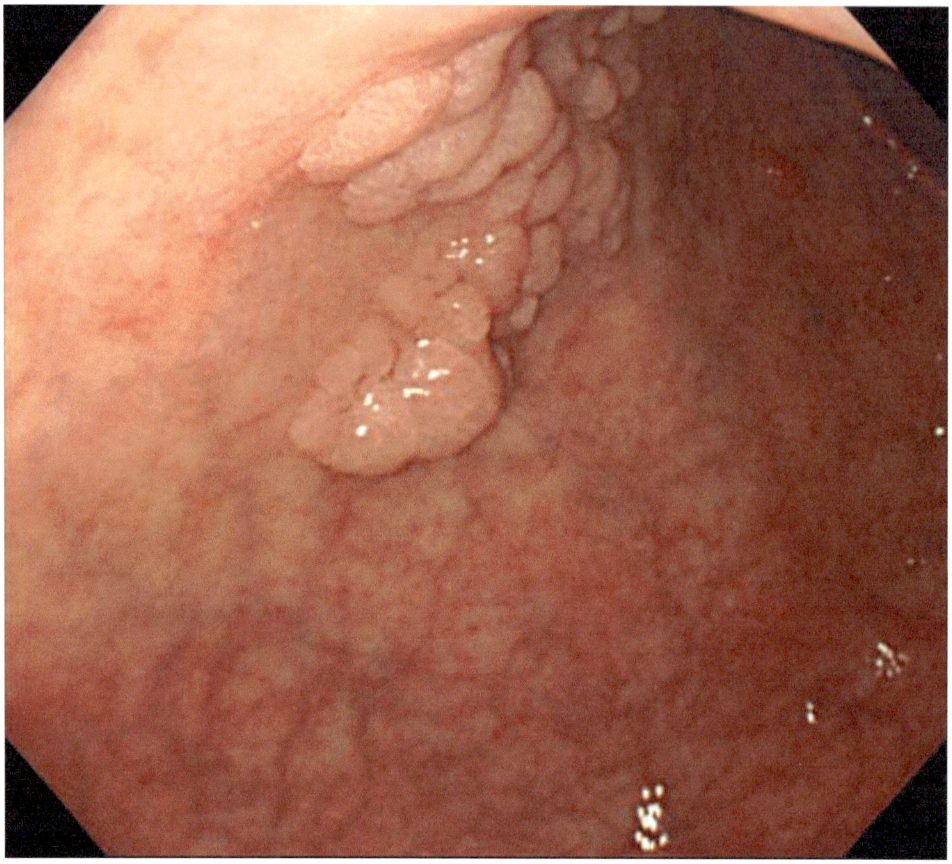

Fig. 20.1 Cancer or adenoma?

Cancer or adenoma? (Fig. 20.1).
Choose your answer from 1 to 3.

(1) WDA (tub1)
(2) MDA (tub2)
(3) Gastric adenoma

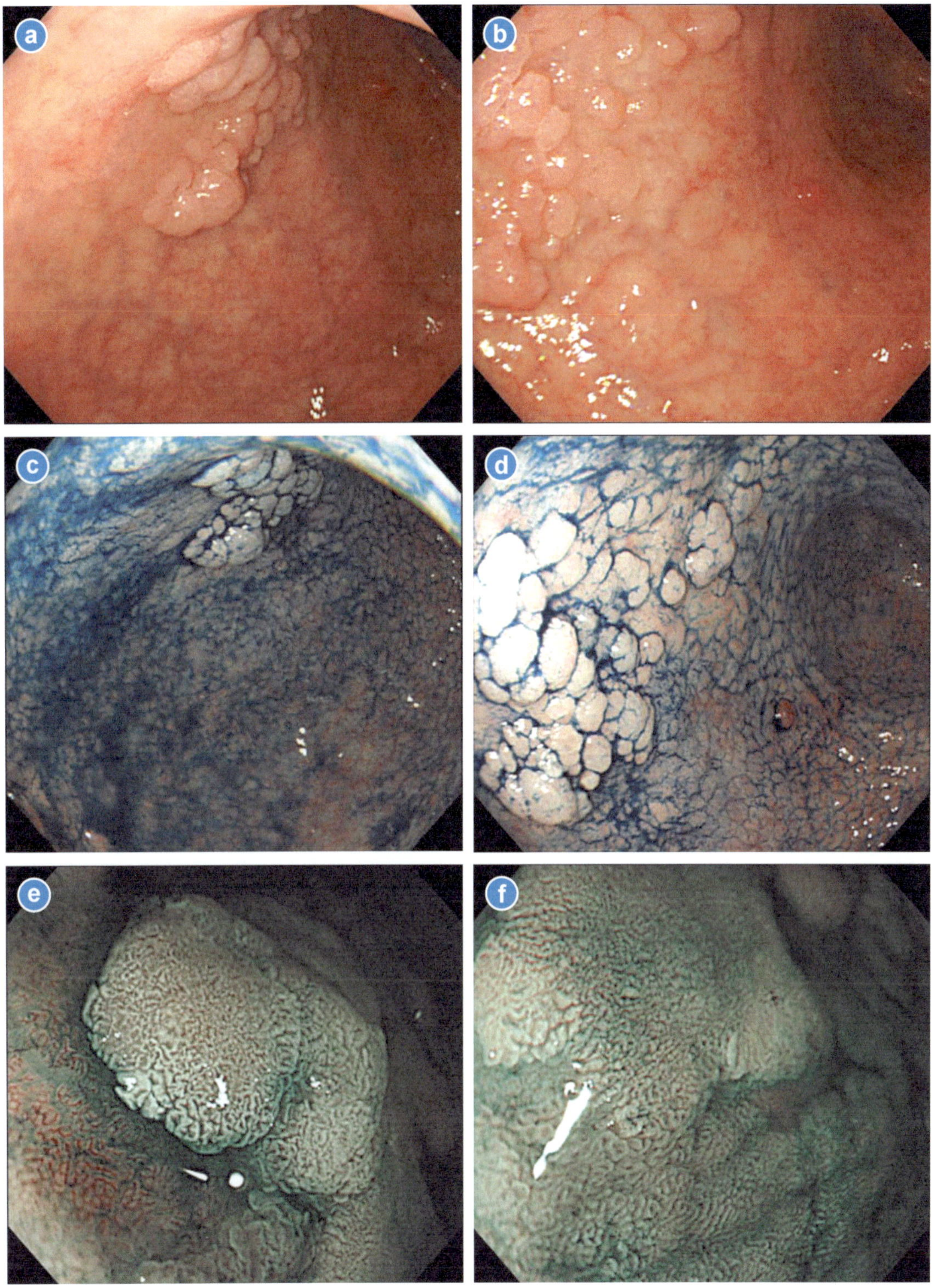

Fig. 20.2 Let's diagnose by observing these six images

20.1 Focus on These Points

20.1.1 Let's Notice Vascular Visibility

- The background mucosa shows markedly visible vessels and disappearance of folds, found in highly atrophic gastritis.
- A whitish protuberant lesion is noted in the anterior wall of the lower gastric body. The whitish lesion is seen as a cluster of multiple nodules of variable sizes. Being of whitish protuberance, the lesion must be differentiated between adenoma and WDA. Although seen as a whitish protuberance, the lesion is diagnosed as WDA (tub1) because of the irregular nodular pattern and variable sizes of the nodules (Fig. 20.3a).

20.1.2 Let's Push the Scope into the Anal Side and Observe the Lateral Extension

- The lesion consisting of a cluster of multiple irregular nodules spreads continuously from the lower body to the anterior wall of the antrum.
- The demarcation of the anal to the greater curvature side of the lesion is unclear because of decreasing height of the lesion becoming almost the same height as the background mucosa.
- The flat part between nodules shows decreased vascular visibility, suggesting presence of flat mucosal (0-IIb) lesion (Fig. 20.3b).

20.1.3 Let's Spray Indigo Carmine for Observing Surface Pattern Well

- Indigo carmine chromoendoscopy enhances the surface pattern and the difference of the elevation clearly.
- In this case, indigo carmine chromoendoscopy reveals the demarcation of the lesion with nodules of variable sizes clearly (Fig. 20.3c).

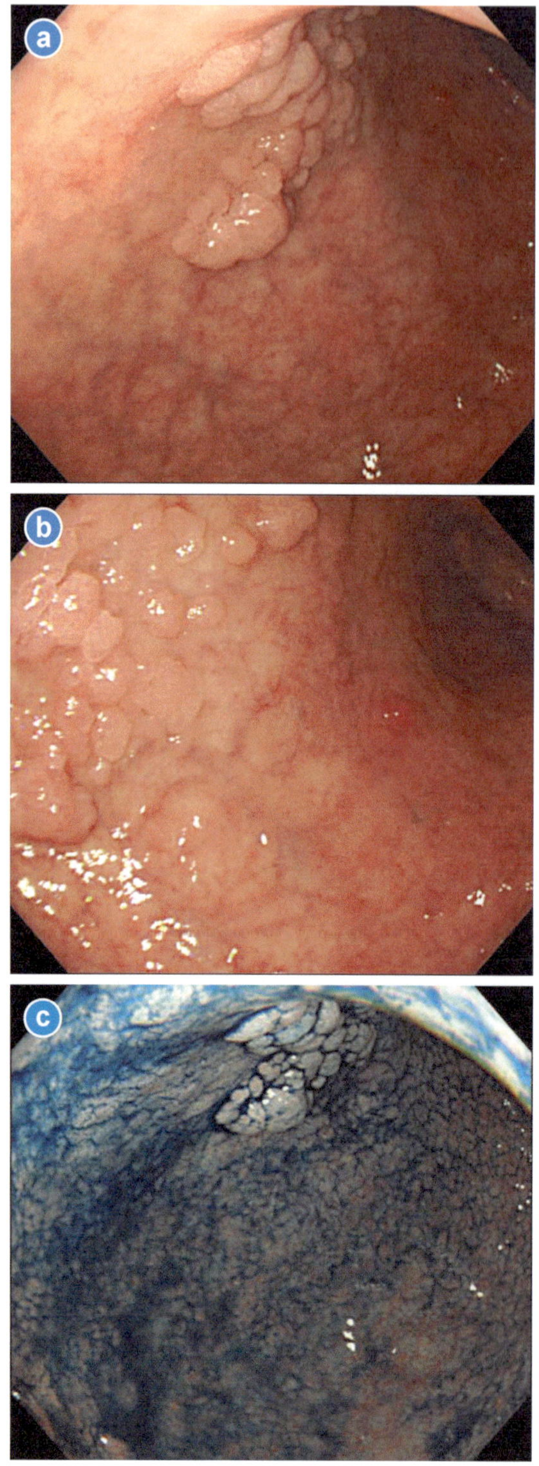

Fig. 20.3 Same images as Fig. 20.2

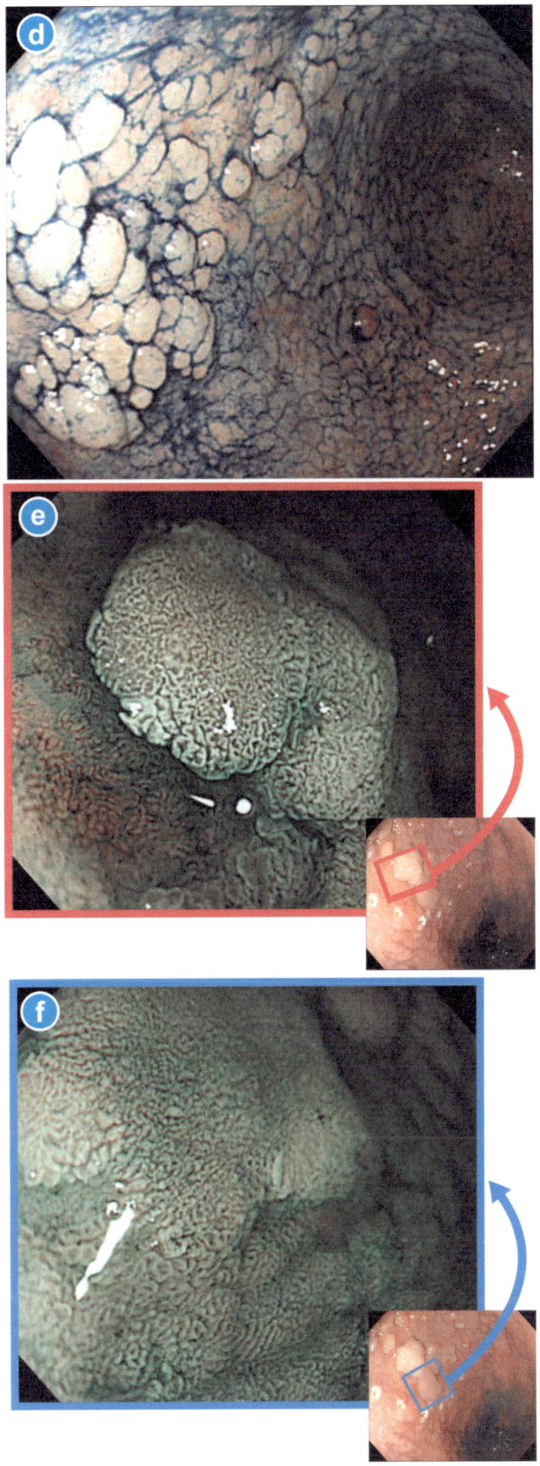

Fig. 20.3 (continued)

20.1.4 Let's Observe the Anal Side of the Lesion

- Indigo carmine chromoendoscopy enhances the irregular nodular pattern and irregular size and shape of the nodules clearly.
- However, the demarcation of the anal to the greater curvature side of the lesion is still unclear (Fig. 20.3d).

20.1.5 Let's Observe the Lesion Using NBI Magnified Endoscopy (1)

- Regularly shaped small round pits are seen in the background mucosa.
- Irregularly shaped dense villi of variable sizes are seen in the protuberant part of the lesion with clear demarcation. The lesion is diagnosed as WDA (Fig. 20.3e).

20.1.6 Let's Observe the Lesion Using NBI Magnified Endoscopy (2)

- The endoscopic image shows the anal side of the lesion.
- The demarcation of the anal side of the lesion is unclear because the height of lesion decreases towards the demarcation, showing little difference in height against the background mucosa.
- However, the demarcation of the lesion can be diagnosed by noting the difference in surface patterns using NBI magnified endoscopy (Fig. 20.3f).

20.2 Let's Compare Fixed Specimens with Resected Specimens

20.2.1 Let's Place Markings to Surround the Lesion

- We marked 3 mm outside surrounding the lesion by the backside of a hook knife with NBI magnified endoscopy (Fig. 20.4).

20.2.2 Let's Examine the Freshly Resected Specimen

- It was impossible to capture the whole lesion in one image by endoscopy. The color points placed on the endoscopic image correspond with the color points placed on the image of the freshly resected specimen.
- The multiple granular nodules of variable sizes are noted on the specimen. The flat part between the nodules has no gap in height with the surrounding mucosa, making the demarcation unclear (Fig. 20.5).

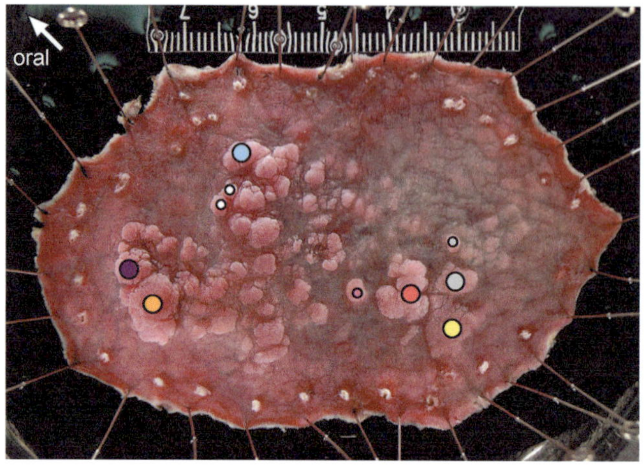

Fig. 20.5 Freshly resected specimen

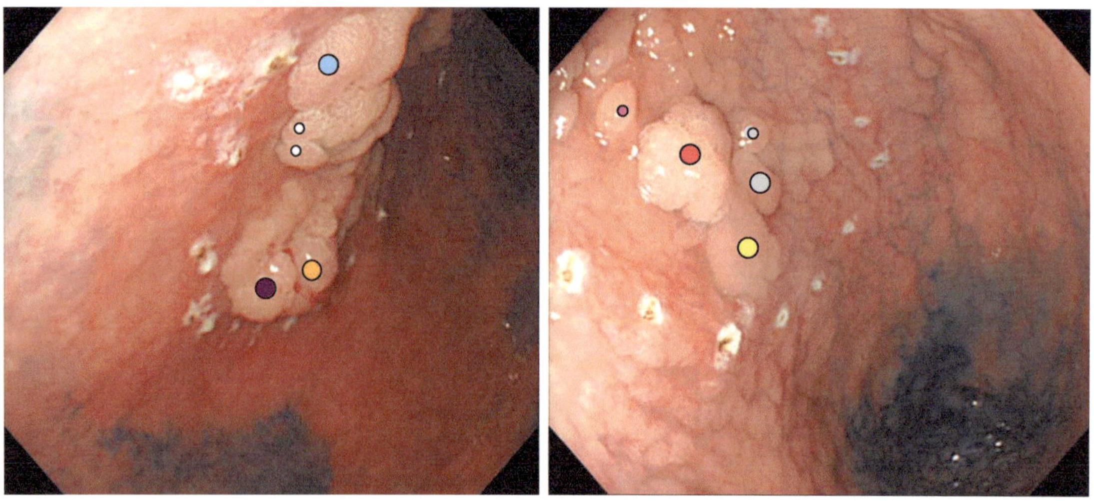

Fig. 20.4 Endscopic image after circumferencial marking

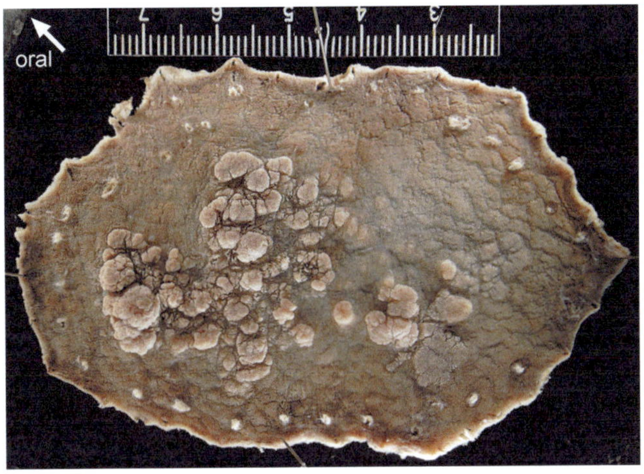

Fig. 20.6 Fixed specimen

20.2.3 Let's Examine the Surface Pattern Further with the Formalin-Fixed Specimen

- This image is of the formalin-fixed specimen.
- The lesion shows irregular nodules of variable sizes, suggesting a diagnosis of WDA.
- The demarcation of the lesion still remains unclear after formalin fixation (Fig. 20.6).

20.2.4 Let's Examine the Histopathological Image

A flat part between nodules is magnified showing histopathology, confirming the diagnosis of WDA (Fig. 20.7a).

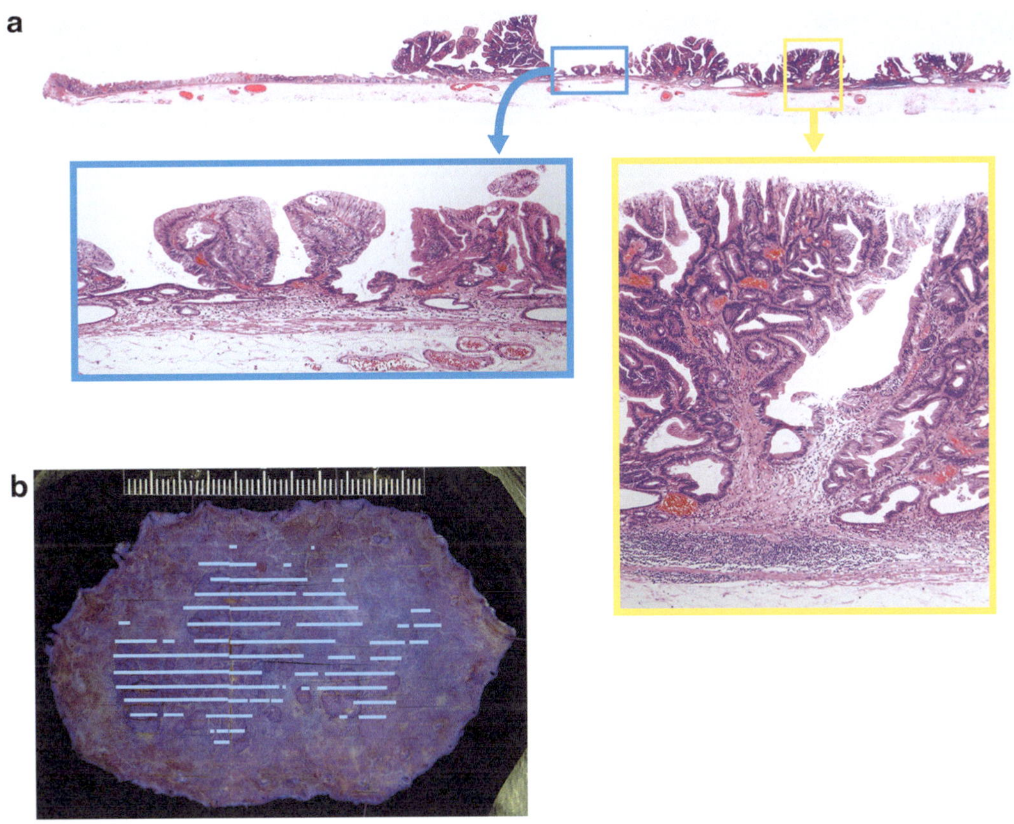

Fig. 20.7 (**a**) Histopathological image of the lesion (**b**) Mapping on the cancer distribution on the specimen

A nodular part is magnified, showing histopathology confirming the diagnosis of WDA. Neoplastic glands noted to form glandular tubules with intact muscularis mucosa confirm the diagnosis of noninvasive cancer (Fig. 20.7b).

Conclusive Diagnosis

Gastric adenocarcinoma, tub1, T1(M), ly0, v0, LM (−), V(−), pType0-IIa + IIb, 59 × 35 mm, L, Ant.

Summary

Although the lesion is whitish and protuberant, it is possible to diagnose the lesion as WDA (tub1) because of the irregular nodular pattern and irregular size of the nodules. The diagnosis of WDA is supported also by NBI magnified endoscopy, showing irregular small villi pattern. In this case, the lesion is likely to be recognized first as a protuberant part, not as a larger lesion exceeding the range caught in one endoscopic view, creating a risk of overlooking the 0-IIb extension. In case of a 0-IIb extension, the lateral border becomes unclear with WL observation as well as with indigo carmine spray. However, the demarcation of the lesion could be recognized as the difference in villi using NBI magnified endoscopy.

20.3 Answer

(1) WDA (tub1).

21 Question 7: Where Is the Horizontal Margin of the Lesion?

Keita Funakawa

K. Funakawa (✉)
Department of Gastroenterology, Kagoshima City Hospital, 37-1, Uearata-Cho, Kagpshima-shi, Kagoshima 890-8760, Japan
e-mail: kfuna@po.synapse.ne.jp

T. Oyama (ed.), *Endoscopic Diagnosis of Superficial Gastric Cancer for ESD*, DOI 10.1007/978-4-431-54469-2_21

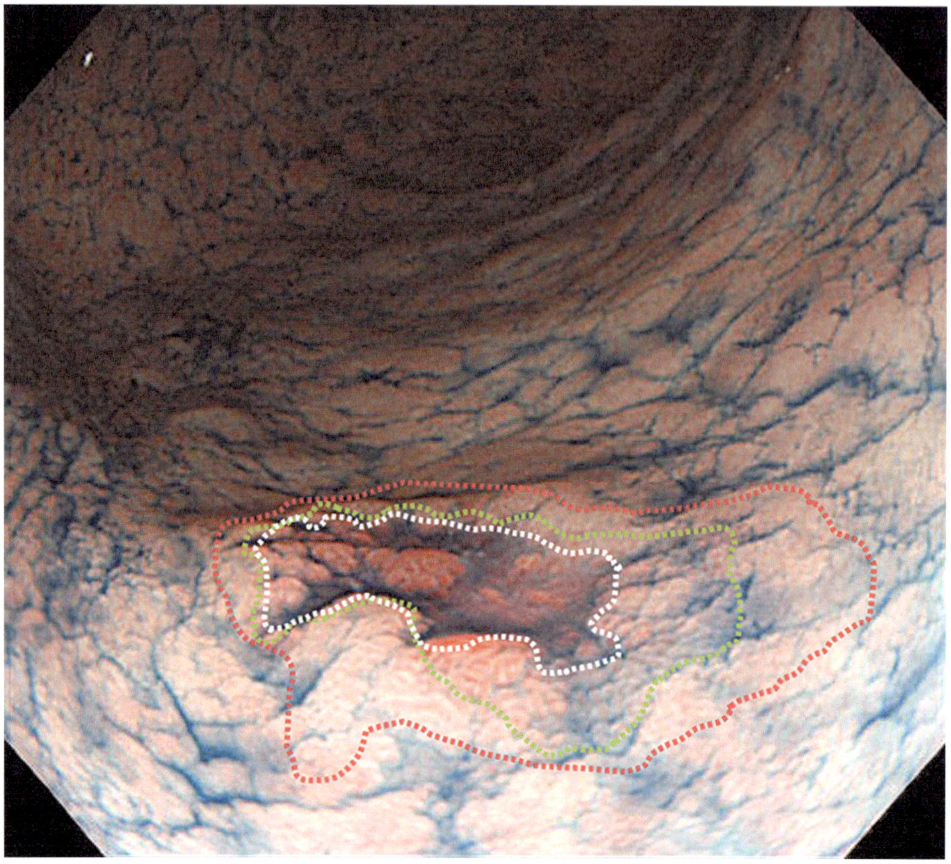

Fig. 21.1 Where is the horizontal margin of the lesion?

Where is the horizontal margin of the lesion (Fig. 21.1)? Choose your answer from 1 to 3.

(1) White dotted line
(2) Green dotted line
(3) Red dotted line

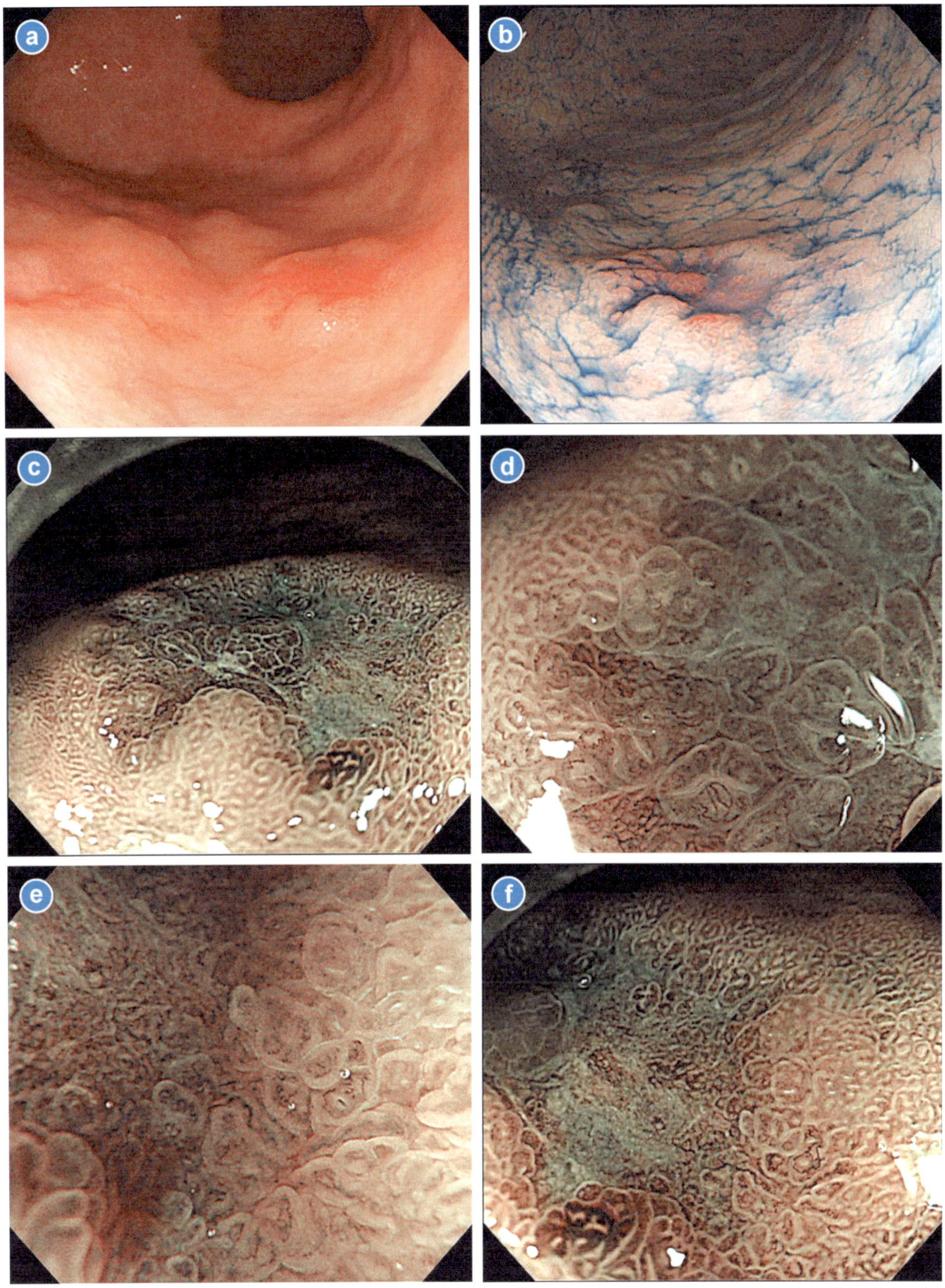

Fig. 21.2 Let's diagnose by observing these six images

21.1 Focus on These Points

21.1.1 Let's Pay Attention to the Depression and the Color Tone

- There is a reddish depressed lesion with marginal protuberance, and at a glance, the borderline of the lesion is clear as the difference of the color tone and the margin of the depression.
- The margin of the depressed lesion is jaggy and irregular like a silkworm-eaten appearance (Fig. 21.3a).

21.1.2 Let's Spray Indigo Carmine

- After spraying indigo carmine, the borderline of the depressed lesion becomes clearer than with usual WL observation. There is a regular gastric areal mucosal pattern around the depressed lesion, but not inside the depressed lesion where coarse nodules and fine granular elevations are seen, but, neither large, high protuberances, nor deep depressions are noted.
- A partial extension of the depressed lesion is seen with a jaggy and irregular margin like a silkworm-eaten appearance.
- The marginal protuberance is smooth as noted by the two black arrows, but the mucosa of the area marked by the blue arrow is granular. The mucosa of the area noted by the red arrow shows a fine granular pattern, and the marginal protuberance is not clear (Fig. 21.3b).

21.1.3 Let's Perform NBI Magnified Endoscopy

- This is a medium-power magnifying endoscopic image.
- The background mucosa has a surface pattern consisting of regular pits and villi, but the mucosa of the depressed lesion has irregular pits and villi of variable sizes and appears more brownish than the background.
- The borderline of the lesion can be clearly detected as noted by the yellow arrows with differences in color and surface structures except for the lower right part of the picture (Fig. 21.3c).

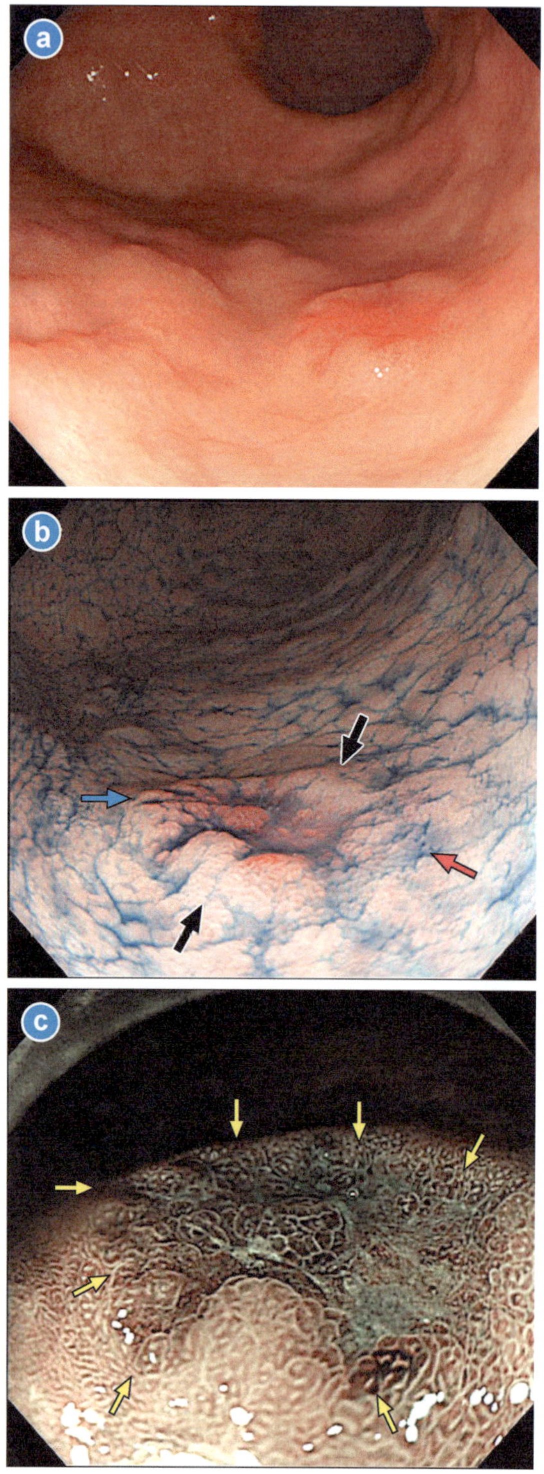

Fig. 21.3 Same images as Fig. 21.2

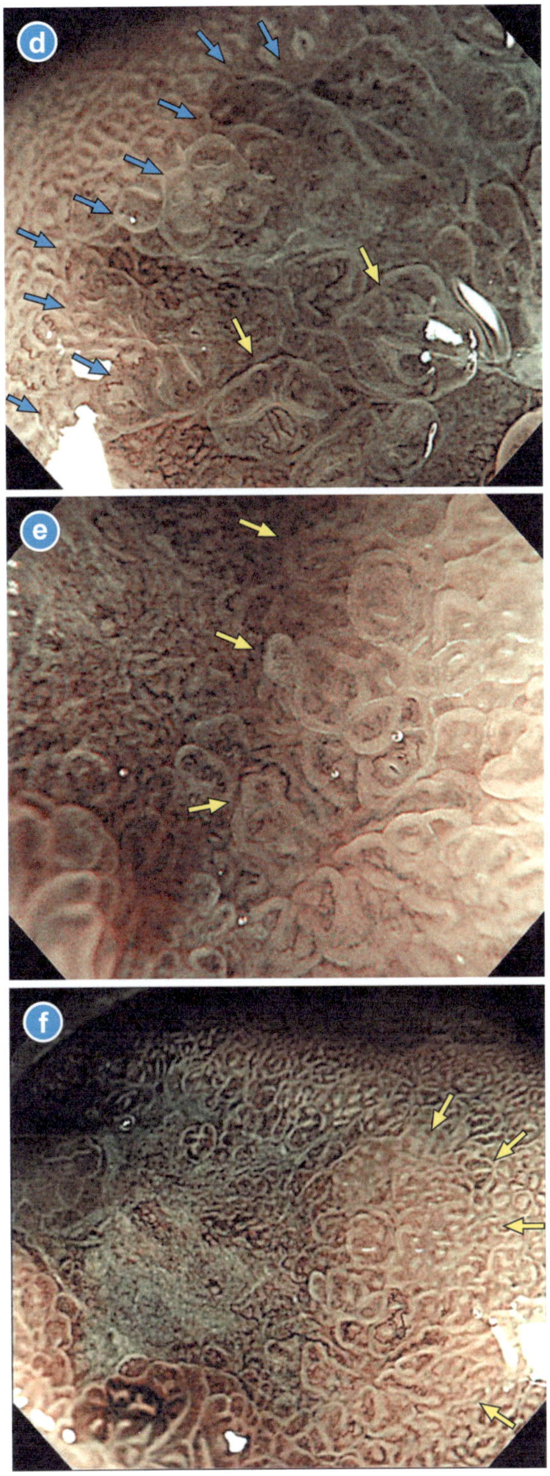

Fig. 21.3 (continued)

21.1.4 Let's Observe the Anal-Side Margin of the Depression Lesion with NBI Magnified Endoscopy

- This is an NBI magnified endoscopic image of the anal-side margin of the depressed lesion (Fig. 21.3d).
- The background mucosa has regular pits and villi pattern.
- The depressed lesion has irregular and variably sized pits and villi and shows fusion of villi as noted by the two yellow arrows.
- The borderline is clearly seen by the difference in the mucosal surface patterns as noted by the blue arrows.

21.1.5 Let's Observe the Oral Side of the Depressed Lesion with NBI Magnified Endoscopy

- This is an NBI magnified endoscopic image of the oral depressed part (Fig. 21.3e).
- The depressed lesion has irregular variably sized villi. In the lesion, the caliber changes of the vessels are mild, but we can see running irregularities of the vessels. Vascular networks are observed partially, but in very few areas as a whole.
- The right side of the yellow arrows is outside of the depression, where irregular villi with variable sizes and fusion are seen. This area also appears suspicious to be a part of a superficial neoplasm. The true demarcation line must be recognized further outside against the background mucosa.

21.1.6 Let's See the Magnifying Endoscopic Image on the Oral Side

- This is the magnifying endoscopic image on the oral side of the lesion.
- Towards the oral side, outside of the depressed lesion, there are irregular, size-variable villi and pitlike patterns, also with fusion of some villi. There is a clear difference with the regular background mucosa as noted by the yellow arrows, supporting diagnosis of this difference as the demarcation line of the lesion.
- Based on these, the lesion can be diagnosed as well-differentiated gastric adenocarcinoma, 0-IIc + IIb, with an invasion depth of M.

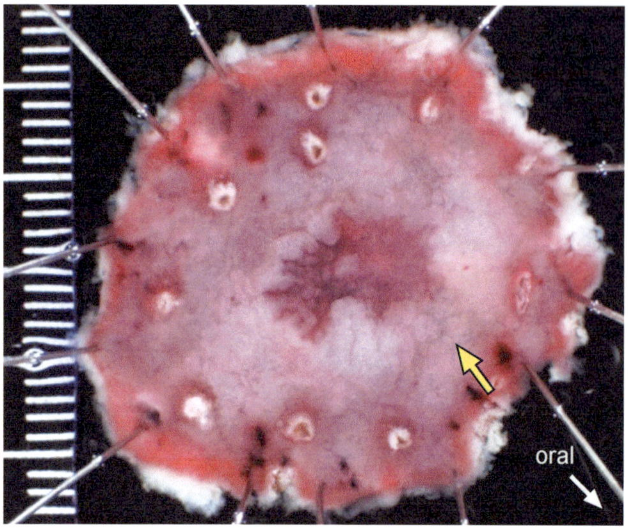

Fig. 21.4 Freshly resected specimen

21.2 Let's Compare Fixed Specimens with Resected Specimens

21.2.1 Let's See the Freshly Resected Specimen

- Strong redness with variably sized irregular granules is noted on the bottom of the depression. The demarcation line can be recognized as the margin of the depression and the difference of color tone.
- The oral extension part of the depression marked by a yellow arrow shows slightly yellowish mucosa compared against the surrounding mucosa, but it is difficult to determine the border of the lesion (Fig. 21.4).

This is the pathological image of the depressed part of the depressed lesion.

This lesion can be diagnosed as WDA based on atypia of the glandular structures and nuclei (Fig. 21.5a).

This is the pathological image of the 0-IIb part.

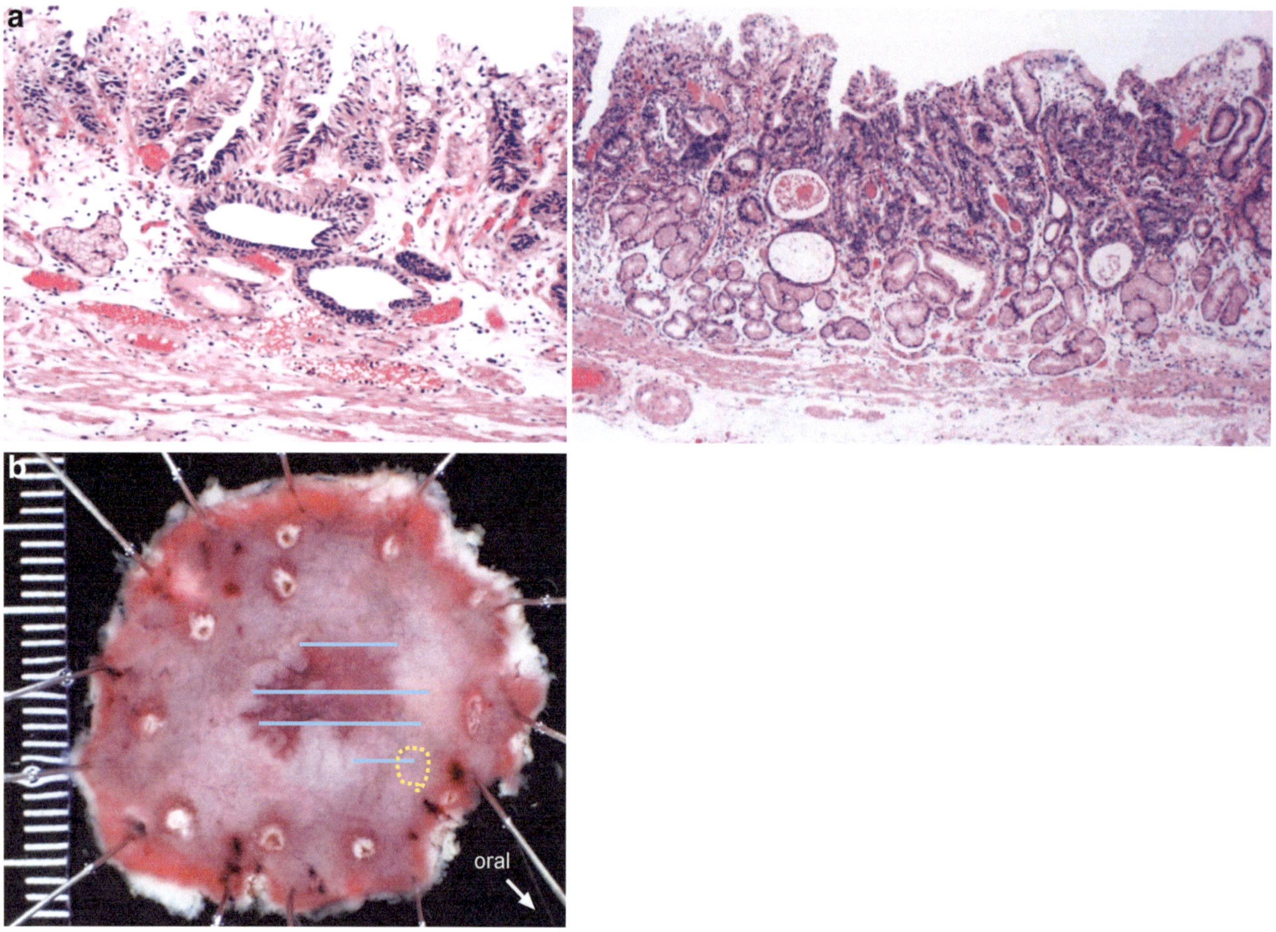

Fig. 21.5 (a) Pathological image of the depressed part of the depressed lesion. (b) Pathological image of the 0-IIb part

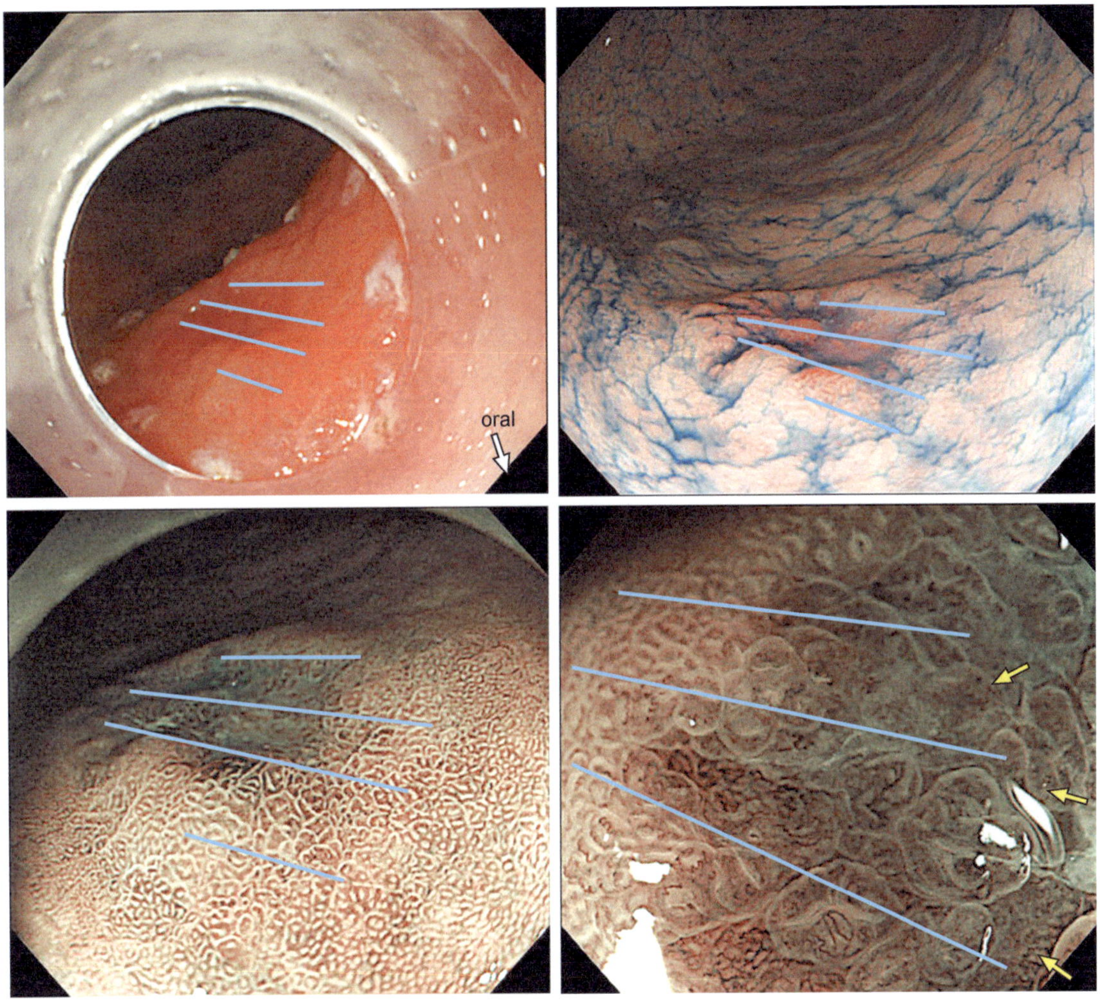

Fig. 21.6 Comparison with the endoscopic images and NBI endoscopic images

This lesion can be diagnosed as WDA based on atypia of the glandular structures and nuclei (Fig. 21.5b).

21.2.2 Let's Compare with the Endoscopic Image

- The mapping of the lesion obtained on the resected image was carefully compared with endoscopic images of usual WL, of indigo carmine dye spray, and of magnified NBI modality and was superimposed on each image.
- The range of the lesion is almost identical to the depressed area except for the oral side, but the lesion extended beyond the depression as a 0-IIb extension of the lesion.
- The 0-IIb extension of the lesion is not visible by WL endoscopy, but can be appreciated as the finely granular mucosa after indigo carmine dye spray. And yet, its horizontal margin remains unclear.
- With NBI magnified image, 0-IIb extension part consists of variably sized irregular villi and pits, and the borderline around the lesion can be clearly recognized as the difference in surface structures (Fig. 21.6).

Conclusive Diagnosis

Gastric adenocarcinoma, tub1 > tub2, T1(M), ly0, v0, LM(−), VM(−), pType 0-IIc, 12 × 8 mm, L, Gre.

Summary
Although the lateral margin of the depressed part can be recognized by difference in color tone and surface structures, the oral extension part of the depression is difficult to detect accurately without NBI magnified endoscopy. NBI magnified endoscopy is useful to diagnose the horizontal margin of the 0-IIb extension.

21.3 Answer

The horizontal margin of the lesion is (2) green dotted line.

Question 8: Where Do You Think Is the Border of This Lesion?

22

Ayako Seki

A. Seki (✉)
Department of Gastroenterology, Nagano Municipal Hospital, 1333-1 Tomitake, Nagano-shi, Nagano 381-8551, Japan
e-mail: ayako_seki@hospital.nagano.nagano.jp

T. Oyama (ed.), *Endoscopic Diagnosis of Superficial Gastric Cancer for ESD*, DOI 10.1007/978-4-431-54469-2_22

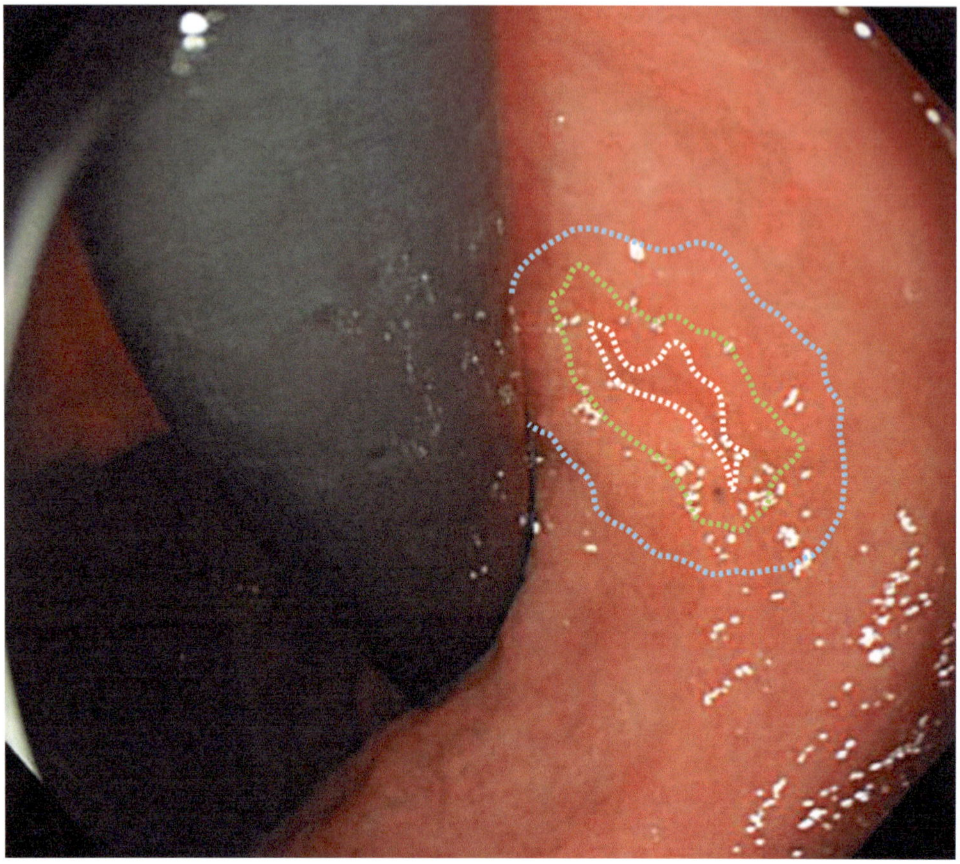

Fig. 22.1 Where do you think is the border of this lesion?

Where do you think is the border of this lesion (Fig. 22.1)?
Choose your answer from 1 to 3.

(1) White dotted line
(2) Green dotted line
(3) Blue dotted line

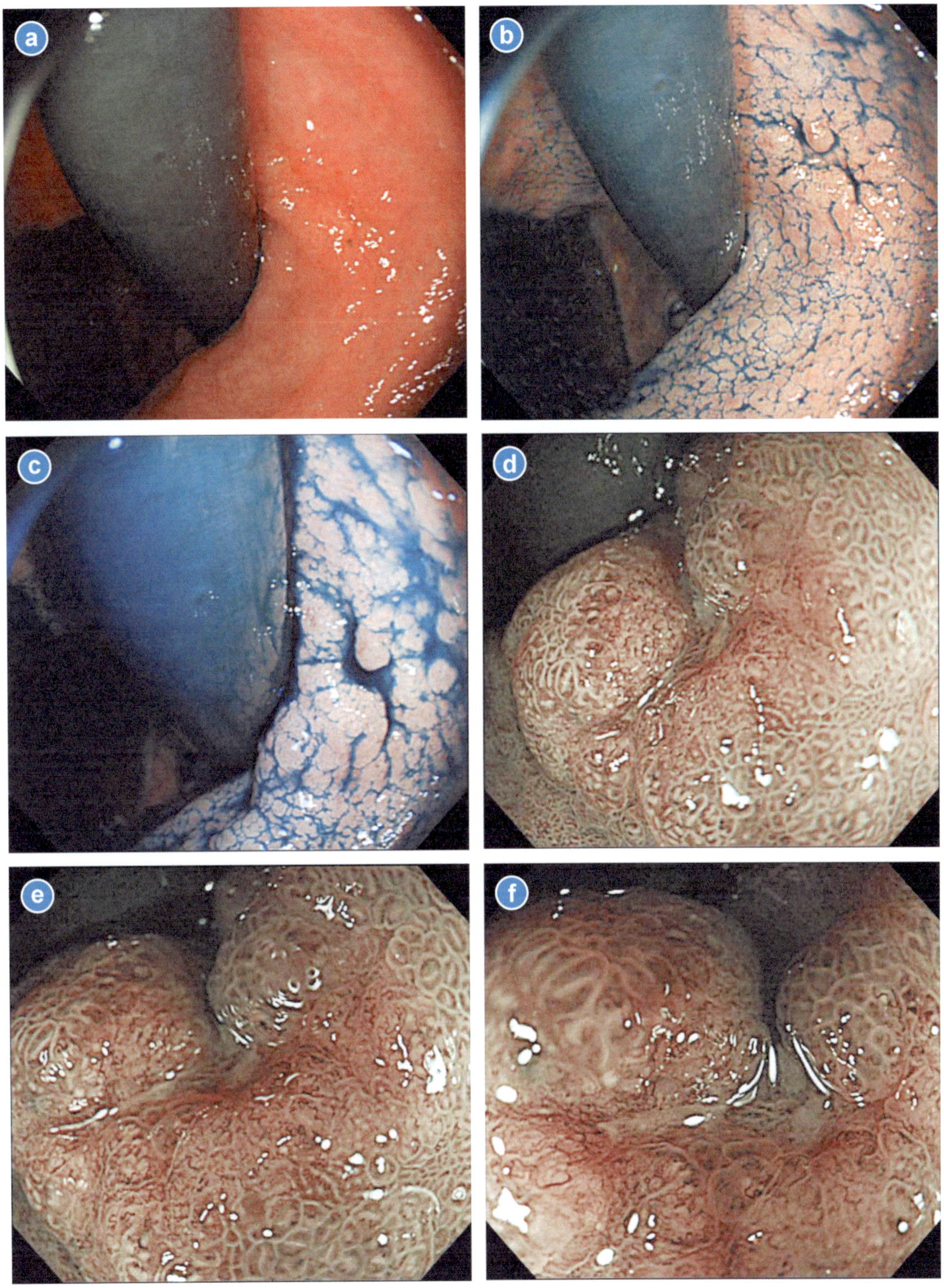

Fig. 22.2 Let's diagnose by observing these six images

22.1 Focus on These Points

22.1.1 Let's Look at the Color and the Shape of the Lesion

- There is a red irregularly shaped, depressed lesion in the lesser curvature of the middle gastric body (Fig. 22.3a).
- The border of the depressed lesion is slightly unclear, and it is surrounded by a paler protuberant area. The irregular shape of the lesion suggests that it is a cancer. But it seems possible that it is a simple erosion because of unclearness of the border.
- To make the border clear, indigo carmine is sprayed.

22.1.2 Let's Spray Indigo Carmine

- The border of the depressed area has become clear with indigo carmine spray, revealing spindle-like extensions (Fig. 22.3b).
- The gastric mucosa outside of the lesion shows a regular surface areal pattern. But the surrounding protuberance has an irregular coarse areal pattern. It is suspected that the cancer is spreading to the surrounding protuberance.
- The color of the depressed area is reddish, and this suggests that the lesion is WDA.

22.1.3 Let's Look at the Mucosal Surface Pattern

- On closing up, an irregular surface pattern extends from the depressed area to halfway up the surrounding protuberance. It is suspected that the range of this cancer includes the depressed area and the surrounding protuberance (Fig. 22.3c).

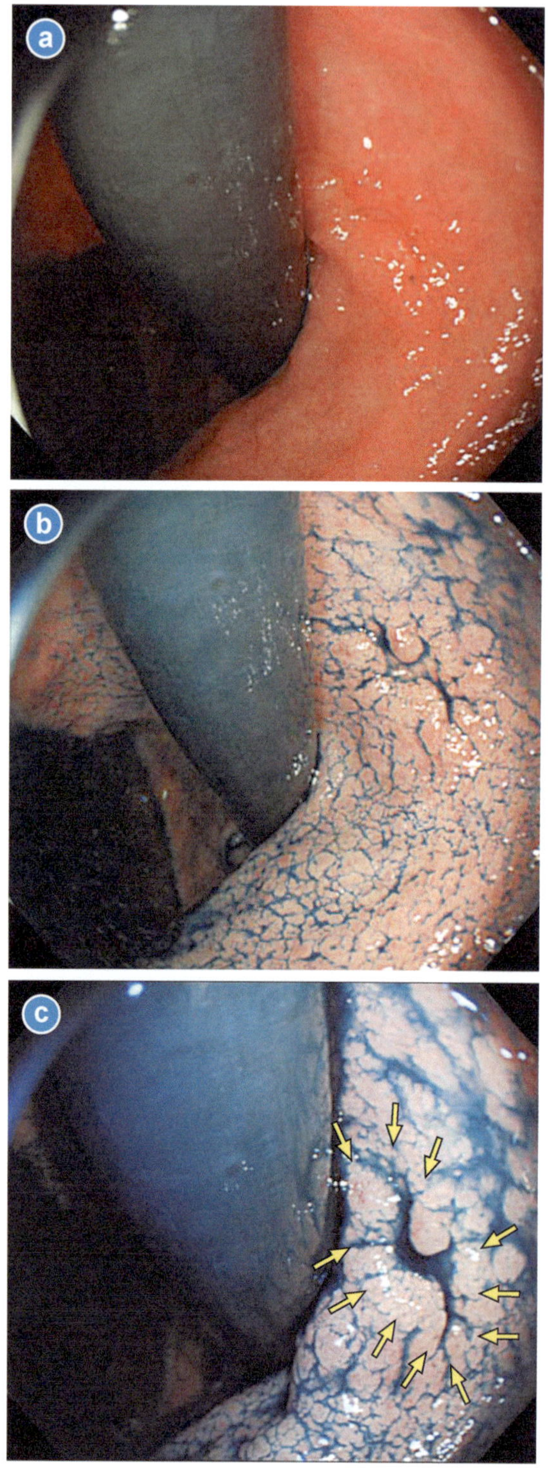

Fig. 22.3 Same images as Fig. 22.2

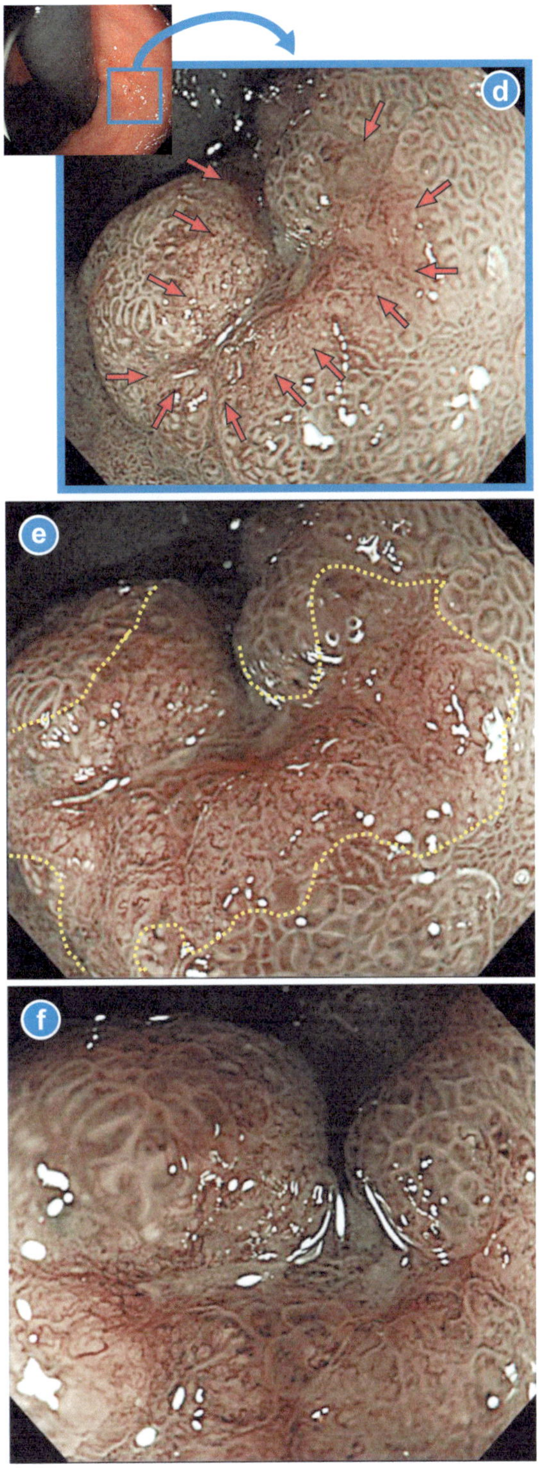

Fig. 22.3 (continued)

22.1.4 Let's Observe with NBI Magnified View

- This is a lower-power NBI magnified view of the posterior wall side of the lesion (Fig. 22.3d).
- The surface fine structure outside of the lesion is mostly pitlike. Villi-like fine structures are seen partially with minimal size variability. They are roundly shaped without irregularities.
- On the other hand, the surface microstructure of the lesion is unclear. The difference between the two is obvious.
- To observe the surface microstructure and vessels in more detail, observation with higher-power NBI magnified view is made.

22.1.5 Let's Look Also at the Surface Vascular Patterns

- This is a middle-power NBI magnified view (Fig. 22.3e).
- In the area of unclear surface patterns, fine vessels with irregular running and caliber changes are noted.
- Some of the surface fine vessels show network patterns, leading to histological typing of well- to moderately differentiated adenocarcinoma.
- The border of the cancer is shown by the yellow dotted line in the left figure, because the difference of the cancer and the normal gastric mucosa is obvious.
- Based on above, the answer is (2).

22.1.6 Let's Magnify the View More and Observe the Lesion in Detail

- This view is obtained with the highest-power magnification NBI (Fig. 22.3f).
- The surface microstructures and vessels in the depressed area are not visible.
- The surface microstructures are unclear in the depressed area and on the surrounding protuberance. And the surface fine vessels show irregular running and caliber changes.

22.2 Let's Compare Fixed Specimens with Resected Specimens

The lesion was diagnosed as WDA, type 0-IIc, with the invasion depth of M. En bloc resection by ESD was performed.

22.2.1 Let's Look at the Color and the Surface Pattern in the Freshly Resected Specimen

- This is the freshly resected specimen (Fig. 22.4).
- The specimen is rotated to be compared with the endoscopic images, with the oral side noted by a black arrow.
- A depressed area with surrounding protuberance is noted in the whitish mucosa with irregular surface.
- The border with the background surface pattern is clearly visible because of the difference in surface patterns.
- Because of the way the specimen has been pinned and fixed, the depressed area of the specimen appears larger than endoscopic images.
- There is a prominent nodule within the depressed area as marked by a yellow arrow.

This pathological image of the depressed area shows structural and nuclear atypia of the glands, confirming the diagnosis of WDA (Fig. 22.5a).

This pathological image of the surrounding protuberance also shows structural and nuclear atypia, confirming the diagnosis of WDA (tub1).

The cancer is shown to the right of the pink arrow, extending halfway up the surrounding protuberance (Fig. 22.5b).

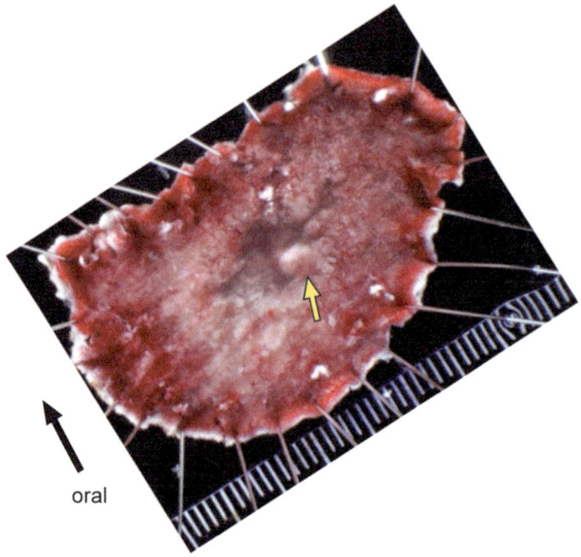

Fig. 22.4 Freshly resected specimen

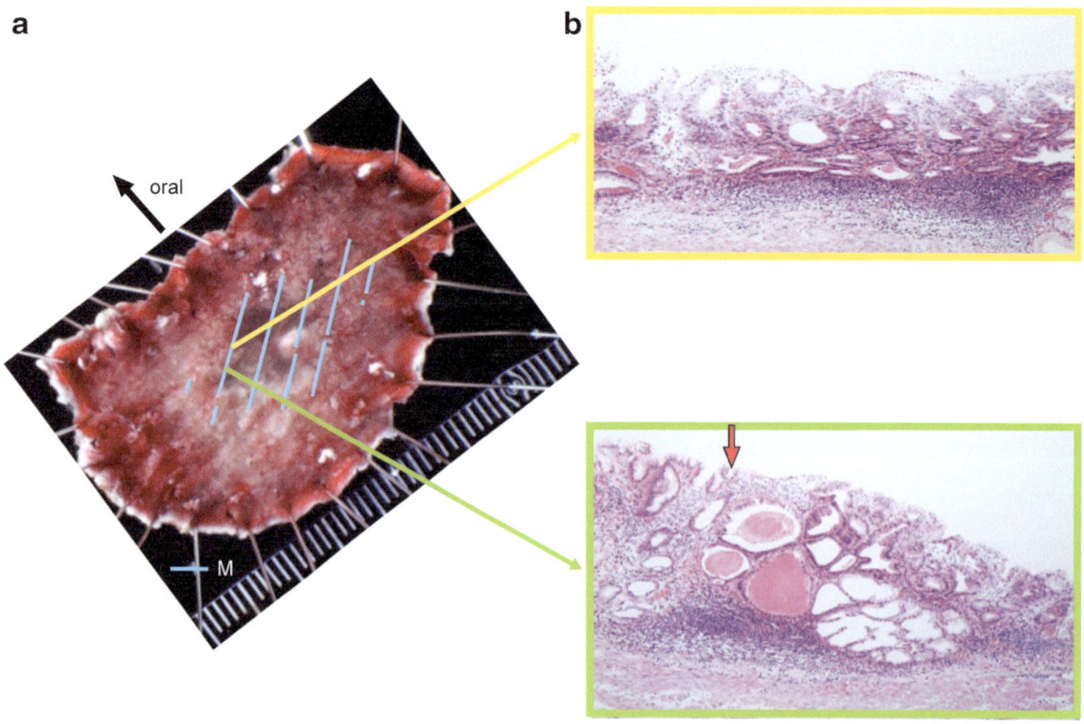

Fig. 22.5 (a) Mapping on the cancer distribution on the specimen (b) The histopathological image of the lesion

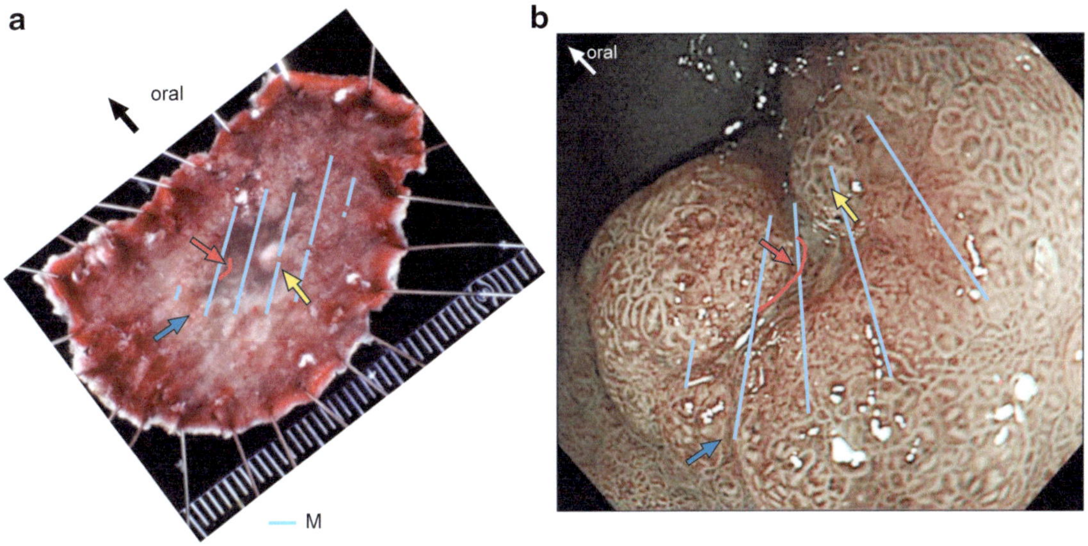

Fig. 22.6 Freshly resected specimen and NBI endoscopic image with mapping of the cancer distribution projected on the specimen

22.2.2 Let's Place Pathological Mapping of the Image on the Freshly Resected Specimen and the NBI Magnified Image

- The left figure shows the mapping on the freshly resected specimen (Fig. 22.6a). The right figure shows the mapping on the NBI magnified image (Fig. 22.6b). The oral side is towards the left upper side in both images.
- The mapping is performed only in the front side of the lesion, because the back could not be seen by the NBI magnified image.
- In both of the figures, yellow arrows point to the raised nodule, red arrows show the curving line of the oral side of the depressed area, and blue arrows correspond with the groove on the left side of the lesion.
- The cancer extends to the surrounding protuberance according to the mapping of the specimen. It corresponds with the area that has irregular surface fine structure and vessels in the NBI magnified images.

Conclusive Diagnosis
Gastric adenocarcinoma, tub1, T1(M), ly0, v0, LM (−), VM(−), pType 0-IIc, 16 × 10 mm, U, less.

Summary
In this case, the cancer was the depressed lesion with surrounding protuberance, and the cancer extends from the depressed area to halfway up the protuberance.

We diagnosed the range of the cancer correctly by using the NBI magnified view.

22.3 Answer

The border of the cancer is (2) green dotted line.

23 Question 9: To What Extent Does the Lateral Extension Reach?

Yuji Nishiyama

Y. Nishiyama (✉)
Department of Internal Medicine, Watanabe Hospital, 539-5,
Tamashimauwanari, Kurashiki, Okayama 713-8101, Japan
e-mail: y-nishiyama@guitar.ocn.ne.jp

T. Oyama (ed.), *Endoscopic Diagnosis of Superficial Gastric Cancer for ESD*, DOI 10.1007/978-4-431-54469-2_23

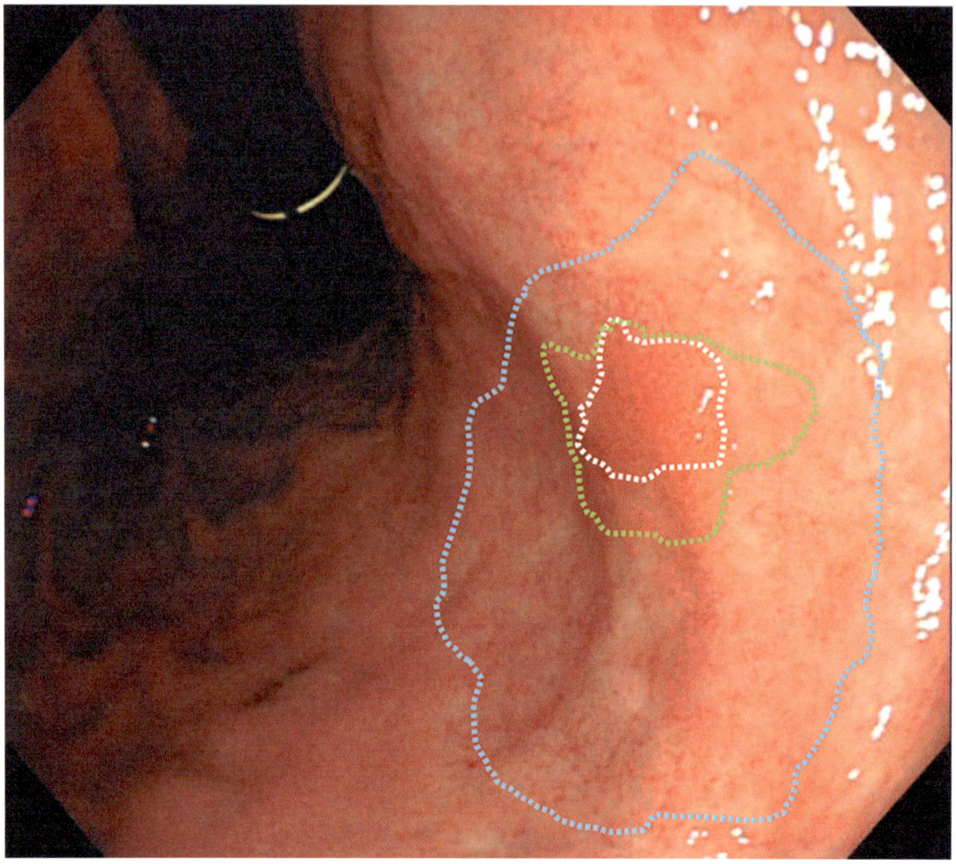

Fig. 23.1 To what extent does the lateral extension reach

To what extent does the lateral extension reach (Fig. 23.1)?
Choose your answer from 1 to 3.

(1) White dotted line
(2) Green dotted line
(3) Blue dotted line

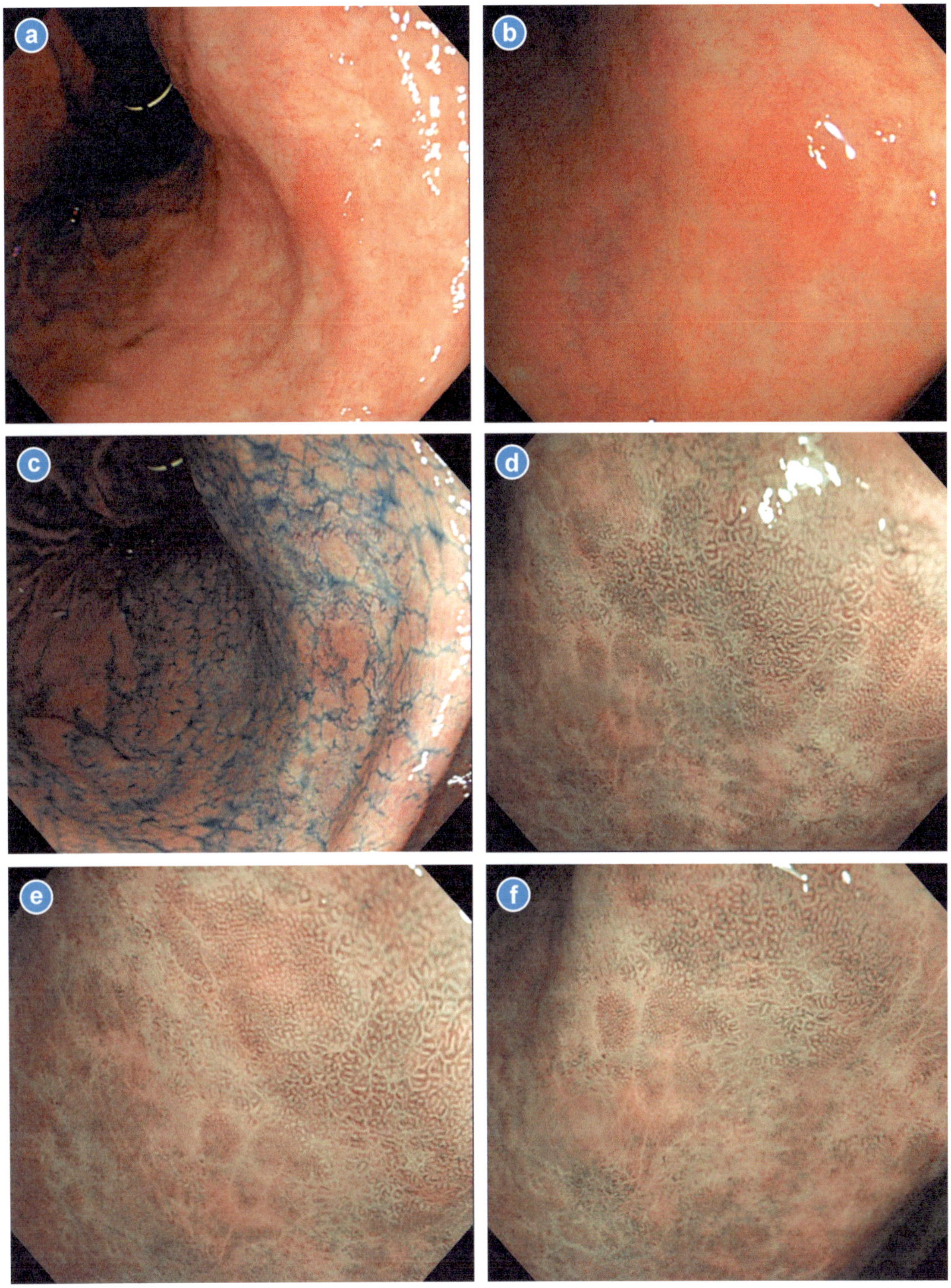

Fig. 23.2 Let's diagnose by observing these six images

23.1 Focus on These Points

23.1.1 Let's Focus on Redness

- As indicated by the yellow arrow, a reddened flat lesion is recognized in the lesser curvature of the lower gastric body. Surface texture of the redness is smooth with ill-defined border.
- An area with a mixture of redness and discoloration is recognized showing its ill-defined border around the redness as indicated by the blue arrows (Fig. 23.3a).

23.1.2 Let's Take a Closer Look

- A close-up image of the reddened area is shown.
- The surface texture of the redness is smooth showing ill-defined border around except for the anal side with a clear border as indicated by black arrows (Fig. 23.3b).

23.1.3 Let's Spray Indigo Carmine

- It is possible to observe the surface texture in detail by spraying indigo carmine.
- While irregularity of the areal pattern is not observed on the surface texture of the mucosa surrounding the lesion, a blurred areal pattern is observed on the site of lesion which repels indigo carmine. However, the border with the site of the lesion is unclear.
- In order to examine further in detail the area with ill-defined border between the redness recognized by usual WL observation and its surrounding area, a NBI--magnified observation is used (Fig. 23.3c).

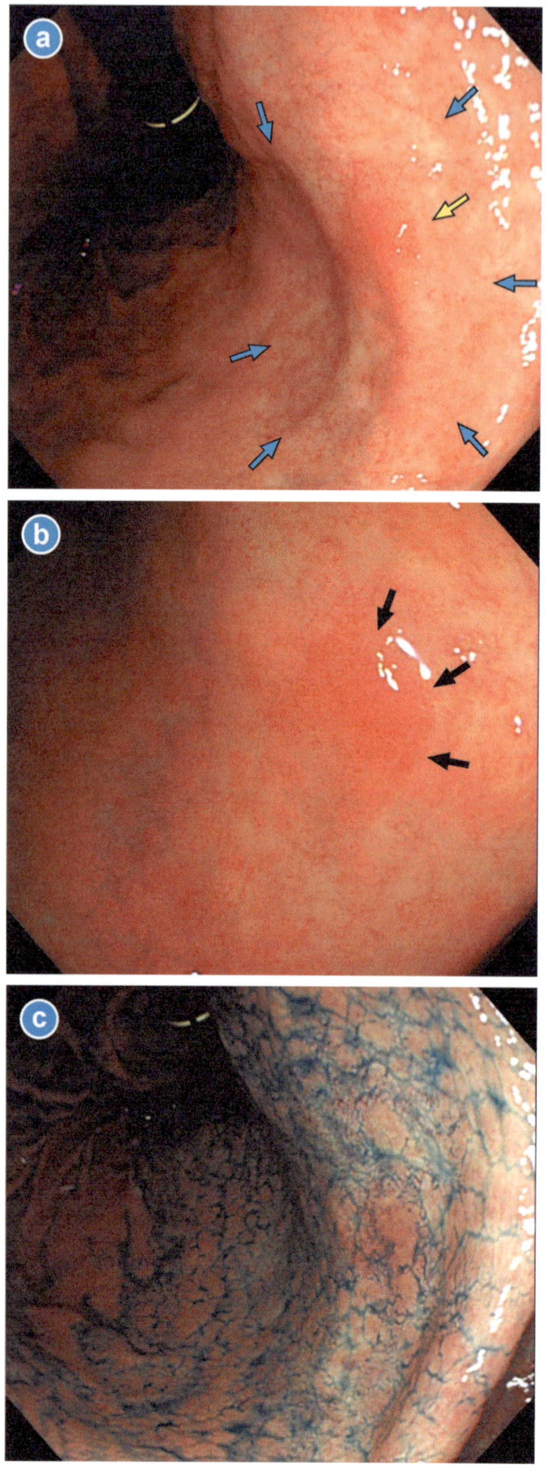

Fig. 23.3 Same images as Fig. 23.2

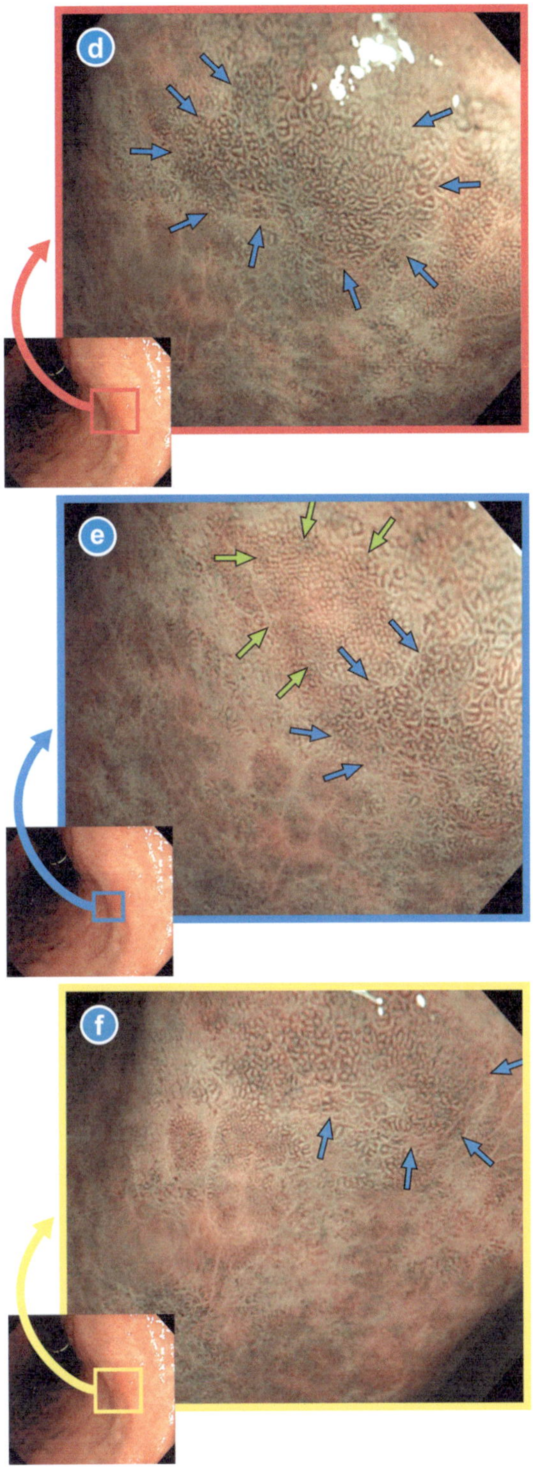

Fig. 23.3 (continued)

23.1.4 Let's Focus on Surface Structures

- This is a lower-power magnified image of NBI of an area recognized as redness by WL observation.
- Pit-like structures are observed on the surface of the reddened site indicated by blue arrows. Even though the degree of irregularity of the pits is mild, difference in size is recognized (Fig. 23.3d).

23.1.5 How Is the Range of Spreading on the Oral Side?

- This is a magnified image of NBI of redness on the oral side (Fig. 23.3e).
- It has been diagnosed to be non-tumor tissue based on the pit-like structures of uniform size and regular shape indicated by green arrows.
- On the other hand, the reddened site indicated by blue arrows has been diagnosed as epithelial tumor based on the pit-like structures with variable sizes and irregular shape.
- Further, the range of lateral extension has been identified by blue arrows based on the difference in pit-like structures.

23.1.6 Let's Examine the Anal Side

- A border on the anal side indicated by blue arrows has been recognized by tracking the spreading of pit-like structures of various sizes back toward the anal side.
- Based on this, the range of tumor spreading has been determined to be the range indicated by blue arrows (Fig. 23.3f).

23.2 Let's Compare Fixed Specimens with Resected Specimens

23.2.1 Let's Perform Marking

- Markings are places outside of the border of cancer diagnosed with magnified NBI (Fig. 23.4).

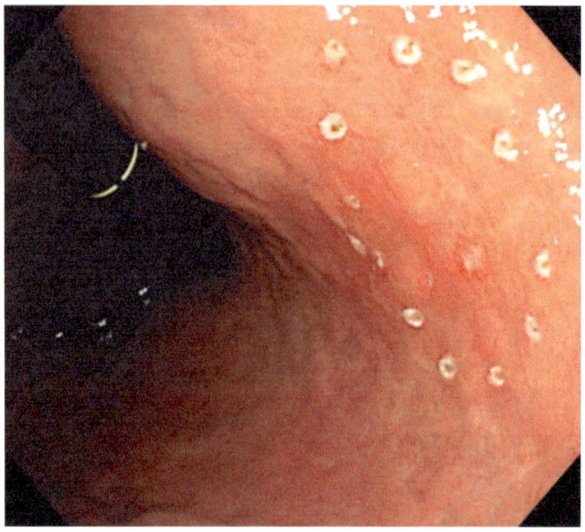

Fig. 23.4 Endscopic image after marking

23.2.2 Let's Take a Look at the Freshly Resected Specimen

- The right side of the figure corresponds to the oral side (Fig. 23.5a).
- A reddened depressed area indicated by red arrows is observed in the center. However, its border is ill-defined.

23.2.3 Let's Take a Look at the Fixed Specimen

- The right side of the figure corresponds to the oral side (Fig. 23.5b).
- Similarly to the case of the fresh specimen, a depressed area indicated by red arrows is also observed in the fixed sample showing its ill-defined border.

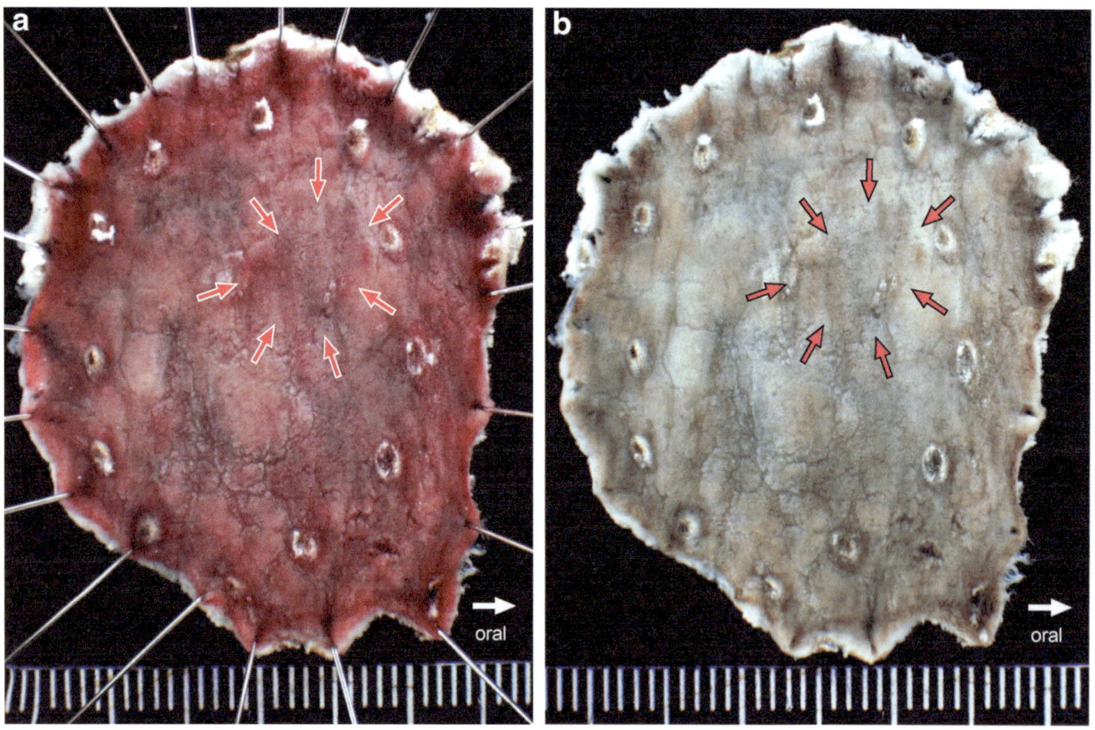

Fig. 23.5 Comparison between the fresh and fixed specimen

This is a histological picture of the site indicated by light blue lines of mapping. With both structural atypia and cellular atypia recognized, it has been diagnosed as WDA (tub1) (Figs. 23.6 and 23.7).

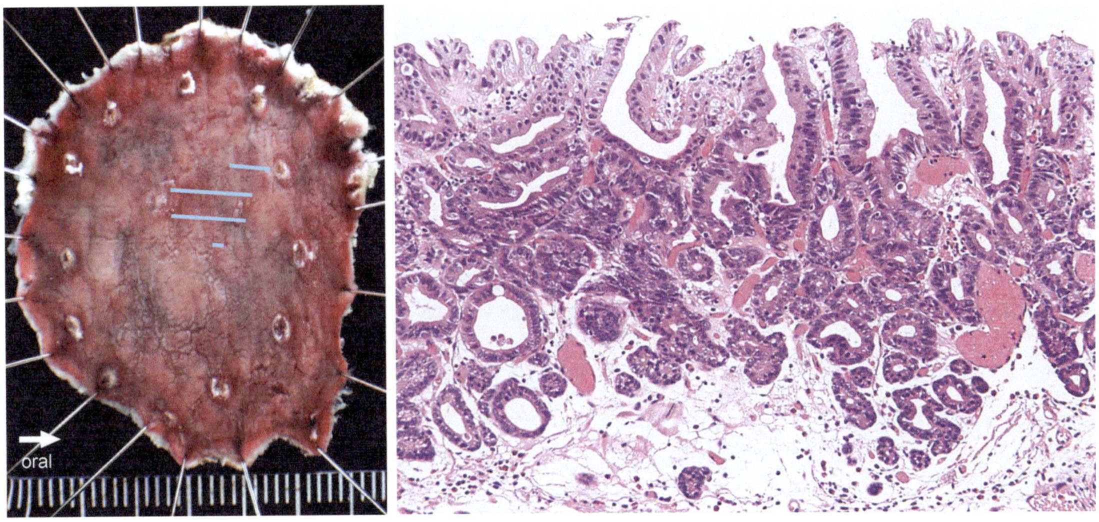

Fig. 23.6 Comparison between the resected specimen and histopathology

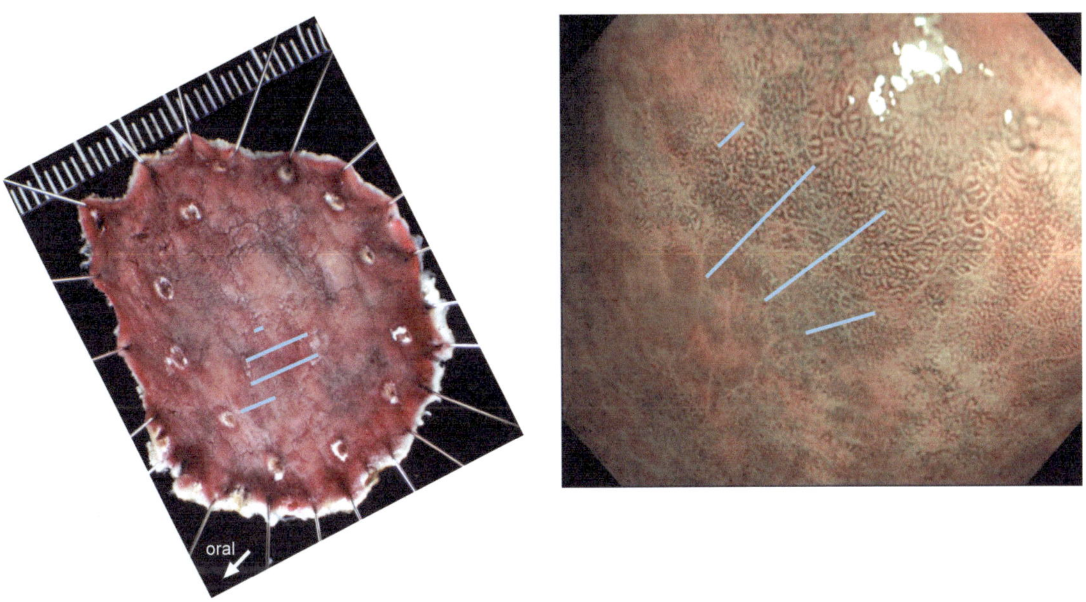

Fig. 23.7 Mapping on the specimen and NBI endoscopy

Conclusive Diagnosis
Gastric adenocarcinoma, tub1, T1 (M), ly0, v0, LM (−), VM(−), p-type 0-IIb, 9 × 7mm, M, less.

Summary
ESD to be performed for the case in other facility has been cancelled due to the ill-defined border. Even though the border was also ill-defined by an ordinary observation at the time of ESD performed in our hospital, the border of the lesion was determined by magnified NBI. Determination of the border of the case was difficult due to the pit-like structure recognized both in the background mucosa and the surface of the cancer part. However, we were able to correctly determine the range of lateral extension by focusing on the irregularity and difference in size of pits.

23.3 Answer

The range of the lateral extension is (1) white dotted line.

Question 10: What Do You Diagnose the Histological Type of This Lesion?

24

Keita Funakawa

K. Funakawa (✉)
Department of Gastroenterology, Kagoshima City Hospital, 37-1, Uearata-Cho, Kagoshima-shi, Kagoshima 890-8760, Japan
e-mail: kfuna@po.synapse.ne.jp

T. Oyama (ed.), *Endoscopic Diagnosis of Superficial Gastric Cancer for ESD*, DOI 10.1007/978-4-431-54469-2_24

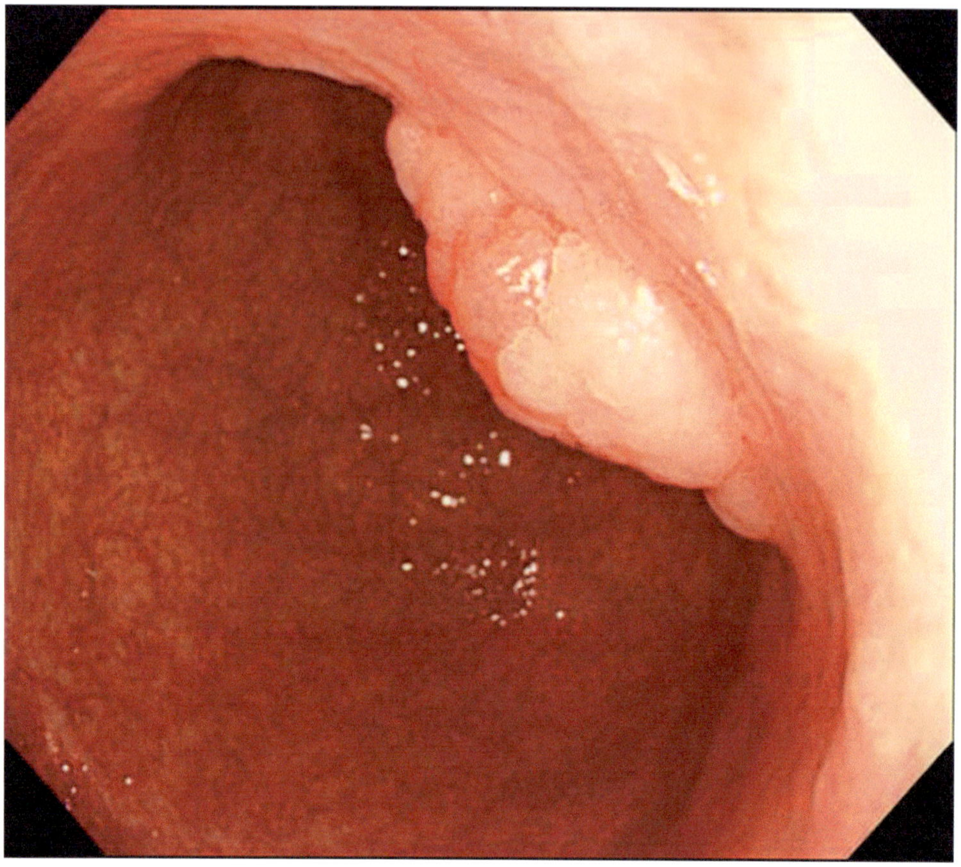

Fig. 24.1 What do you diagnose the histological type of this lesion

What do you diagnose the histological type of this lesion (Fig. 24.1)?
Choose your answer from 1 to 4.

(1) Adenoma
(2) Tubular adenocarcinoma
(3) Papillary adenocarcinoma
(4) The mixed type of tubular and papillary adenocarcinoma

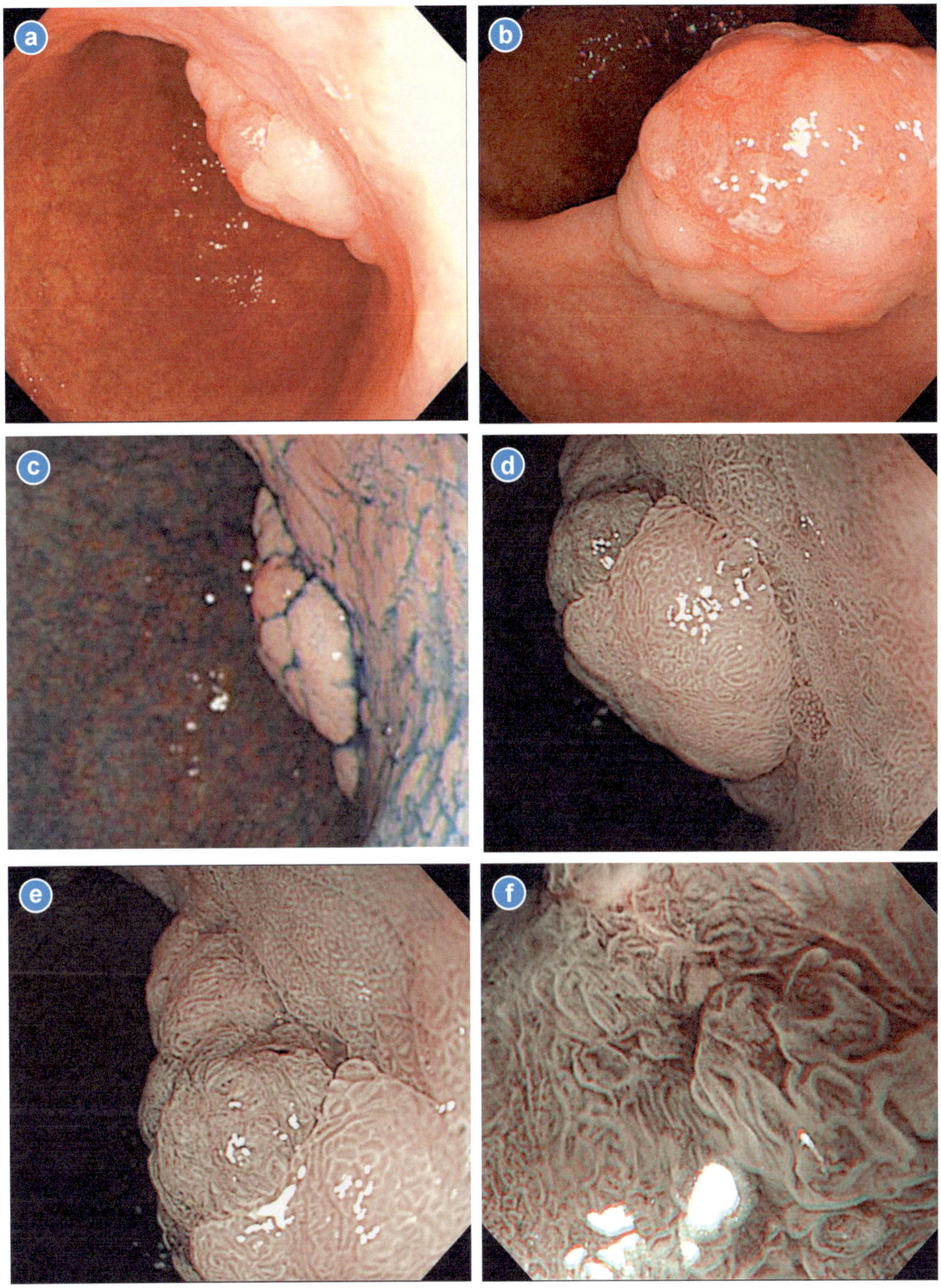

Fig. 24.2 Let's diagnose by observing these six images

24.1 Focus on These Points

24.1.1 The Shape of the Lesion

- The steeply elevated lesion is recognized at the posterior side of the lesser curvature of the angular incisures (Fig. 24.3a).
- The lesion consists of a cluster of variously sized nodules and each nodule appears relatively smooth.
- The lesion is well demarcated, suggesting it is an epithelial tumor.

24.1.2 The Color of the Nodules

- Each nodule shows various colors: reddish, pinkish, and whitish (Fig. 24.3a).
- The colors of the whitish part (marked with a blue arrow) and reddish part (marked with a red arrow) are clearly different, which indicates the possible difference in histological characteristics.

24.1.3 The Shape and Color of the Lesion Observed in Retroflex View

- The marginal part of the lesion consists of whitish, round, and variously sized nodules (Fig. 24.3b).
- The apex part as noted by a red arrow has reddish and rough surface.
- The lesion is highly elevated, but has neither swollen nor depressed changes often recognized in submucosal massively invasive adenocarcinomas.

24.1.4 The Edge and Surface Characteristics of the Lesion Are Recognized by Spraying Indigo Carmine

- The edge of the lesion is visualized more clearly by collected indigo carmine solution (Fig. 24.3c).
- Each of the nodules has a smooth surface repelling indigo carmine unlike the surrounding mucosa with mesh-like pattern.

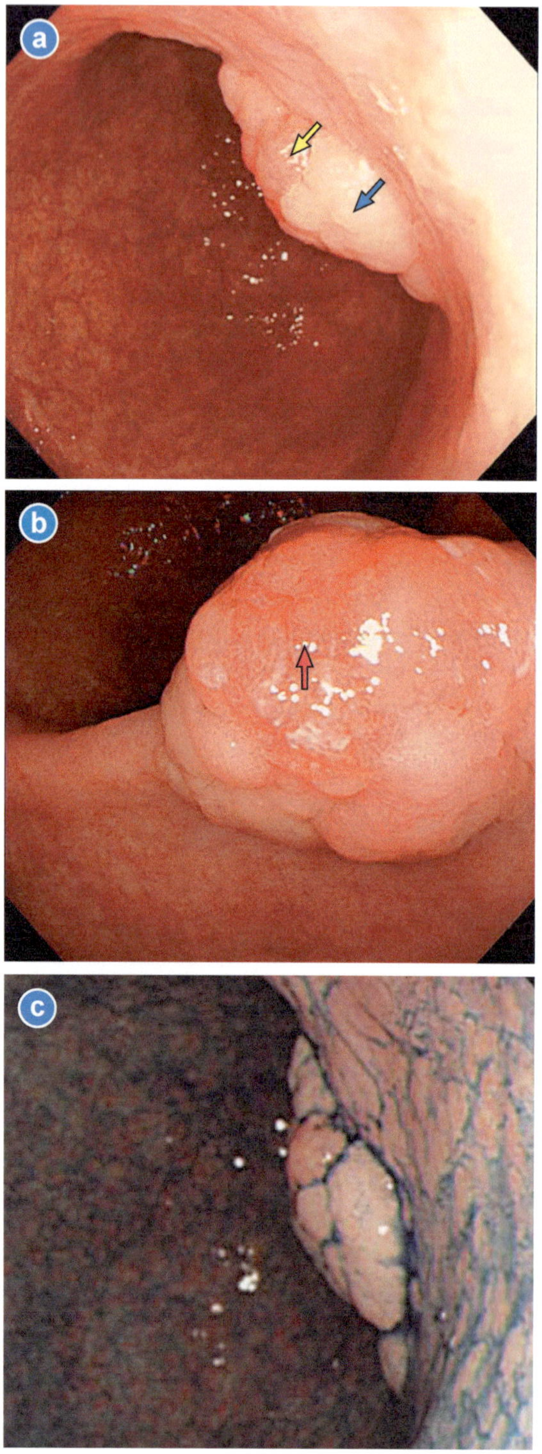

Fig. 24.3 Same images as Fig. 24.2

24.1.5 What Should We Do Next?

- We check the differences of superficial mucosal microstructure and capillary architecture between whitish and reddish parts by using NBI magnified endoscopy (Fig. 24.3c).

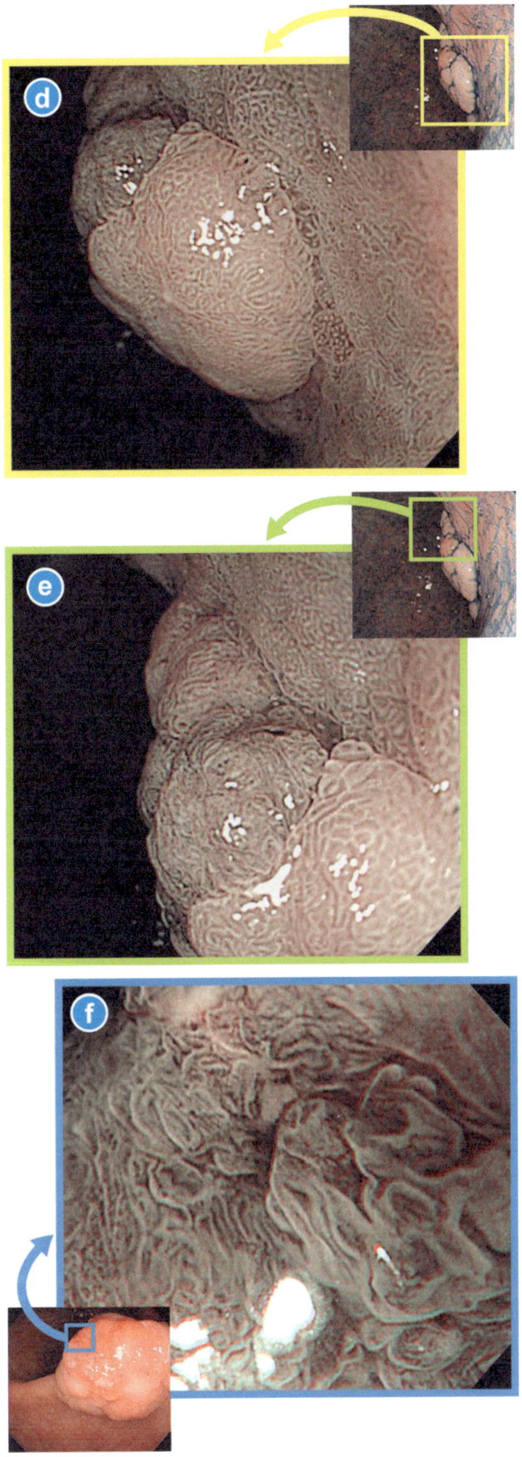

Fig. 24.3 (continued)

24.1.6 Let's Pay Attention to the Whitish Part of the Oral Side of the Elevation

- The surrounding mucosa has homogeneously sized and shaped villi-like and pit structures (Fig. 24.3d).
- NBI magnified endoscopy of the marked part with the blue arrow in Fig. 24.3a reveals homogeneous sized villi-like structure with irregular arrangement but almost homogeneous shape.
- These findings suggest this whitish part is neoplastic with a mild histological atypia.

24.1.7 Let's Pay Attention to the Reddish Part of the Oral Side of the Lesion

- NBI magnified endoscopy of the marked part with the yellow arrow in Fig. 24.3a reveals heterogeneously sized and irregularly shaped villi-like structures, whose contours are unclear compared with the marked part with blue arrow shown in Fig. 24.3a.
- These findings indicate the histological atypia of the reddish part is more severe than that of the whitish part (Fig. 24.3e).

24.1.8 Let's Focus on the Central Reddish Site

- NBI magnified endoscopy of the marked part with the red arrow in Fig. 24.3b reveals heterogeneously sized and irregularly shaped villi-like structure, indicating the papillary proliferation of neoplastic glands (Fig. 24.3f).

24.1.9 How Should We Diagnose?

- This elevated lesion is well demarcated and irregularly shaped, and the color and surface pattern are both heterogeneous in WL endoscopy. NBI Magnified endoscopy reveals variably sized and irregularly shaped villi-like structures. Via both types of endoscopy, this lesion can be diagnosed as a gastric adenocarcinoma (type 0I) (Fig. 24.3e).
- The lesion is tall but has neither tightly swollen appearance, nor markedly raised or depressed sites, indicating the invasion depth is intramucosal. Variously colored and shaped sites are recognized in the lesion by WL endoscopy, and NBI magnified endoscopy reveals heterogeneously sized and irregularly shaped villi-like structure, whose irregularity degree is different by sites in the lesion, suggesting the mixture of tubular and papillary adenocarcinomas.

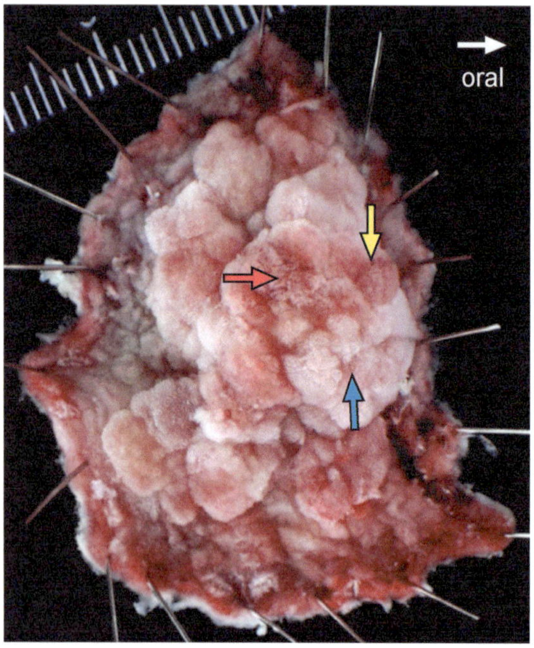

Fig. 24.4 Freshly resected specimen

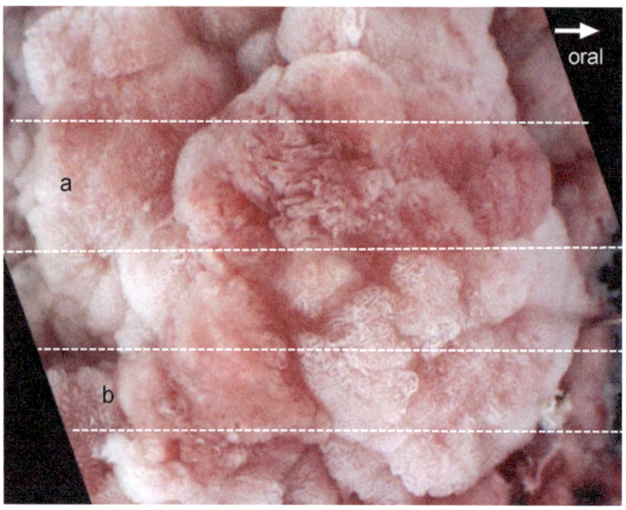

Fig. 24.5 Magnified view of the elevated part

24.2 Let's Compare Fixed Specimens with Resected Specimens

24.2.1 Let's Note the Shape and Color of the Elevated Part

- The lesion consists of multiple nodules, and the lesion is well demarcated.
- The surface structure is kept, and the whitish site (marked with a blue arrow) and reddish site (marked with a yellow arrow) of the oral side of the lesion have rough surface.
- The central reddish site (marked with a red arrow) shows a fuzzy appearance (Fig. 24.4).

24.2.2 Let's Focus on Superficial Microstructures of the Elevated Part

- Magnifying view of the site marked with the red arrow reveals swollen villi-like structures of various sizes and severely irregular shapes.
- Magnifying view of the site marked by the blue arrow reveals small villi-like structures with heterogeneous size and mildly irregular shapes.
- Magnifying view of the site marked with yellow arrow reveals small villi-like structures with unclear contour.
- The differences in the mucosal microstructures visualized with NBI magnified endoscopy are also recognized in the freshly resected specimen.
- The specimen was cut to investigate histological characteristics of each analyzed part (Fig. 24.5).

24.2.2.1 Histological Findings of Segment A: The Central Reddish Part Marked with the Red Arrow

The glandular epithelium shows papillary growth with focal fusion and thick intervening parts between crypts, diagnosed as papillary adenocarcinoma. This histological characteristic is reflected in the NBI magnified endoscopic findings showing variably sized and irregularly shaped villi-like structures (Fig. 24.6a).

24.2.2.2 Segment A: High-Power Magnification

High-grade hyperemia is recognized in the stromal tissue, which is considered as the cause of reddish appearance (Fig. 24.6b).

24.2.2.3 Histological Findings of Segment A: The Reddish Part of the Oral Side of the Lesion Marked with the Yellow Arrow

The neoplastic tubular glands grow long, tortuously, and densely, and the openings of the crypts are unclear, diagnosed as WDA (tub1). The histological feature is reflected in NBI magnified endoscopic finding showing irregularly shaped and unclearly contoured villi-like structures (Fig. 24.7a).

24.2.2.4 Histological Findings of Segment B: The Whitish Part of the Oral Side of the Lesion Marked with the Blue Arrow

The structural atypia of the neoplastic epithelium is mild, and the openings of the crypts are well kept, compared with the prior figure. This histological feature is reflected in NBI magnified endoscopic finding showing almost homo-

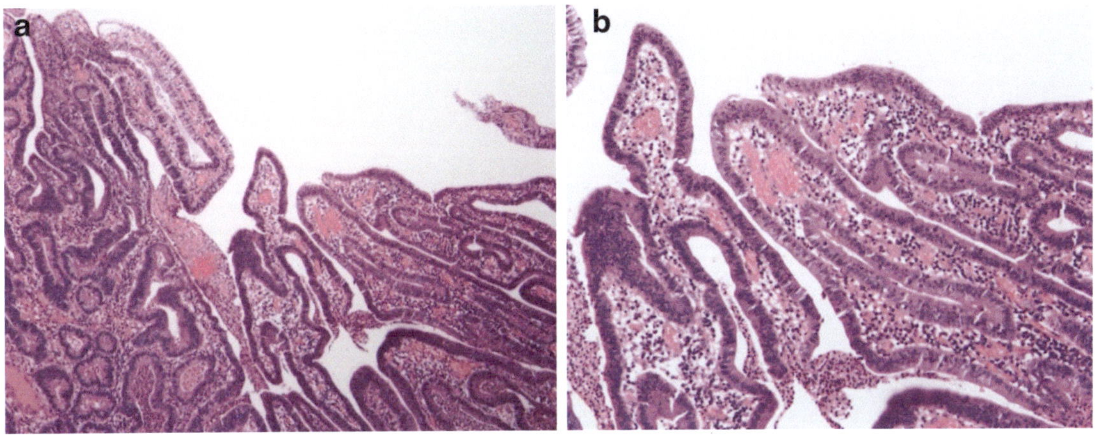

Fig. 24.6 (**a**) Histological image of the central reddish part marked with the *red arrow* (**b**) High-power magnification image

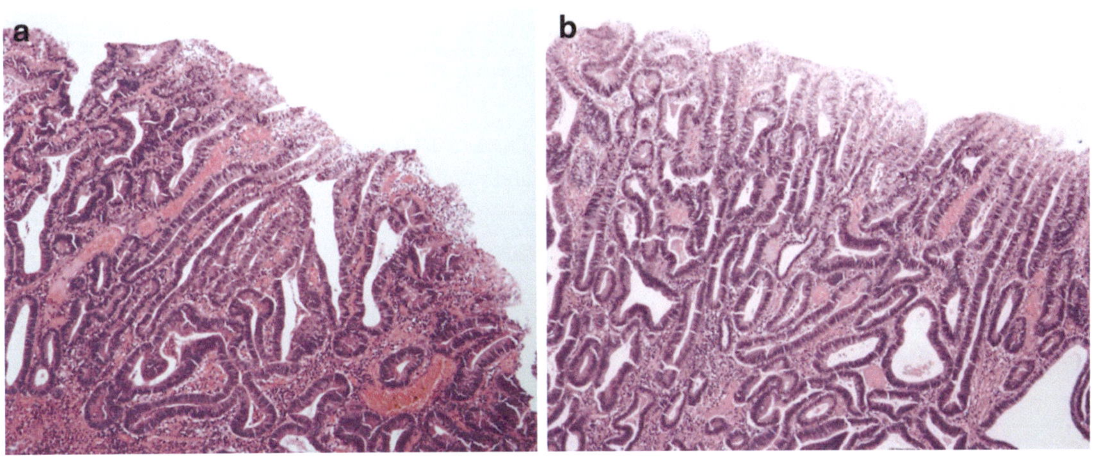

Fig. 24.7 (**a**) Histological image of the reddish part of the lesion marked with the *yellow arrow* in Fig. 24.5 (**b**) Histological image of the reddish part of the lesion marked with the *blue arrow* in Fig. 24.5

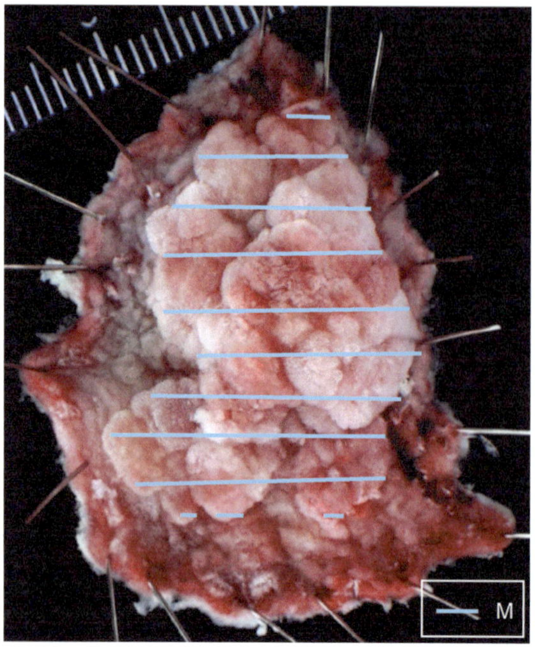

Fig. 24.8 Mapping of the cancer distribution projected on the freshly resected specimen

geneously shaped and clearly contoured villi-like structures (Figs. 24.7b and 24.8).

Conclusive Diagnosis
Gastric adenocarcinoma, tub1 > pap, T1(M), ly0, v0, LM(−), VM(−), p-type 0I, 30 × 23 mm, M, less.

Summary
Predicting histological characteristics of gastric neoplasms via endoscopic findings is very important for determining therapeutic strategy. In this case, WL endoscopy shows three different sites in color and mucosal pattern, and NBI magnified endoscopy leads us to predict histological type of each site, which has been confirmed also by detailed histological analysis of the resected specimen.

24.3 Answer

The correct histological type is (4) the mixed type of tubular and papillary adenocarcinoma.

25 Question 11: Where Is the Horizontal Margin of the Lesion?

Keita Funakawa

K. Funakawa (✉)
Department of Gastroenterology, Kagoshima City Hospital, 37-1, Uearata-Cho, Kagoshima-shi, Kagoshima 890-8760, Japan
e-mail: kfuna@po.synapse.ne.jp

T. Oyama (ed.), *Endoscopic Diagnosis of Superficial Gastric Cancer for ESD*, DOI 10.1007/978-4-431-54469-2_25

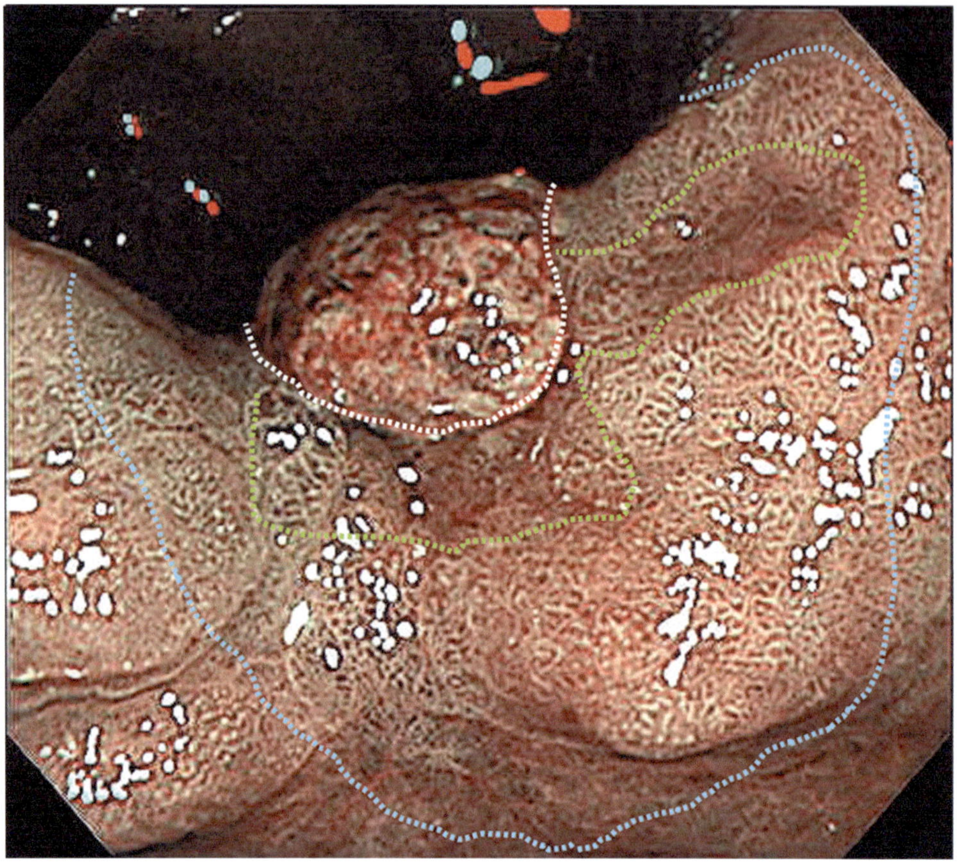

Fig. 25.1 Where is the horizontal margin of the lesion?

Where is the horizontal margin of the lesion? (Fig. 25.1)
Choose your answer from 1 to 3.

(1) White dotted line
(2) Green dotted line
(3) Blue dotted line

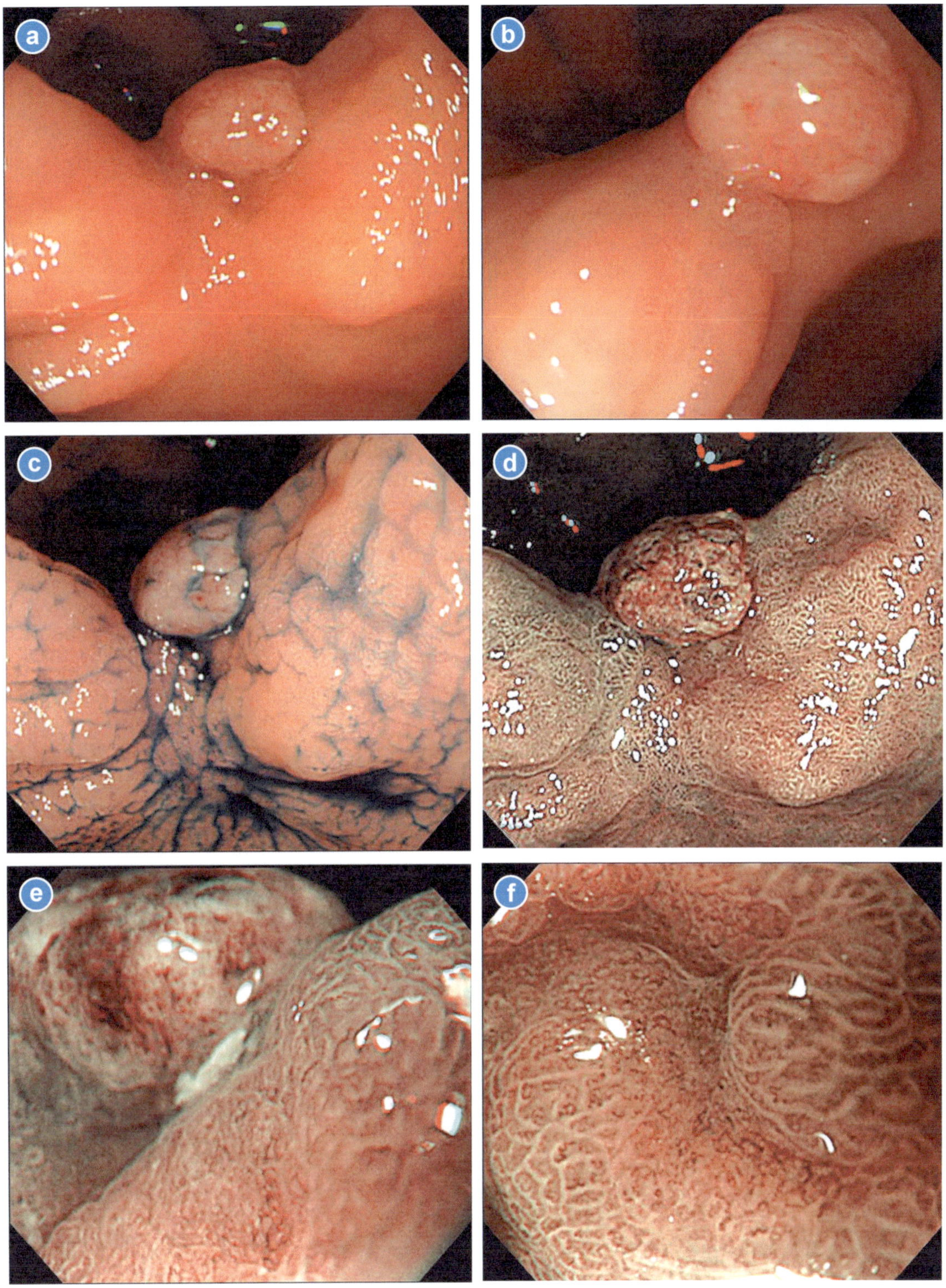

Fig. 25.2 Let's diagnose by observing these six images

25.1 Focus on These Points

25.1.1 Let's Pay Attention to the Depression and the Protuberance

- A reddish depressed lesion with mucosal convergence is noted at the lesser curvature of the gastric angle. The gastric angle is deformed, and there is an Isp-like reddish protuberance at the center of the depression (Fig. 25.3a).

25.1.2 Let's Pay Attention to the Folds

- The mucosal convergence is observed not toward one point but for the whole plain of depression.
- The mucosal folds taper and disappear gradually near the protuberance, and there was neither disruption nor fusion of mucosal folds.

The cause of mucosal convergence is fibrosis of submucosal layer, and a common cause of fibrosis is an ulcer or an invasion of cancer to the submucosal layer. Because there is neither thickness nor fusions of the folds that indicate an invasion to the submucosal layer, the mucosal convergence is caused by ulcer scarring. The mucosa converges to multifocal points, so we recognize that the ulcer relapsed very often, and was treated many times, and multifocal mucosal convergences reflect the therapeutic course (Fig. 25.3a).

25.1.3 Let's Pay Attention to the Depression

- Although the borderline of the reddish depression is unclear, we can see the borderline of the depression as marked by the yellow arrow (Fig. 25.3b).

25.1.4 Let's Pay Attention to the Protuberance at the Anterior Wall

- The central protuberance grows precipitously and its borderline is clear. The color tone is mixed with redness and a faded color, and several irregular elevations and depressions are noted on the surface (Fig. 25.3b).
- No obvious depression appears at the anterior wall of the protuberance. A granular protuberance I noted as marked by blue arrows and the borderline as the margin of the protuberance.

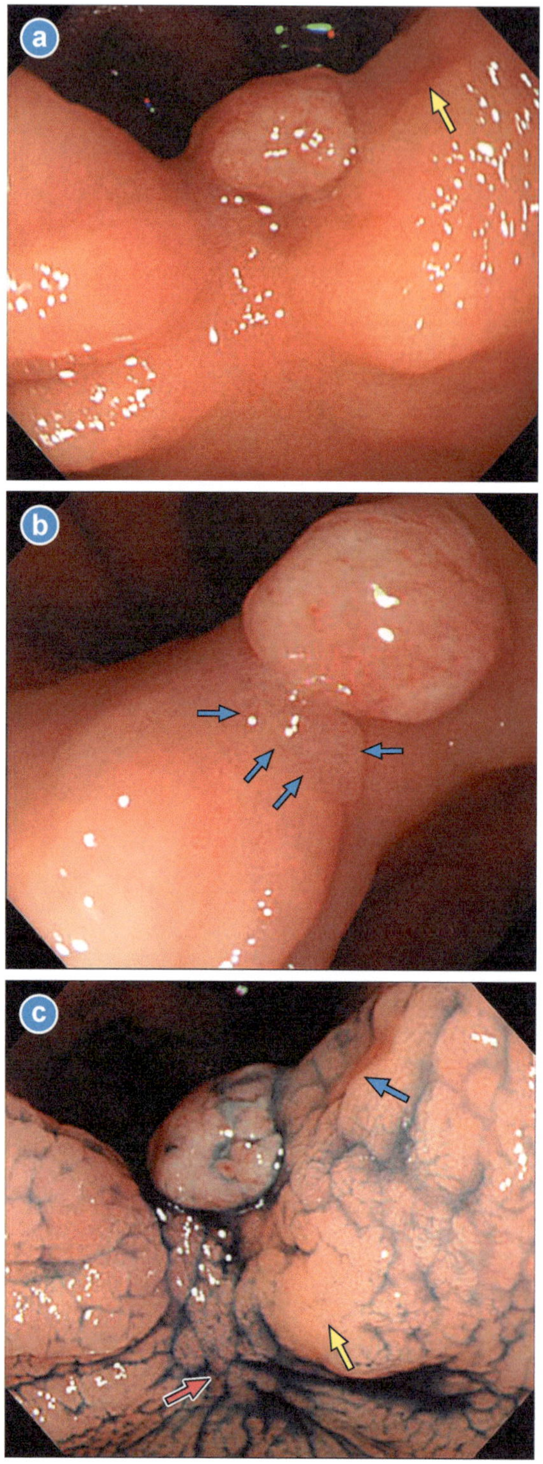

Fig. 25.3 Same images as Fig. 25.2

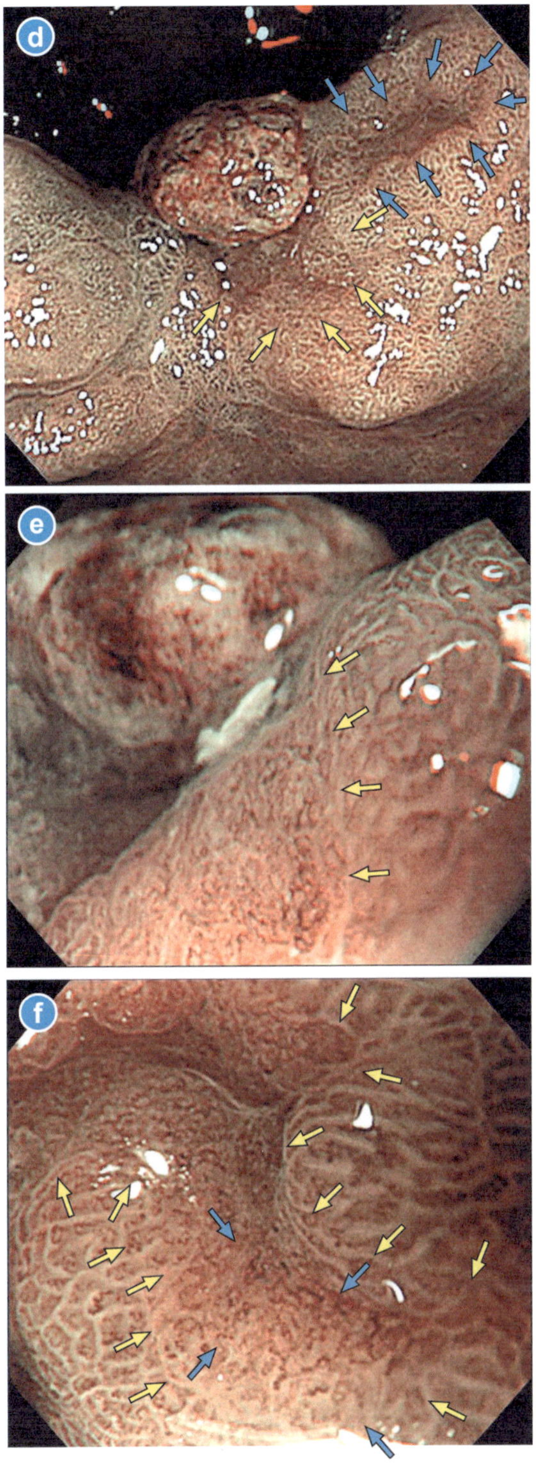

Fig. 25.3 (continued)

25.1.5 Let's Spray Indigo Carmine

- After indigo carmine spraying, a regular surface areal pattern is noted in the background (Fig. 25.3c).
- The depression is noted at the posterior wall of the protuberance, but its borderline is unclear as marked by the blue line. In the anal side, there is an area without clear areal patterns as marked by the yellow arrow. A fold convergence with surrounding depression is noted by the red arrow. However, no apparent borderline is noted around the depressed area and the area is diagnosed as nonneoplastic.
- Further observation was performed with NBI magnified endoscopy.

25.1.6 Let's Perform NBI magnified endoscopy

- This is a low-power magnification image (Fig. 25.3d).
- Despite the image with low-power magnification, we can see a regular pit and villi pattern in the background, but Part A marked with yellow arrows and Part B marked with blue arrows are brown in color and slightly depressed.

25.1.7 Let's See a Proximal Image of Part A

- This is a NBI magnified image of the anal to the posterior wall of the protuberance (Fig. 25.3e).
- The left side of the picture is the depression and the yellow arrows trace its margin.
- Regular pits with low density are noted to the right of these arrows. The surface pattern is different across the borderline of the depression. On the left side of the borderline marked by the arrows, there are highly dense, irregular, and fine pits, with some areas of unclear surface patterns.
- The lesion is diagnosed as well to MDA.

25.1.8 Let's See a Proximal Image of Part B

- This is a NBI magnified endoscopic image of the depressed part at the posterior wall of the protuberance (Fig. 25.3f).

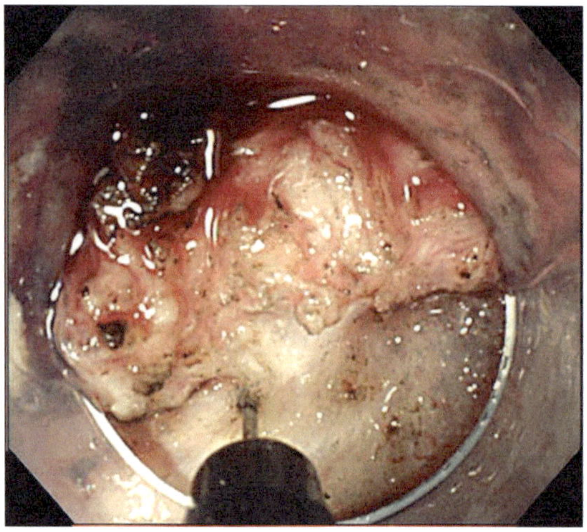

Fig. 25.4 Endoscopic image while performing ESD

25.2 Let's Compare Fixed Specimens with Resected Specimens

25.2.1 Let's Perform ESD

- This is the endoscopic image while performing ESD; it was hard to dissect the lesion because of strong fibrosis. We performed one-half circumferential incision and dissection from the anterior wall side after marking and dissected toward the posterior wall side (Fig. 25.4).
- And then, we performed another one-half circumferential incision and dissection from the posterior wall side and dissected toward the anterior wall side.
- Although the muscle layer was partially exposed because of the severe fibrosis in the scar, we could achieve en bloc resection without complications.

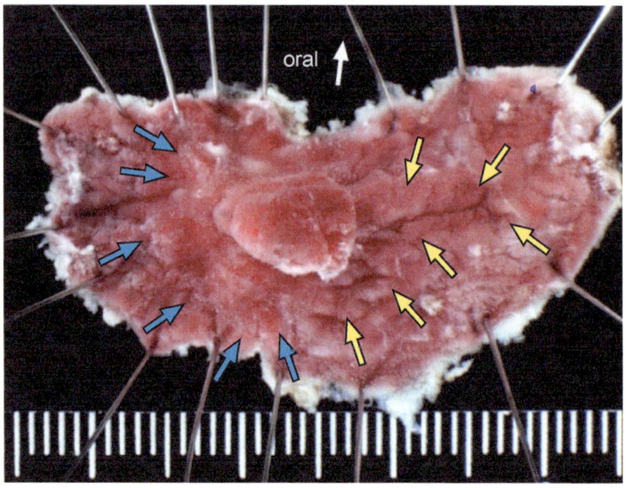

Fig. 25.5 Freshly resected specimen

25.2.2 Let's Pay Attention to the Surface Pattern and the Color Tone

- The upper side of the image is the oral side (Fig. 25.5).
- There is a reddish precipitous protuberance at the center of the lesion, and the borderline is clearly the margin of the protuberance.
- There is a flat elevation with reddish and discolored parts at the anterior wall side of the protuberance, but the demarcation line is unclear.
- Coarse areal patterns are noted at the anal to the posterior wall sides of the central protuberance, but the borderline is unclear.
- The background around the depression shows an almost regular pit- and villi-like pattern. On the other hand, the surface pattern of the depressed part is a variably sized pit-like pattern and the surface pattern of the area noted by blue arrows is unclear. There are abnormal vessels with running irregularity, caliber changes, and network formations.
- Based on these, the lesion is diagnosed as well to MDA.
- To summarize, the protuberance and its orally located depression and posteriorly located depression are cancer and the endoscopic diagnosis is gastric adenocarcinoma, cType 0-I+IIc, and tub1-2.

25.2.3 Let's See the Pathological Image

- The left picture shows the pathological image of the central protuberance. Based on structural and cellular atypia, the lesion is diagnosed as MDA (tub2). The right picture shows the submucosal layer with severe fibrosis and a partially resected muscle layer (Fig. 25.6).

Based on mapping images of the freshly resected and fixed specimens, mapping is placed on the endoscopic image (Fig. 25.7).

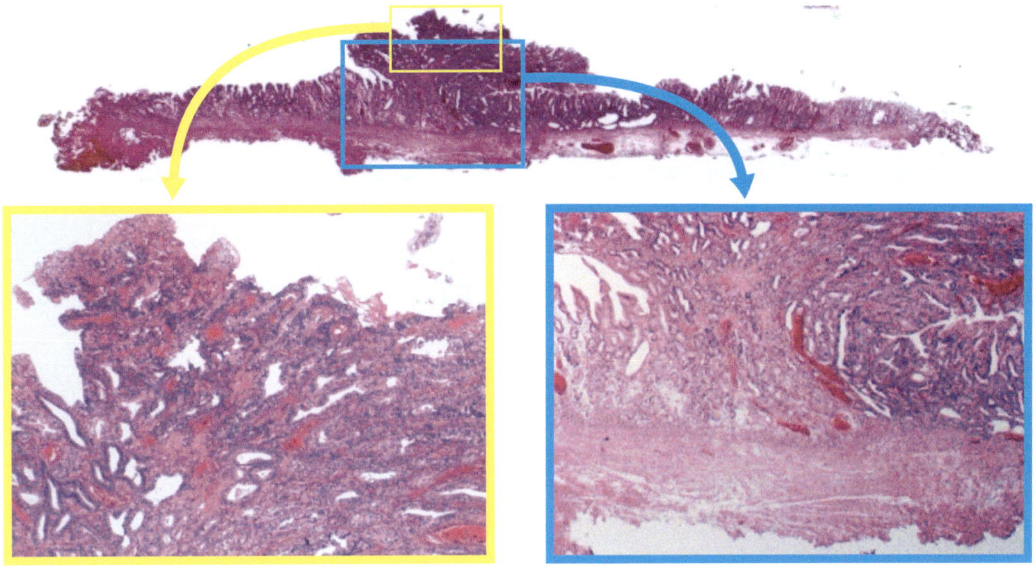

Fig. 25.6 Histological image of the resion

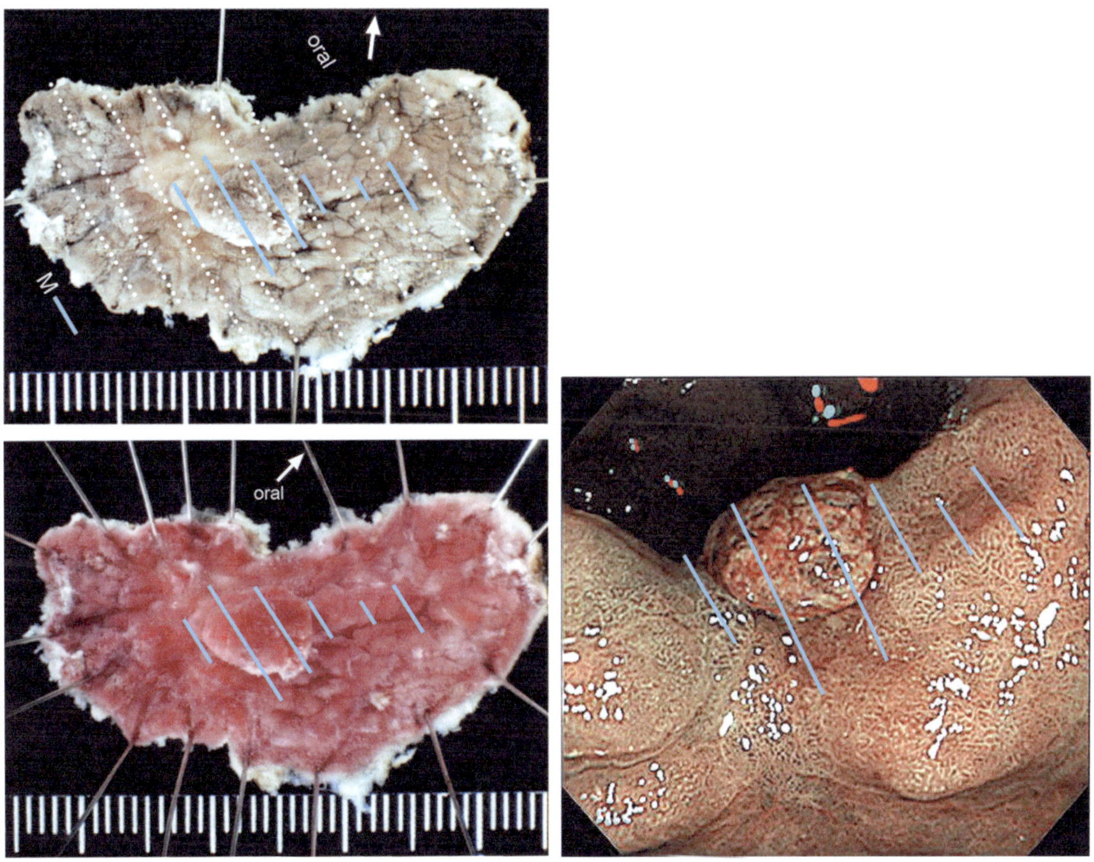

Fig. 25.7 Fixed and freshly resected specimen and NBI magnified endoscopic image with mapping of the cancer distribution projected on the specimen

Conclusive Diagnosis
Gastric adenocarcinoma, tub1>tub2, T1(M), ly0, v0, LM(−), VM(−), pType 0-I+IIc, ML, Less, 19×10mm, CurEA.

Summary
This was a case with a recurrent 0-IIa lesion after EMR and APC (argon plasma coagulation). We can see the irregular protrusion at the center of the mucosal convergence, and we can easily recognize this part as cancer. On the other hand, it was hard to detect the 0-IIc lesion around the protuberance with WL, but we could detect the borderline of the lesion with NBI. The cause of the local recurrence for this case is the initial misdiagnosis of a horizontal extension range; it is very important to pay attention to the 0-IIb extension.

25.3 Answer

The horizontal extension range is (2) green dotted line.

Question 12: What Do You Diagnose the Histological Type of This Lesion?

26

Kotaro Shibagaki

K. Shibagaki (✉)
Department of Endoscopy, Shimane University Faculty of Medicine,
1060 Nishikawatsu-cho, Matsue, Shimane 690-8504, Japan
e-mail: shibagaki@zb.wakwak.com

T. Oyama (ed.), *Endoscopic Diagnosis of Superficial Gastric Cancer for ESD*, DOI 10.1007/978-4-431-54469-2_26

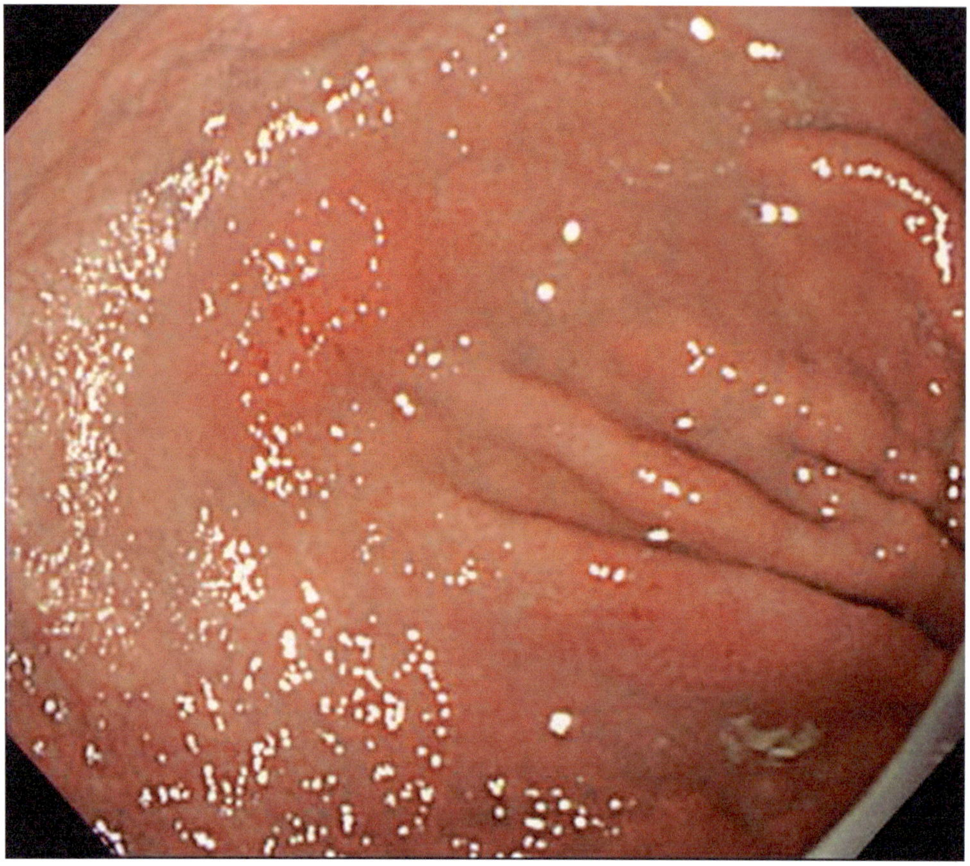

Fig. 26.1 What do you diagnose the histological type of this lesion?

What do you diagnose the histological type of this lesion? (Fig. 26.1)
Choose your answer from 1 to 3.

(1) WDA (tub1)
(2) MDA (tub2)
(3) PDA (por)

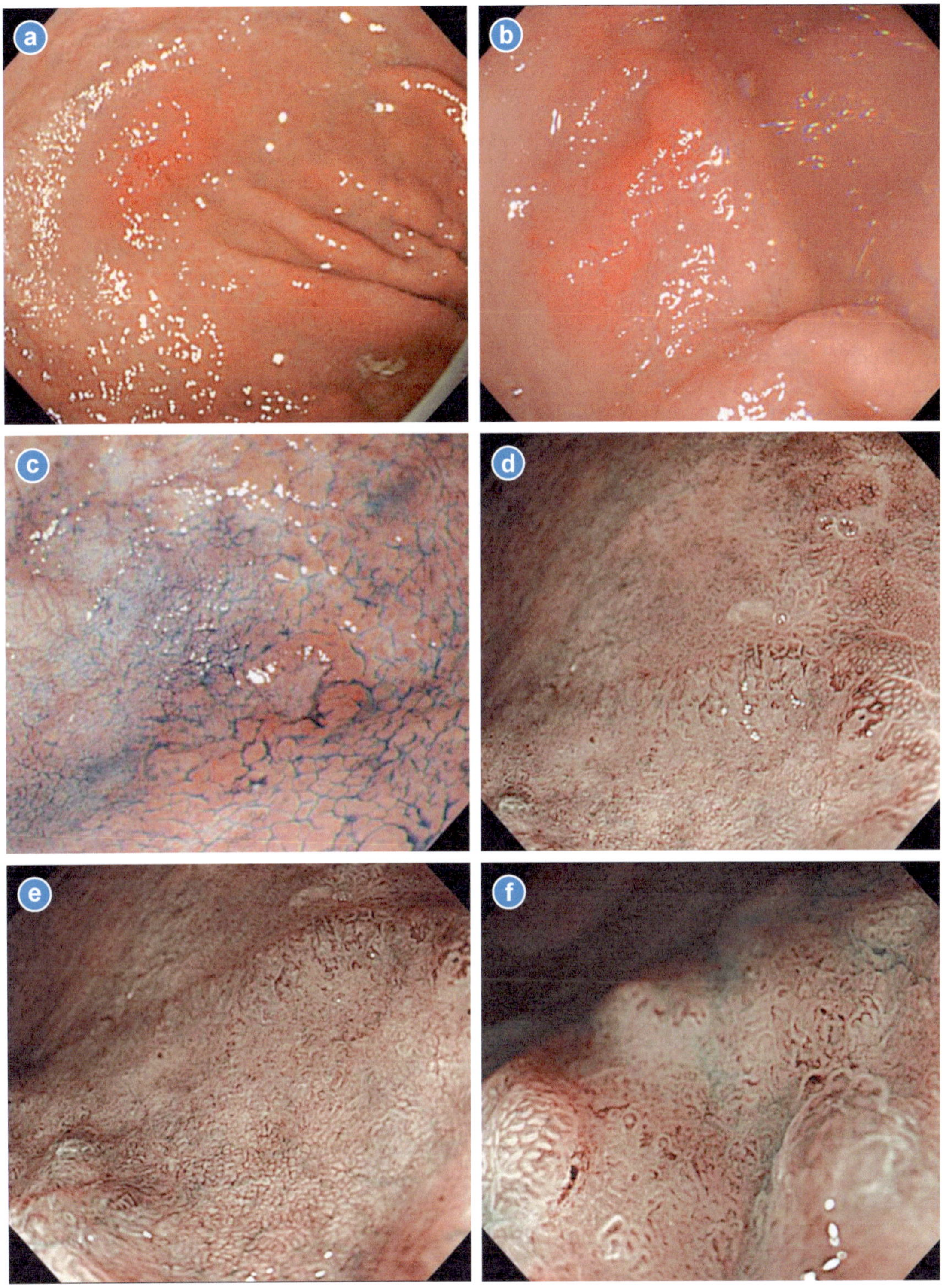

Fig. 26.2 Let's diagnose by observing these six images

26.1 Focus on These Points

26.1.1 Let's Pay Attention to the Reddish Part

- A reddish and slightly elevated lesion is recognized at the greater curvature of the fornix. The lesion is irregularly shaped, unclearly demarcated, and depressed in the central part (Fig. 26.3a).

26.1.2 Let's Pay Attention to the Depressed Part

- The depressed part is flat, whitish, and well demarcated on the posterior and anal side (Fig. 26.3a).

26.1.3 How Should We Interpret?

- The depressed lesion is an irregularly shaped, partially well-demarcated, whitish lesion surrounded with unevenly spread reddish elevation. These endoscopic findings indicate that this lesion is an epithelial neoplastic lesion, but an inflammatory lesion or an extra-nodal marginal zone lymphoma of a mucosa-associated lymphoid tissue type should be ruled out (Fig. 26.3a).

26.1.4 Suctioning Air Is Useful for Approaching a Lesion

- It is often difficult to approach a lesion located at the greater curvature of the fornix, but suctioning air reduces the distance between the scope and the lesion to enable a closer observation.
- By approaching the lesion, we can easily recognize the anterior and anal edge of the depressed lesion (marked with blue arrows). Moreover, granular light reflex is visualized on the depressed site (marked with a yellow arrow), which informs us that it has a granular mucosal structure (Fig. 26.3b).

26.1.5 Let's Confirm the Mucosal Surface Pattern of the Depressed Site

- Indigo carmine spraying shows an unclear mucosal surface pattern and its demarcation line on the anterior and anal side encroaching upon the surrounding mucosa (marked with red arrows).

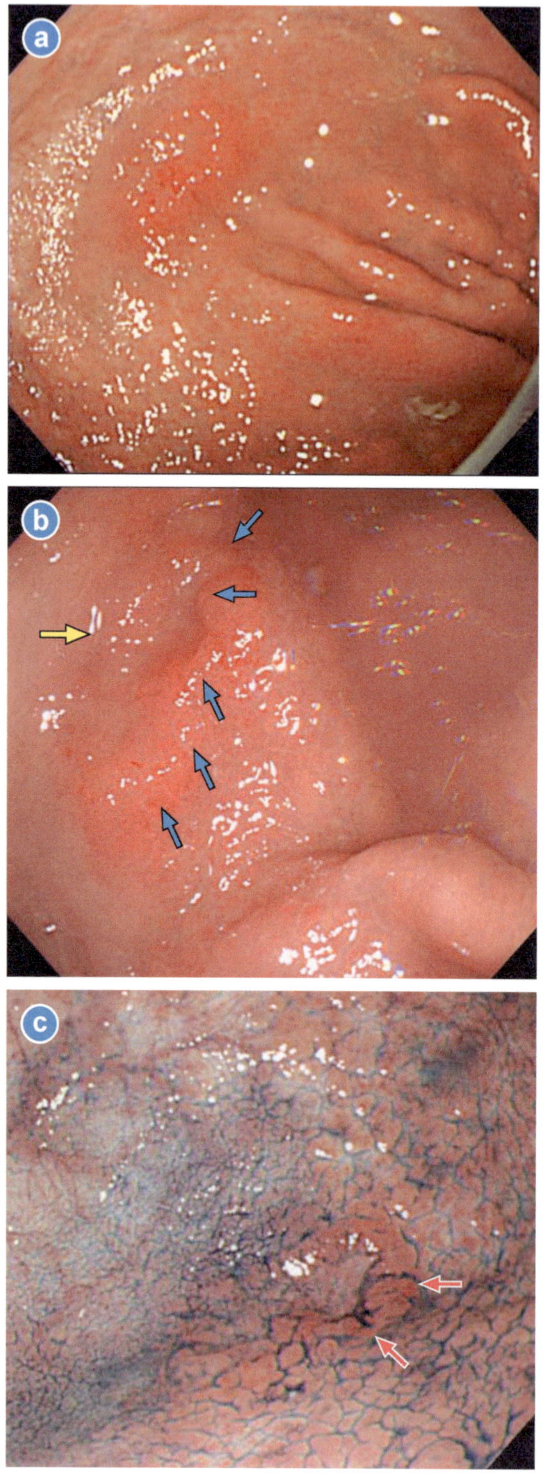

Fig. 26.3 Same images as Fig. 26.2

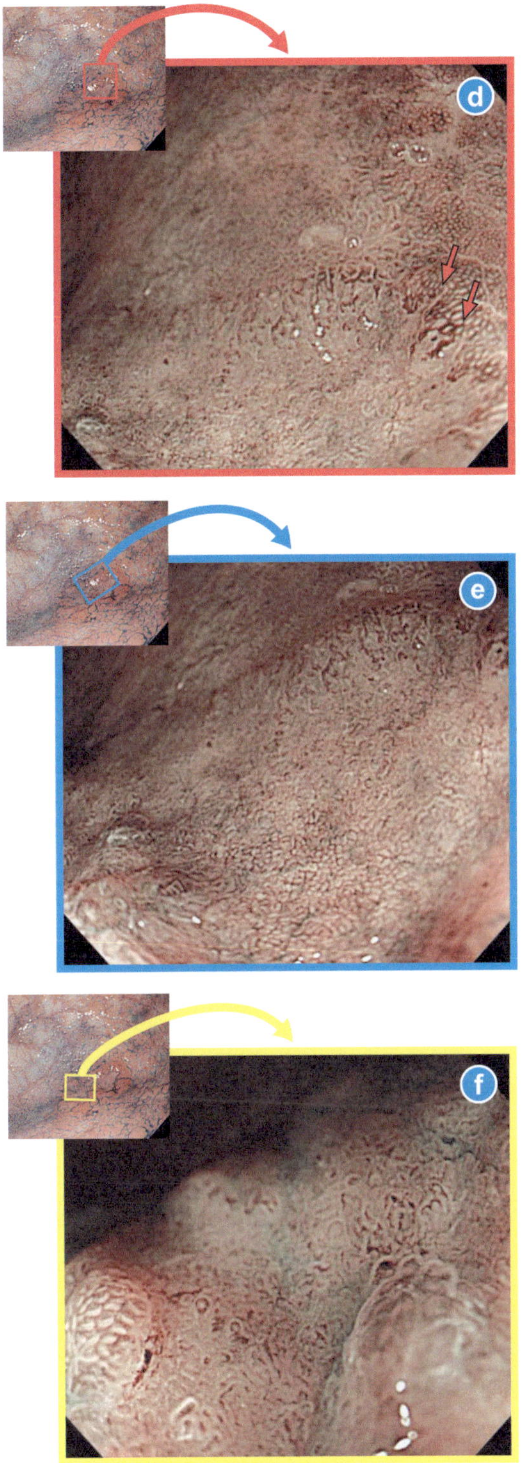

Fig. 26.3 (continued)

- Via these endoscopic findings, this lesion is suspected of a depressed type of superficial adenocarcinoma, and the invasion depth is considered to be mucosal layer because the depressed site shows neither thickened nor further depressed changes on it. This lesion has a granular mucosal pattern with a reactive hyperplastic change in surrounding mucosa, indicating a differentiated adenocarcinoma. However, as this lesion is whitish and partially has unclear mucosal surface pattern, we should rule out an undifferentiated adenocarcinoma.
- NBI magnified endoscopy is performed to analyze the histological type and laterally extending range of the lesion (Fig. 26.3c).

26.1.6 Let's Focus on the Anterior Side of the Lesion

- The surrounding mucosa has evenly sized and shaped pit- and villi-like structures. On the other hand, the lesion shows an unclear mucosal microstructure with clear demarcation from the surrounding mucosa.
- The "worm-eaten appearance" of a cancerous microinvasive feature is identified on the edge marked with red arrows (Fig. 26.3d).

26.1.7 Let's Observe Superficial Microvessels Within the Depressed Lesion

- On the anterior and the anal part of the lesion, the abnormal vessels with irregular extension, dense growth, and mildly variable vessel calibers form irregular mesh-like networks (Fig. 26.3e).

26.1.8 Let's Observe the Posterior Side of the Lesion

- The surrounding mucosa is slightly elevated and has homogeneously sized and shaped pit structure. On the other hand, the lesion has heterogeneously sized and irregularly shaped villi-like structures with dense growth and is well demarcated from the surrounding mucosa, which proves that the edge of the depressed site

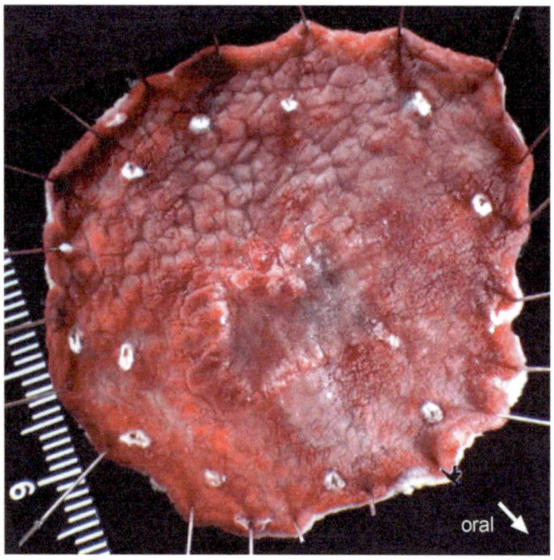

Fig. 26.4 Freshly resected specimen

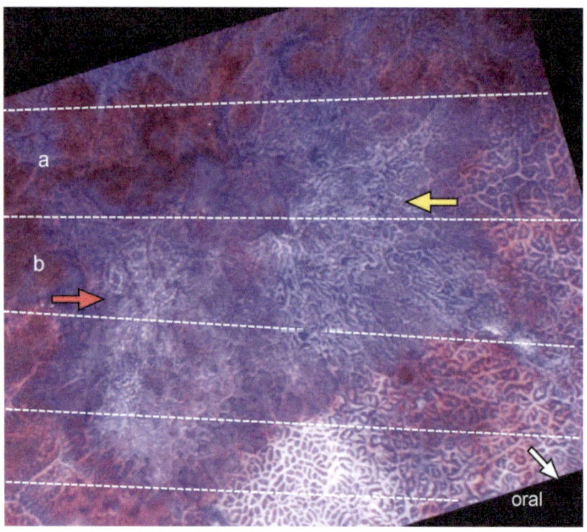

Fig. 26.5 Magnified image of the depressed lesion stained by crystal violet

recognized by WL endoscopy corresponds to the demarcation line visualized by NBI magnified endoscopy.

- The capillaries of the lesion show heterogeneous vessel caliber and irregular distribution.
- Via these endoscopic findings, we diagnose this lesion as a differentiated adenocarcinoma (Fig. 26.3f).

26.2 Let's Compare Fixed Specimens with Resected Specimens

26.2.1 Let's Pay Attention to the Depressed Lesion

- In the center of the resected specimen, we can recognize a whitish and irregularly shaped depressed lesion well demarcated from the surrounding mucosa. The lesion is flat and evenly depressed and has a granular mucosal pattern (Fig. 26.4).

26.2.2 Let's Note the Superficial Mucosal Microstructures

- By crystal violet staining, we can recognize the heterogeneously sized, irregularly shaped, and densely growing pit structures in the anterior side marked with a red arrow and heterogeneously sized and irregularly shaped villi-like structure in the posterior side marked with a yellow arrow. As the mucosal microstructure is kept throughout the lesion, this lesion is thought to consist only of differentiated-type adenocarcinoma.
- The specimen is sectioned along the white dotted lines (Fig. 26.5).

26.2.2.1 Histologic Finding of Segment B, the Site Presenting pit Structure Marked with Red Arrow

The neoplastic glands grow straightly and densely, and the stromal tissue is filled with capillary blood vessels diagnosed as WDA (tub1). The openings of the neoplastic glandular crypts are very small on the superficial part (Fig. 26.6a).

26.2.2.2 Histologic Finding of Segment A, the Site Presenting Villi-Like Structure Marked with Yellow Arrow

The neoplastic epithelium shows tortuous and papillary growth, and the stromal tissue has the capillaries with heterogeneous vessel caliber and distribution. The neoplastic glands are widely opened on the superficial part (Fig. 26.6b).

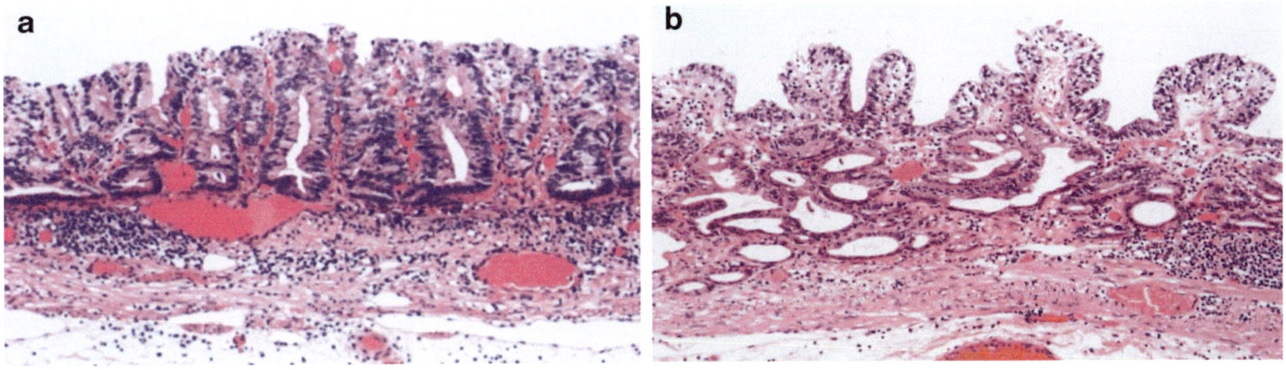

Fig. 26.6 (**a**) Histological image of pit structure marked with *red arrow* in the Fig. 26.5 (**b**) Histological image of villi-like structure marked with *yellow arrow* in the Fig. 26.5

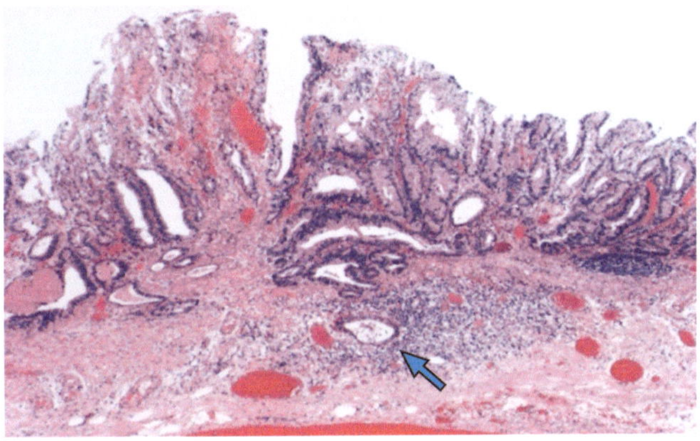

Fig. 26.7 Histological image of the carcinomatous submucosal microinvasion in segment (a) in the Fig. 26.5

26.2.2.3 Histologic Finding of Segment A, the Site of the Carcinomatous Submucosal Microinvasion

Neoplastic epithelium is slightly noted to invade into the submucosal layer as marked with a blue arrow without destruction of the mucosal muscle (Fig. 26.7).

26.2.2.4 Comparison Between the Resected Specimen and WL Endoscopic Findings

By comparing the resected specimen and endoscopic finding, the histological mapping can be drawn from the endoscopic image (Fig. 26.8).

26.2.2.5 Comparison Between Histologic Finding Shown in Fig. 26.6a and NBI Magnified Endoscopic Finding

The white dotted line of segment b shown on the left page is corresponding to the white dotted line shown in the upper figure, and the histological feature of the green dotted line is shown in Fig. 26.6a.

Figure 26.6a shows small openings of the neoplastic glands and stromal tissue filled with a lot of capillaries. This histological feature is reflected to the NBI magnified endoscopic finding presenting an unclear mucosal microstructure and the capillary vessels densely growing and forming mesh-like networks (Fig. 26.9a).

26.2.2.6 Comparison Between Histologic Finding Shown in Fig. 26.6b and NBI Magnified Endoscopic Finding

The white dotted line of segment a shown on the left page is corresponding to the white dotted line shown in the upper figure, and the histological feature of the blue line is shown in Fig. 26.6b.

Figure 26.6b shows the neoplastic epithelium with papillary growth and wide openings of glandular crypts, and the abnormal capillaries with heterogeneous vessel caliber and distribution are recognized in the stromal tissue. This histological feature is reflected to the NBI magnified endoscopic finding presenting the irregular villi-like structure and abnormal capillary pattern (Fig. 26.9b).

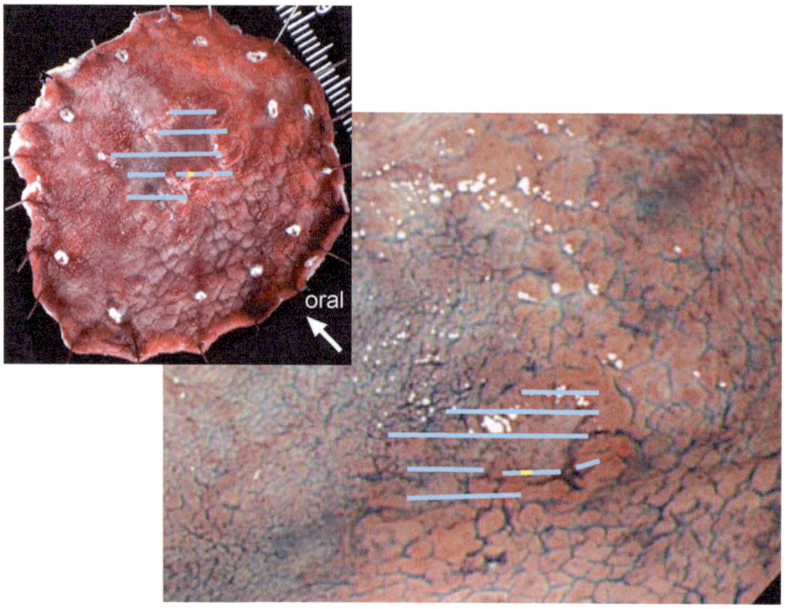

Fig. 26.8 Comparison between resected specimen and WL endoscopic image with mapping on the cancer distribution on the specimen

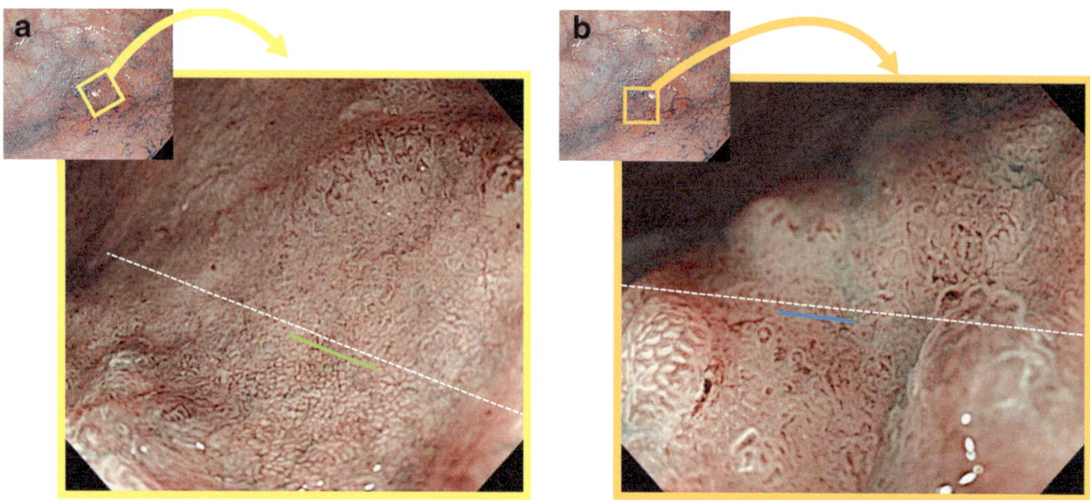

Fig. 26.9 (**a**) Comparison between histologic finding shown in Fig. 26.6a and NBI magnified endoscopic finding (**b**) Comparison between histologic finding shown in Fig. 26.6b and NBI magnified endoscopic finding

Conclusive Diagnosis

Gastric adenocarcinoma, tub1 > pap, T1a (SM1, invasion depth:140 μm, invasion width: 210 μm), ly0, v0, LM(−), VM(−), pType 0IIc, 16 × 11 mm, U, Gre.

Summary

It is difficult to predict the histological type of this lesion with WL endoscopy, but NBI magnified endoscopy enables it by visualizing the superficial mucosal microstructure pattern and capillary pattern. Moreover the lateral extending range is also well recognized, which enables an infallible en bloc resection.

26.3 Answer

The correct histological type is (1) WDA (tub1).

Question 13: What Is the Histological Type of This Lesion?

27

Ayako Seki

A. Seki (✉)
Department of Gastroenterology, Nagano Municipal Hospital, 1333-1
Tomitake, Nagano-shi, Nagano 381-8551, Japan
e-mail: ayako_seki@hospital.nagano.nagano.jp

T. Oyama (ed.), *Endoscopic Diagnosis of Superficial Gastric Cancer for ESD*, DOI 10.1007/978-4-431-54469-2_27

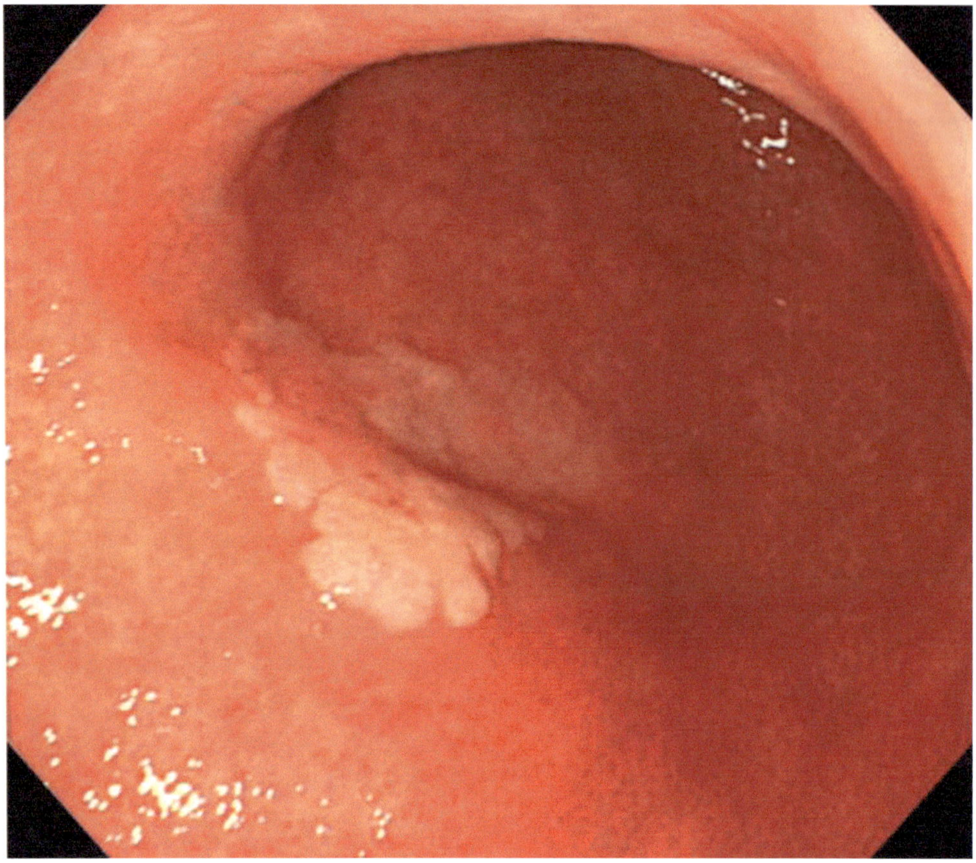

Fig. 27.1 What is the histological type of this lesion?

What is the histological type of this lesion? (Fig. 27.1) Choose your answer from 1 to 3.

(1) Adenoma
(2) WDA
(3) Mixed type of WDA and PDA

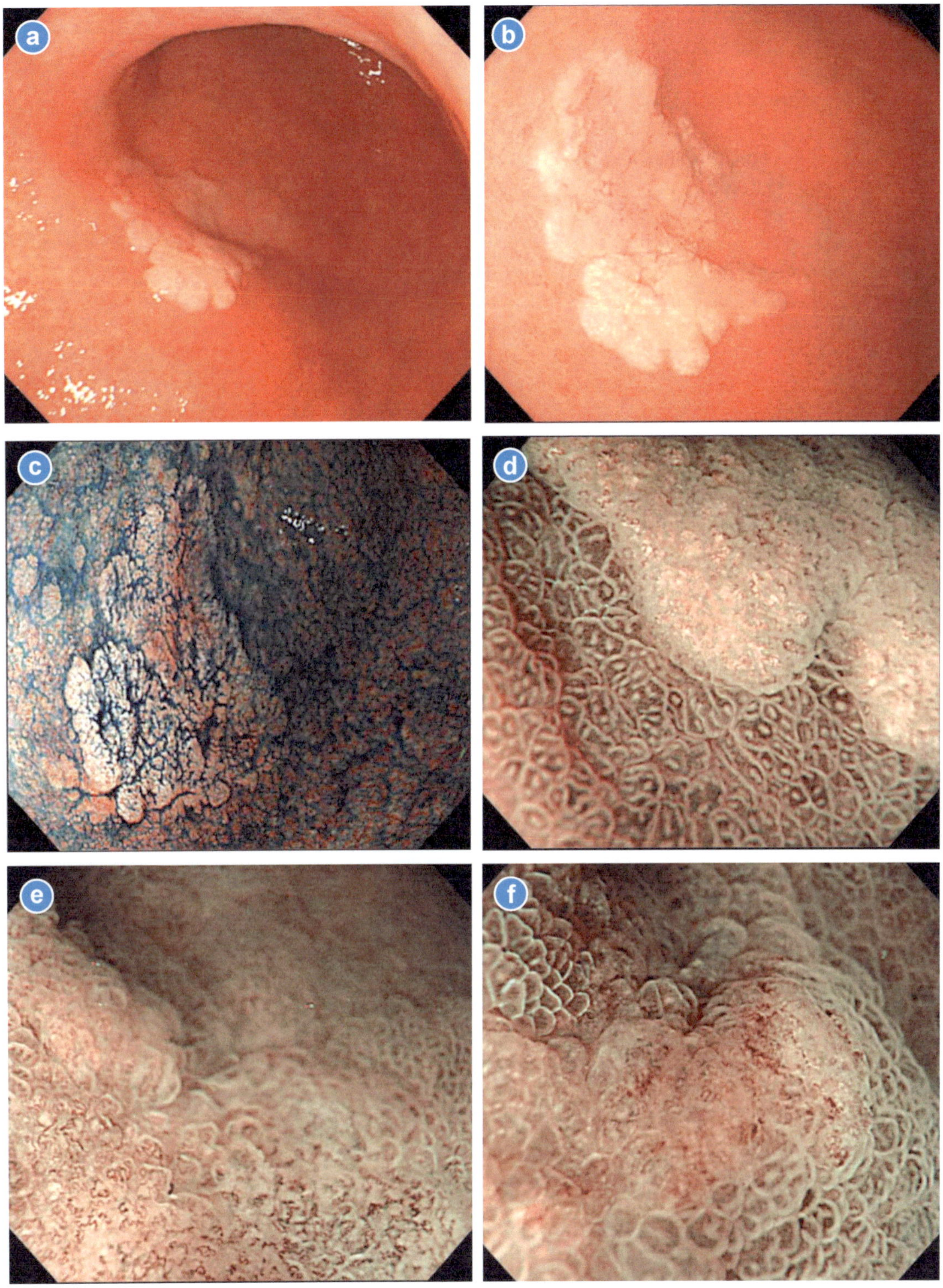

Fig. 27.2 Let's diagnose by observing these six images

27.1 Focus on These Points

27.1.1 Let's Take an Overview Look at the Lesion from a Distance

- There was a flat elevated lesion with a clear border in the greater curvature of the antrum.
- The main color of the protuberance is whitish and yellowish, but some parts are reddish.
- Generally, a whitish protuberance with a clear border is suspected that it's an adenoma. But this lesion had reddish area in some part of it, so it might be accompanied by adenocarcinoma (Fig. 27.3a).

27.1.2 Let's Observe Closely

- The lesion is roughly classified into three parts.
- The oral side designated as Part A is a whitish flat elevated area with yellowish granules suggesting this to be a xanthoma as marked by a yellow arrow.
- The anterior side designated as Part B has a slightly unclear border and has a reddish depressed area (shown by red arrows). Besides, the anal side named Part C is almost flat and has slightly whitish and unclear areas (Fig. 27.3b).

27.1.3 How Do You Interpret These Findings?

- This lesion has three parts with each showing distinctively different colors and features. It is suggested that each of them has a different histological characteristic.
- Based on these observations, this lesion is suspected to contain carcinoma in adenoma or a differentiated adenocarcinoma that has three different components (Fig. 27.3b).

27.1.4 Let's Spray Indigo Carmine

- After indigo carmine spraying, the mucosal surface shows many small granules of variable size. The size and shape of them were irregular.
- And the lesion didn't contain any regular smooth nodules like an adenoma, so we suspected that it was the whole differentiated adenocarcinoma rather than adenoma (Fig. 27.3c).

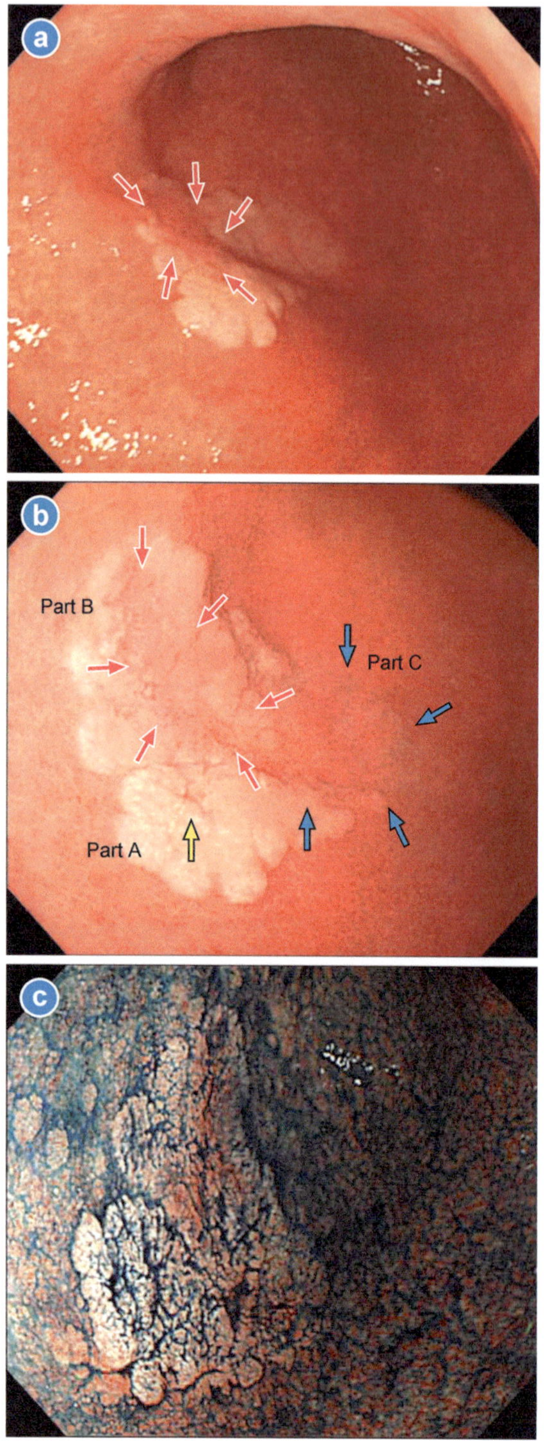

Fig. 27.3 Same images as Fig. 27.2

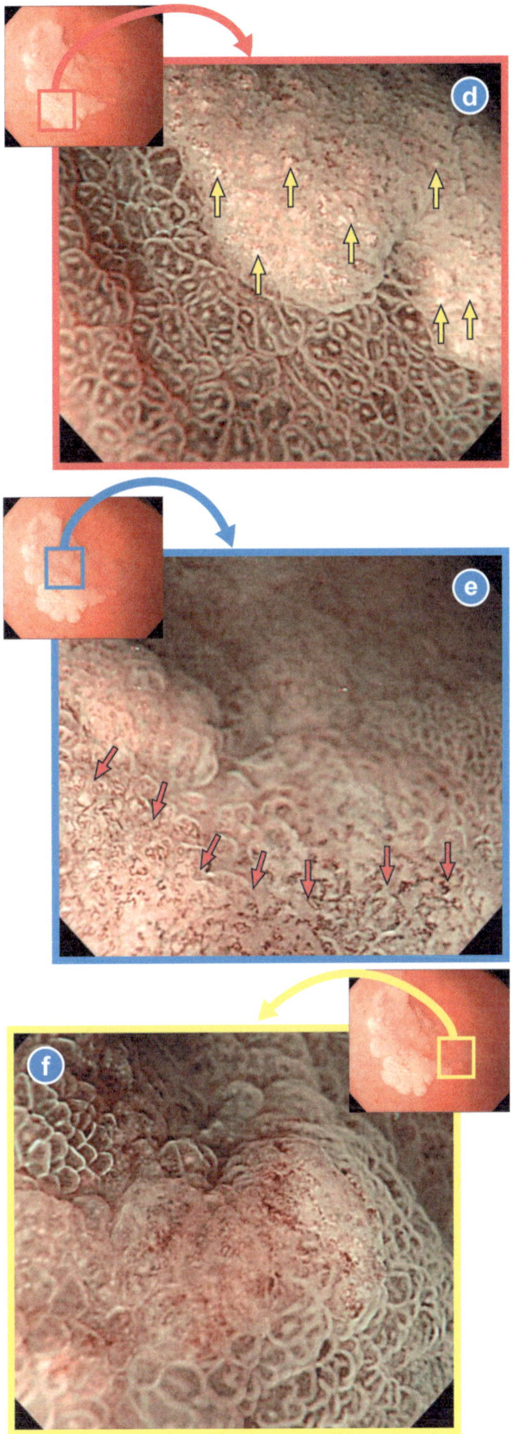

Fig. 27.3 (continued)

27.1.5 Let's Observe the Oral Side of the Lesion (Part A in Fig. 27.3b) with NBI Magnified Endoscopy

- The surrounding mucosa shows regular round pitlike structures (Fig. 27.3d).
- In Part A, the surface fine structures are unclear, and the surface fine vessels show irregular running and caliber changes.
- By observation with NBI magnified view, we suspected that it might not be an adenoma because of the unclearness of the surface microstructure and the abnormality of the fine vessels on the area. The reason is that an adenoma generally has densely regular pitlike or villi-like fine structures.
- As shown by yellow arrows, many whitish and yellowish granules are noted within the elevated lesion. It is suspected to be accompanying xanthomas.

27.1.6 Let's Observe Inside the Lesion (Part B in Fig. 27.3b) with Magnified NBI

- In Part B, there are distorted villi-like fine structures, and they are unclear below the red arrows. And the surface fine vessels showed irregular running and caliber change (Fig. 27.3e).
- Based on severe atypia of the surface microstructures and vessels, the histological type of Part B is diagnosed as MDA.

27.1.7 Let's Observe the Anal Side of the Lesion (Part C in Fig. 27.3b) with Magnified NBI

- The surrounding mucosa shows round villi-like structures (Fig. 27.3f).
- The surface fine structures and vessels at the center of Fig. 27.5 are more unclear than Parts A and B.
- Typical abnormalities like corkscrew vessels are absent in this area, but the histological type is suspected to be PDA because of marked structural unclearness of Part C.

27.2 Let's Compare Fixed Specimens with Resected Specimens

- Based on endoscopic observations, the lesion was diagnosed as gastric cancer with xanthomas, 0-IIa + IIc, moderately to PDA.
- Its invasion depth was diagnosed as intramucosal, because there was neither depression nor protuberance in the lesion which appeared without thickness to suggest submucosal invasions. Finally, we performed en bloc resection by ESD.

27.2.1 Let's Observe the Freshly Removed Specimen

- The freshly resected specimen is rotated to be compared with the endoscopic images. The oral side is the left lower side of the specimen as shown by a black arrow.

Part A: A flat elevated area with many whitish and yellowish granules with clear border

Part B: A reddish, slightly elevated area with slightly unclear border

Part C: A whitish flat area with unclear border (Fig. 27.4)

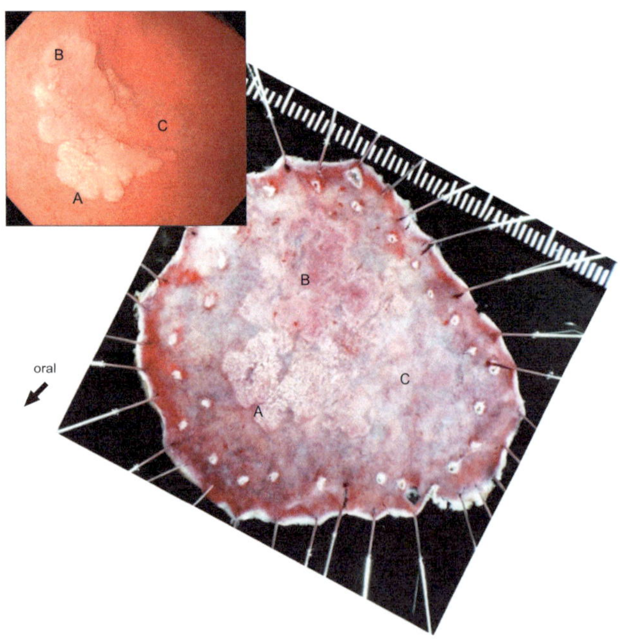

Fig. 27.4 Endoscopic image and freshly resected specimen of the lesion

27.2.2 Let's Perform Histological Mapping of the Freshly Resected Specimen

- As the mapping on the image of the freshly resected specimen shows, there are three histological types noted in the lesion (Fig. 27.5).

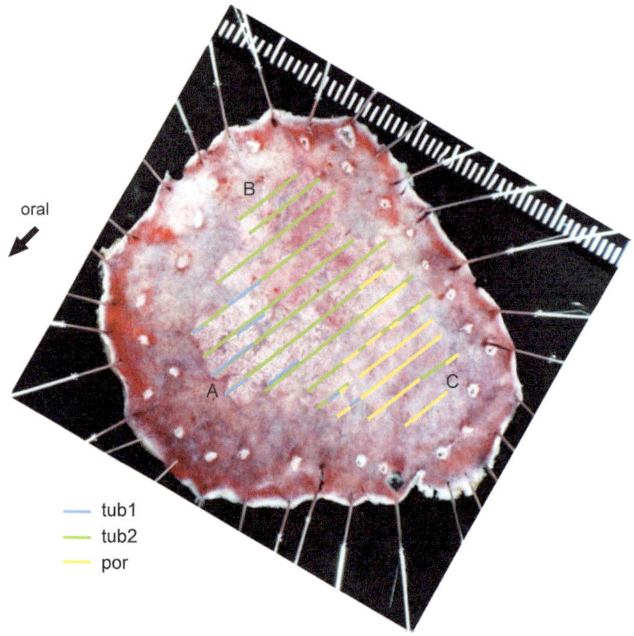

Fig. 27.5 Endoscopic image and freshly resected specimen of the lesion

27.2.3 Let's Compare NBI Magnified Images with the Histological Images

This is a histological picture of the blue line in Part A (Fig. 27.6a). In the mucosa, there are abnormal glands with structural atypia and horizontal connections. This part is diagnosed as WDA, and its invasion depth is in intramucosa. There are foamy cells in the stroma as shown in the blue lined box. The whitish and yellowish granules in the endoscopic images are clusters of foamy cells.

Unclearness of the surface structures by NBI magnified view is likely caused by cancer glands so dense that the orifices of the glands are too narrow to be seen.

This is a histological image of the green line in Part B (Fig. 27.6b). There are small glands showing horizontal connections in the area that we observed distorted villi-like

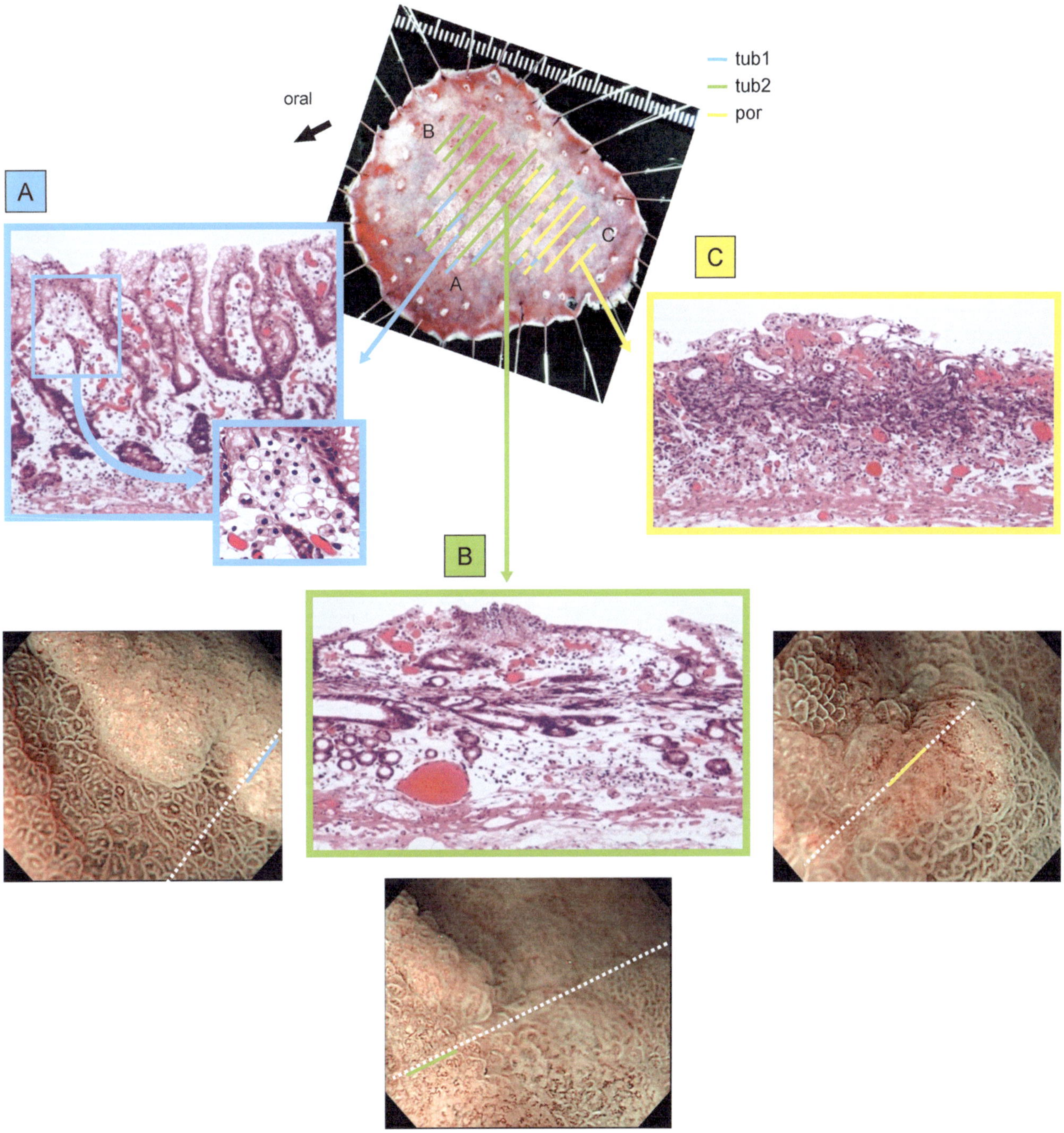

Fig. 27.6 Comparison between NBI magnified endoscopic images with the histological images

fine structures and abnormal fine vessels by NBI magnified view. This part is diagnosed as MDA, and its invasion depth is intramucosal.

This is a histological image of the yellow line in Part C (Fig. 27.6c). There is an increase of cancer cells in the area that shows unclearness of the surface structures and vessels with NBI magnified view. Most of the cancer cells don't form glands. Only a few of them form small glands. The part is diagnosed as PDA and its invasion depth is intramucosal.

Conclusive Diagnosis

Gastric adenocarcinoma, tub2>por>tub1, T1(M), ly0, v0, LM(−), VM(−), pType 0-IIa, 35 × 27 mm, M, Ant, Gre.

Summary

This lesion is a mixed tissue type adenocarcinoma with xanthomas.

With magnified NBI, we were able to diagnose before ESD that the lesion is a cancer consisting of various histological features.

Finally, we decided that it was the contraindication, because the major axis of the PDA was over 2 cm.

Additional surgical excision was performed, but there was no lymphatic metastasis in the surgical specimen.

27.3 Answer

The histological type of this lesion is (3) mixed type of WDA and PDA.

28 Question 14: Where Is the Lateral Extension of This Gastric Lesion?

Akiko Takahashi

A. Takahashi (✉)
Division of Endoscopy, Saku Central Hospital, 197 Usuda, Saku,
Nagano 384-0301, Japan
e-mail: aurevoireurope@yahoo.co.jp

T. Oyama (ed.), *Endoscopic Diagnosis of Superficial Gastric Cancer for ESD*, DOI 10.1007/978-4-431-54469-2_28

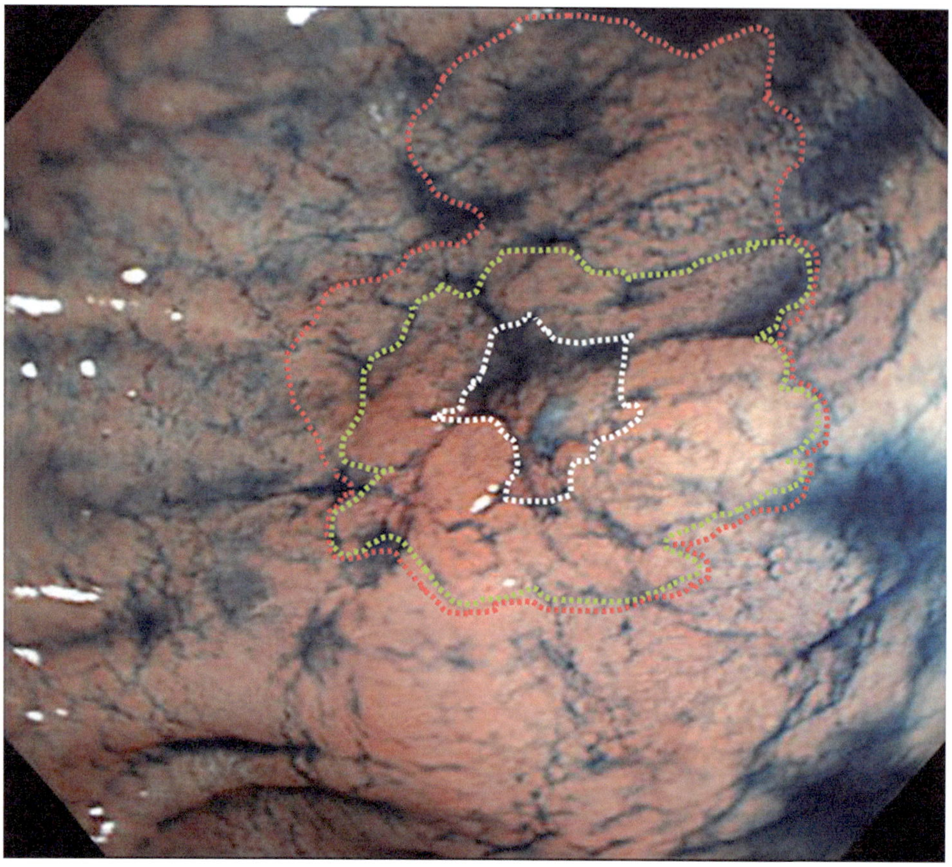

Fig. 28.1 Where is the lateral extension of this gastric lesion?

Where is the lateral extension of this gastric lesion? (Fig. 28.1)
Choose your answer from 1 to 3.

(1) White dotted line
(2) Green dotted line
(3) Red dotted line

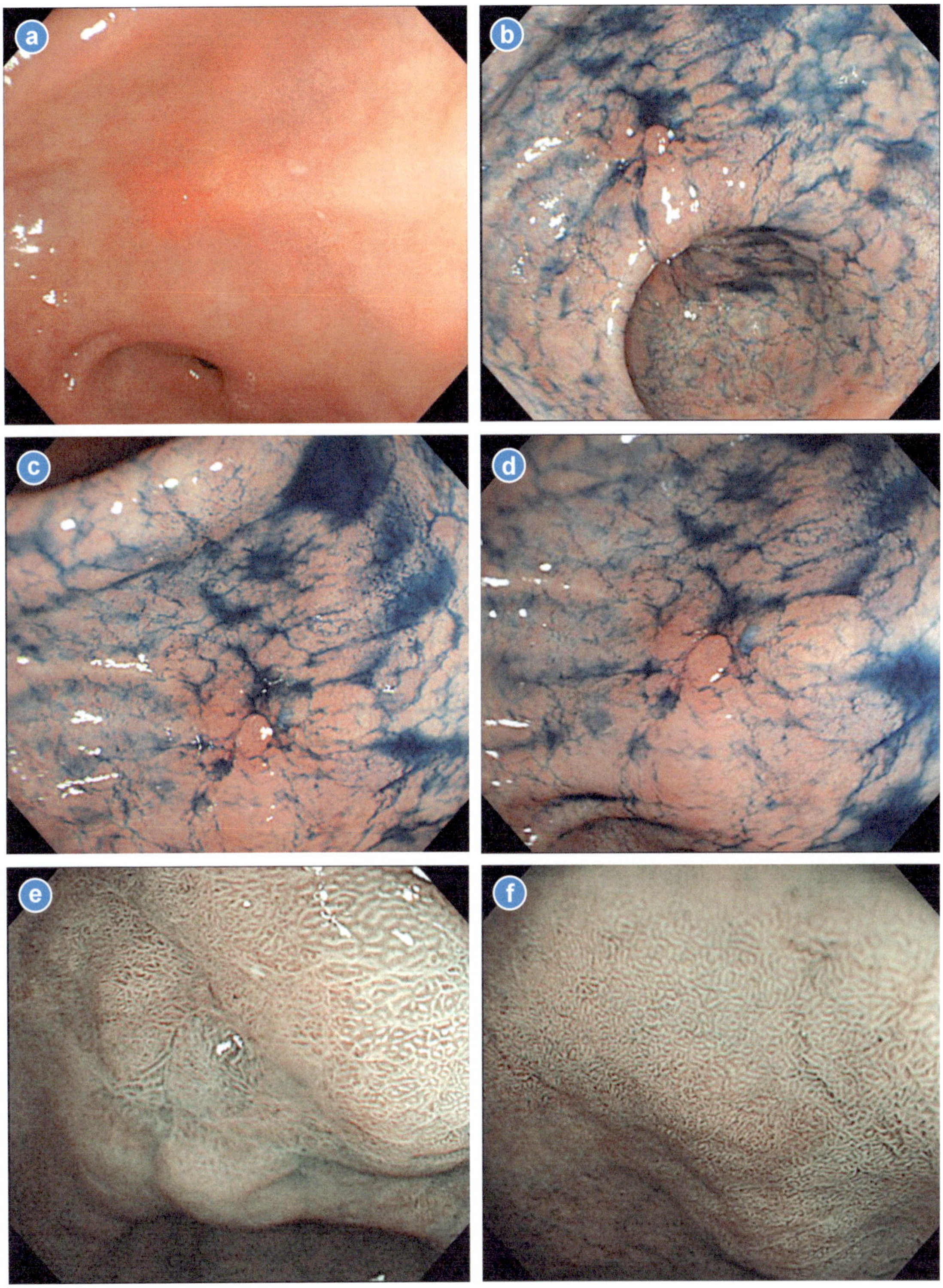

Fig. 28.2 Let's diagnose by observing these six images

28.1 Focus on These Points

28.1.1 Let's Note the Reddish Mucosa

- WL endoscopy shows an irregularly uneven and reddish area with unclear margin on the lesser curvature of the gastric antrum (Fig. 28.3a).
- WL endoscopy shows an unclear margin. Therefore, to distinguish between cancer and noncancer (such as inflammatory changes) is difficult.

28.1.2 Let's Check the Depressed Part and Surrounding Area

- Chromoendoscopy using indigo carmine shows an irregular depression with a clear margin. However, it doesn't show a worm-eaten appearance on its margin suggestive of cancer (Fig. 28.3b).
- Also, chromoendoscopy using indigo carmine shows an irregular areal pattern spreading in the surrounding area but without clear margins.

28.1.3 Let's Observe the Lesion Closely

- The mucosa surrounding the depression is observed with a close-up view (Fig. 28.3c).
- Only the posterior margin of the lesion can be traced with irregularity of areal patterns as marked by green arrows. The margin on other sides is unclear.
- At this stage, the depressed part traced with a yellow dotted line is thought of as cancer. However, the lateral extension of the lesion is unclear.
- The posterior margin of the depressed part is observed further with moderately NBI magnified endoscopy to determine the lateral extension.

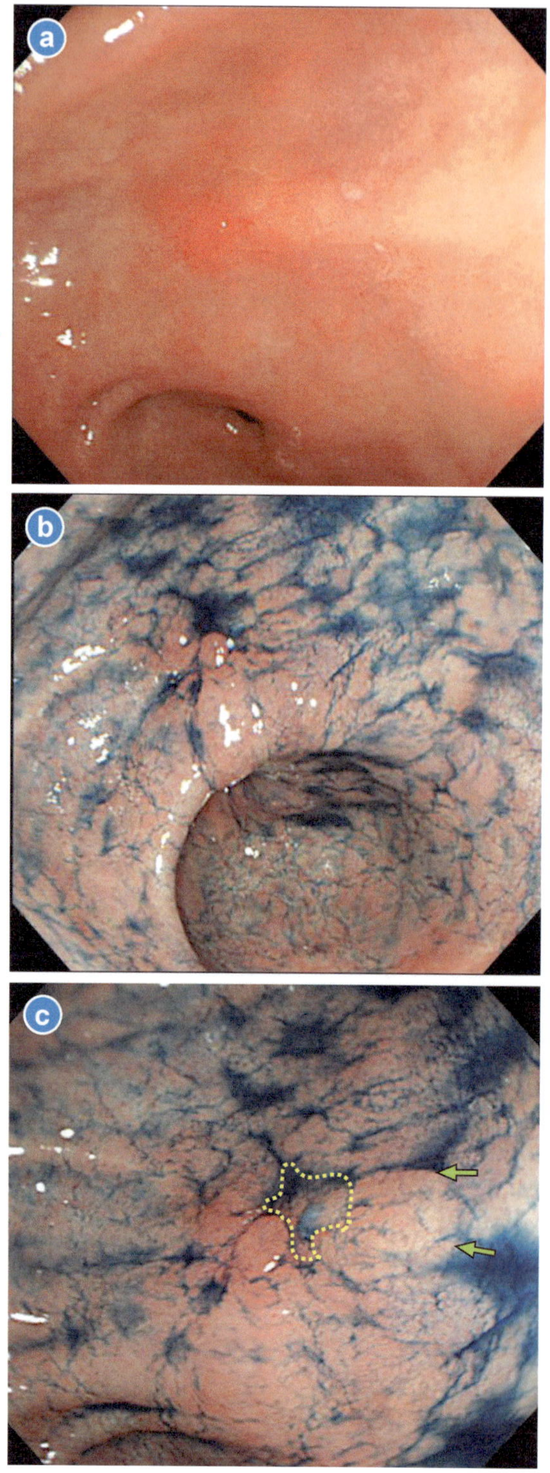

Fig. 28.3 Same images as Fig. 28.2

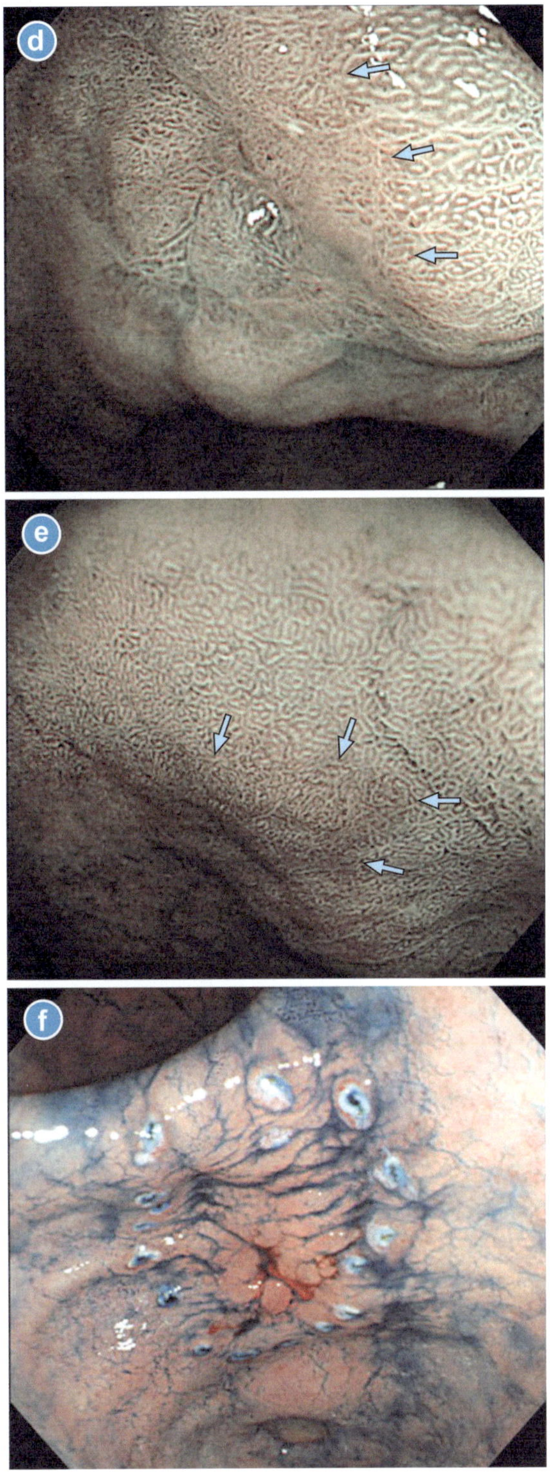

Fig. 28.3 (continued)

28.1.4 Let's Check the Background Mucosa

- The background mucosa on the posterior side of the depressed part shows a pitlike pattern with evenly sized pits without irregularity (Fig. 28.3d).

28.1.5 Let's Check the Posterior Wall of the Lesion

- NBI magnified endoscopy on the posterior wall of the lesion shows a mixture of pitlike pattern and villous pattern with variable sizes and high density.
- No vascular patterns are recognized. And the area marked with light blue arrows is determined as the margin of the lesion by differences in surface pattern compared to the background mucosa (Fig. 28.3d).

28.1.6 Let's Check the Oral Side of the Lesion

- NBI magnified endoscopy shows a mixture of highly dense and variably sized pits and villi in the oral side of the depressed part (Fig. 28.3e).
- NBI magnified endoscopy of the background mucosa shows regular villous pattern. The area marked by light blue arrows is the margin of the lesion by difference of this surface pattern.
- Therefore, the lesion extended not only to the depressed part but also the oral side. It is diagnosed as WDA, T1a-M, 0-IIc + IIb. After placing markings by NBI magnified endoscopy the lesion was resected en bloc by ESD (Fig. 28.3f).

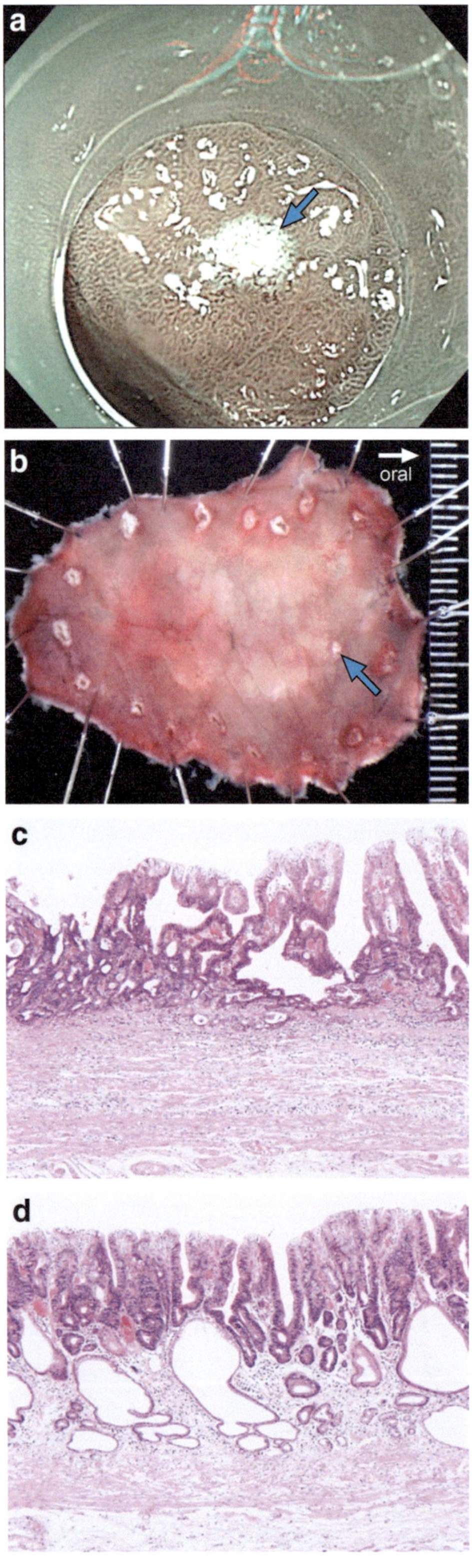

Fig. 28.4 Endoscopic image and freshly resected specimen of the lesion

28.2 Let's Compare Fixed Specimens with Resected Specimens

- A landmark marking was placed to the oral margin as noted by a blue arrow to confirm the diagnosis of the lateral extension (Fig. 28.4a).

28.2.1 Let's Check a Freshly Resected Specimen

- The right side of the picture is the oral side (Fig. 28.4b).
- The freshly resected specimen shows a reddish depression on the anal side with a surrounding flat elevation spreading orally.
- In addition, the fresh specimen shows a whitish mucosa on the oral side continuously (landmark: blue arrow).

28.2.2 Let's Observe Pathological Findings

- This picture shows pathological findings on HE stained of the reddish depressed part.
- Cells with enlarged nuclei are forming neoplastic tubular glands.
- This picture shows structural atypia and, in part, small tubular glands' formation leading to diagnosis of MDA.
- The submucosal layer itself is intact, and the lesion is diagnosed as mucosal cancer (Fig. 28.4c).
- The pathological evaluation shows regular neoplastic tubular formation in the flat and whitish part extending toward the oral side, and the lesion is diagnosed as WDA (Fig. 28.4d).
- The pathological evaluation shows nonneoplastic tubular formation in the deeper part of the mucosal layer. The mucosal structure, therefore, has a double layer formation of the surface neoplasm and the deeper nonneoplastic glands (Fig. 28.4d).

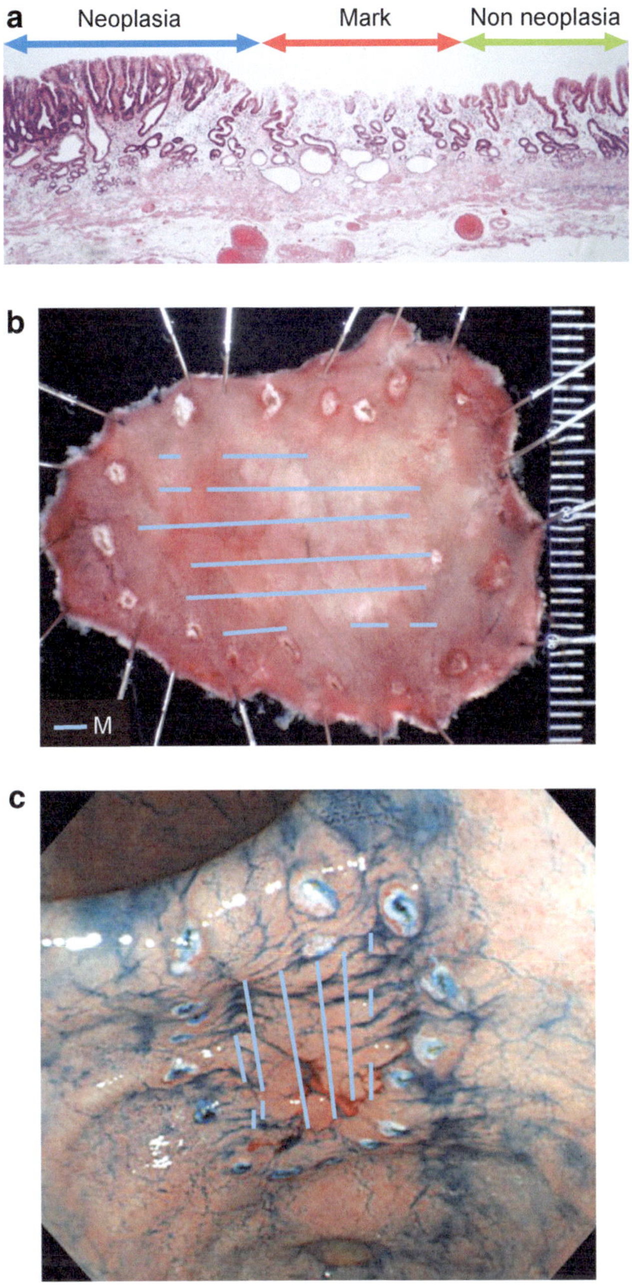

Fig. 28.5 (**a**) Histopathology of the lesion (**b**) The resected specimen with mapping of the cancer distribution (**c**) WL endoscopic image with mapping of the cancer distribution on the specimen

A marking had been intentionally placed to inspect the diagnosis of the lateral extension on the oral side. The left and the right sides of the mark are neoplasia and nonneoplasia, respectively. Therefore, the diagnosis of the lateral extension by NBI magnified endoscopy was confirmed accurate (Fig. 28.5a).

A histological mapping is placed on the endoscopic picture after marking. This picture shows that the flat whitish part extending toward the oral side from the depressed area continuously is cancer (Fig. 28.5b, c).

Conclusive Diagnosis

Gastric adenocarcinoma, tub1> > tub2, T1(M), ly0, v0, LM(−), VM(−), pType 0-IIc + IIb, 22 × 15 mm, L, less.

Summary

Conclusive diagnosis is gastric well-differentiated to MDA, T1a-M, pType 0-IIc + IIb, 22 × 15 mm, L, Less. Lymph duct and venous invasions are negative. Lateral and vertical margins are negative.

Initially, only the depressed part appeared as cancer by WL endoscopy and chromoendoscopy using indigo carmine. It is possible to diagnose 0-IIb extension of the oral side by differences of surface pattern by NBI magnified endoscopy.

It is necessary to suspect a IIb extension anytime a lesion is noted and to observe the surrounding mucosa of the main lesion in detail.

28.3 Answer

The lateral extension of the lesion is (3) red dotted line.

29 Question 15: Which Line Demarcates This Lesion Best?

Shigetaka Yoshinga

S. Yoshinga (✉)
Endoscopy Division, National Cancer Center Hospital, 5-1-1 Tsukiji,
Chuo-ku, Tokyo 104-0045, Japan
e-mail: shiyoshi@ncc.go.jp

T. Oyama (ed.), *Endoscopic Diagnosis of Superficial Gastric Cancer for ESD*, DOI 10.1007/978-4-431-54469-2_29

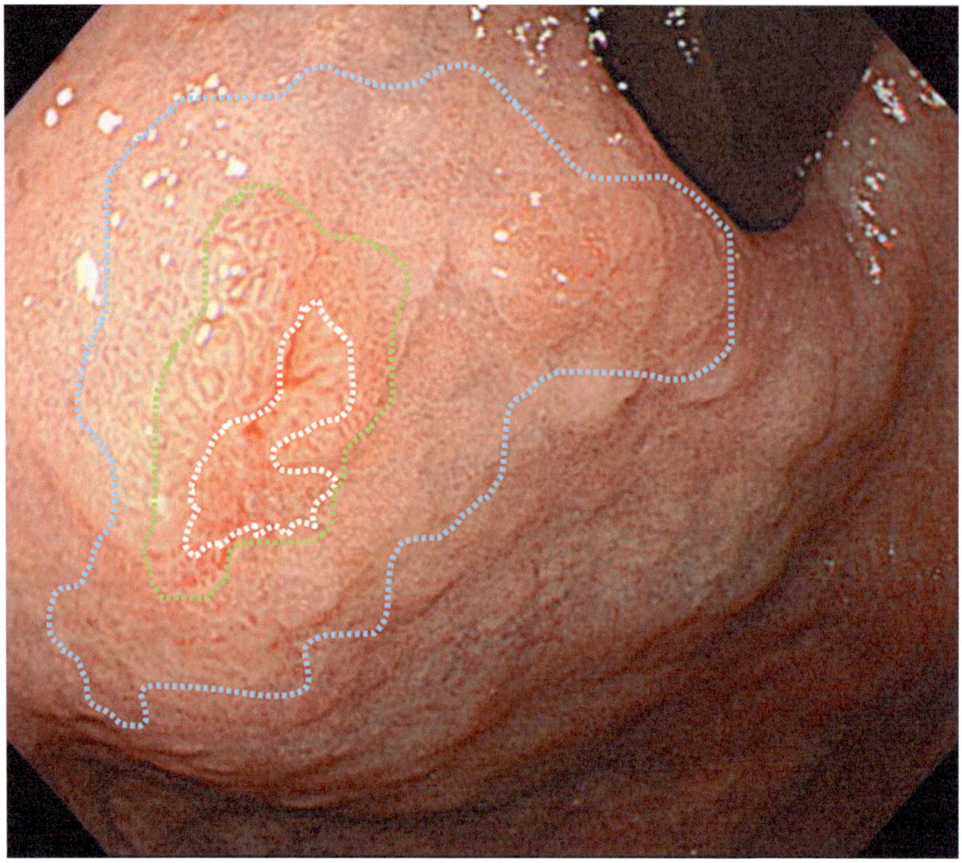

Fig. 29.1 Which line demarcates this lesion best?

Which line demarcates this lesion best? (Fig. 29.1)
Choose your answer from 1 to 3.

(1) White dotted line
(2) Green dotted line
(3) Blue dotted line

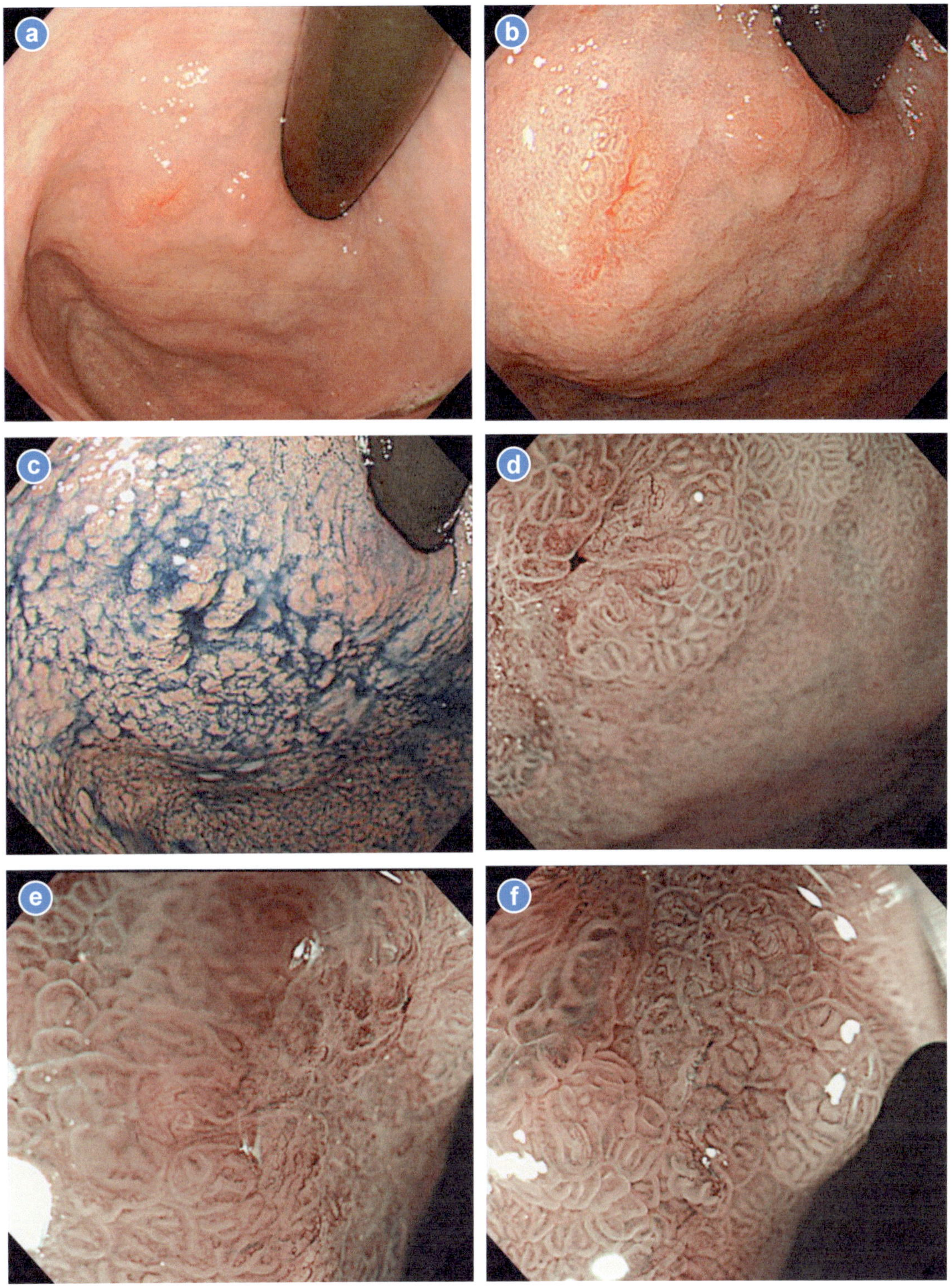

Fig. 29.2 Let's diagnose by observing these six images

29.1 Focus on These Points

29.1.1 Let's Pay Attention to Bleeding

- This is an endoscopic image of the cardia in the retroflexed view.
- Multiple reddish areas are seen around the cardia as marked by yellow arrows. One of those areas, located on the greater curvature near the posterior wall in the fornix, is accompanied by bleeding as marked by a red arrow.
- Compared with the size of the endoscope, this reddish area is about 10 mm in size, and it is more defined than any other reddish areas (Fig. 29.3a).

29.1.2 Let's Pay Attention to the Reddish Area

- This is a close-up endoscopic image taken of a relatively more reddish area with bleeding (Fig. 29.3b).
- In this view, a slightly longitudinal and irregular depression with a surrounding reddish elevation is seen just at the bleeding point.
- The demarcation of reddish area is clear, and the surface of this mucosa is relatively more irregular than the surrounding mucosa.
- A surface of the surrounding mucosa is slightly rough, and RAC (regular arrangement of collecting venules) and atrophic mucosa are not seen.
- Demarcations of other reddish areas are not clear, and there is no remarkable change between surfaces of those areas and surrounding mucosa. Therefore, these areas are caused by inflammation.

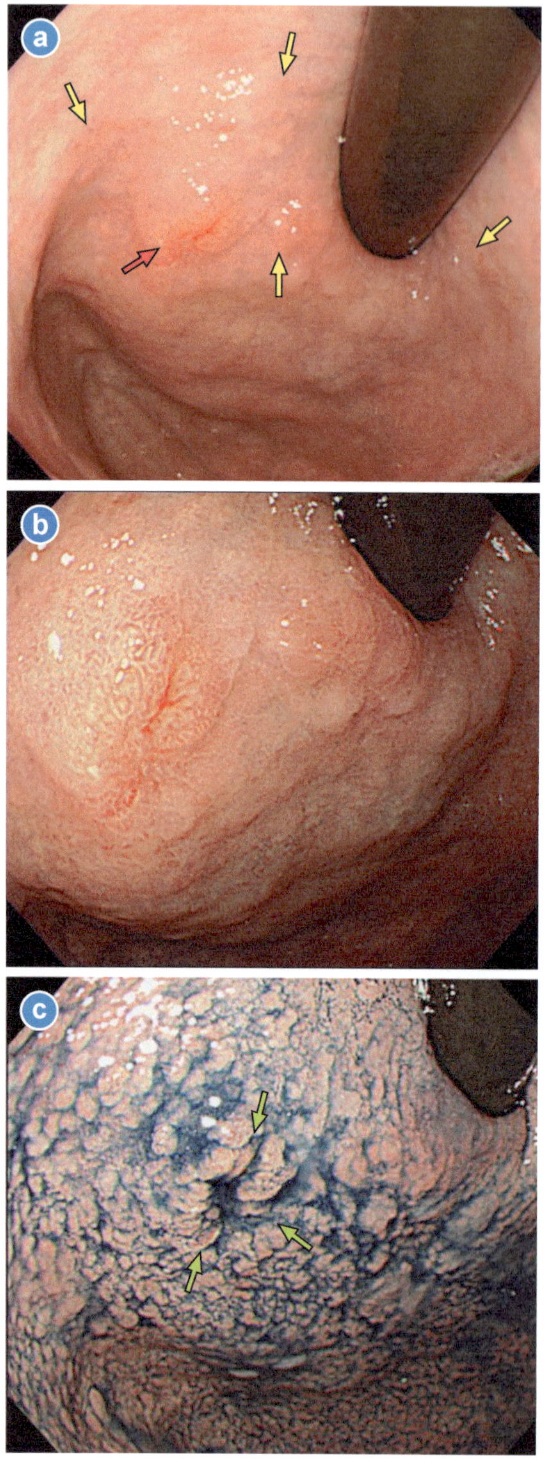

Fig. 29.3 Same images as Fig. 29.2

29.1.3 Let's Pay Attention to the Depression

- After application of indigo carmine dye, a demarcation of the central irregular depression becomes clear, and threadlike troughs are seen around this depression as marked by green arrows (Fig. 29.3c).
- A demarcation of the surrounding elevation is not clear; therefore, the true lesion appears to be the depression only.
- Although there is some pooling of indigo carmine around this lesion, the demarcation of the surrounding elevations is not clear.

29.1.4 What Is the Next Step to Better Define the Lesion?

- NBI magnified endoscopy is performed in order to evaluate this lesion more precisely (Fig. 29.3c).

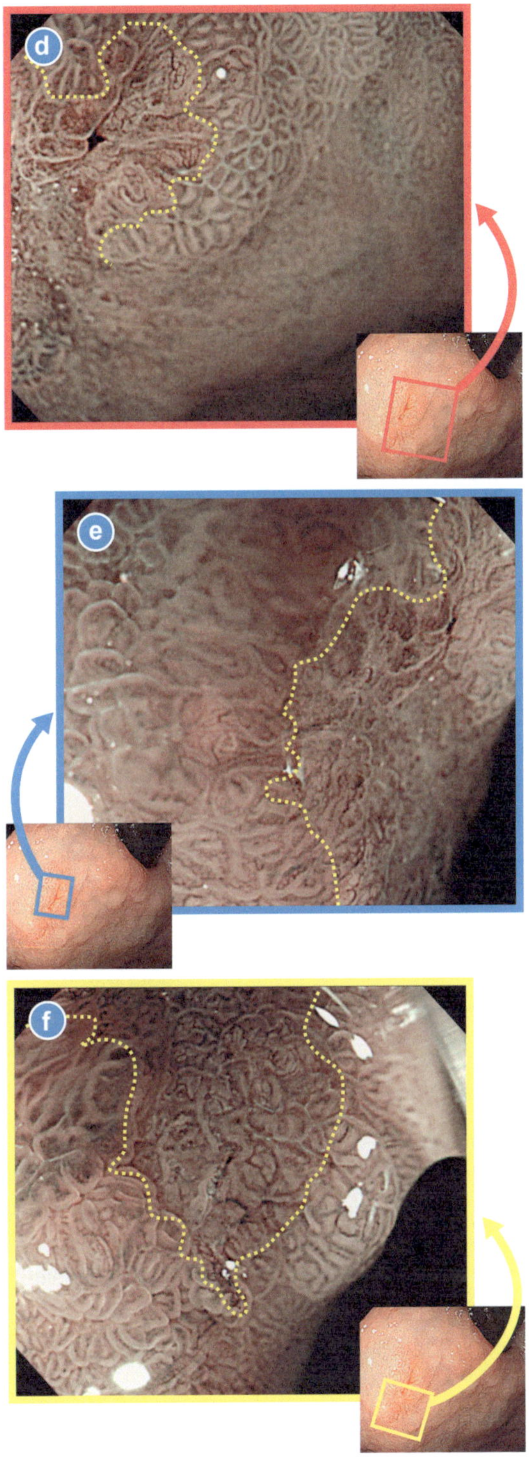

Fig. 29.3 (continued)

29.1.5 Let's Pay Attention to the Surface Pattern on the Oral Side

- This is an endoscopic image of the oral side of the reddish lesion with a depression observed with magnified NBI (Fig. 29.3d).
- Though regular pits and villi are seen on the right side of the yellow dotted line, irregular villi-like structure is seen on the left side.

29.1.6 Let's Pay Attention to the Vascular Pattern

- Irregular vascular patterns are seen just on the irregular surface on the left side. So-called fine network patterns are seen only in the small area of the lesion (Fig. 29.3d).
- According to these findings, the demarcation of this lesion is shown by a yellow dotted line, and we diagnose this lesion is spreading from the depression to the surrounding elevation slightly.

29.1.7 Let's Pay Attention to the Surface Pattern of the Posterior Side

- This is an endoscopic image of the center to the posterior side of the reddish lesion with a depression observed by magnified NBI (Fig. 29.3e).
- Though regular pits and villi are seen on the left side of the yellow dotted line, irregular villi-like structures are seen, and some parts of this become unclear on the right side.

29.1.8 Let's Pay Attention to the Vascular Pattern

- Though an irregular vascular pattern is also seen just on the irregular surface on the right side, the vascular pattern is not clear compared with the previous image (Fig. 29.3e).
- According to these findings, the demarcation of this lesion is shown by the yellow dotted line. This lesion is seen spreading from the depressed area and slightly into the surrounding elevation.

29.1.9 How About the Surface Pattern on the Anal Edge?

- This is an endoscopic image of the anal side of the reddish lesion with a depression observed with magnified NBI (Fig. 29.3f).
- An irregular and variably sized pitlike structure is seen.

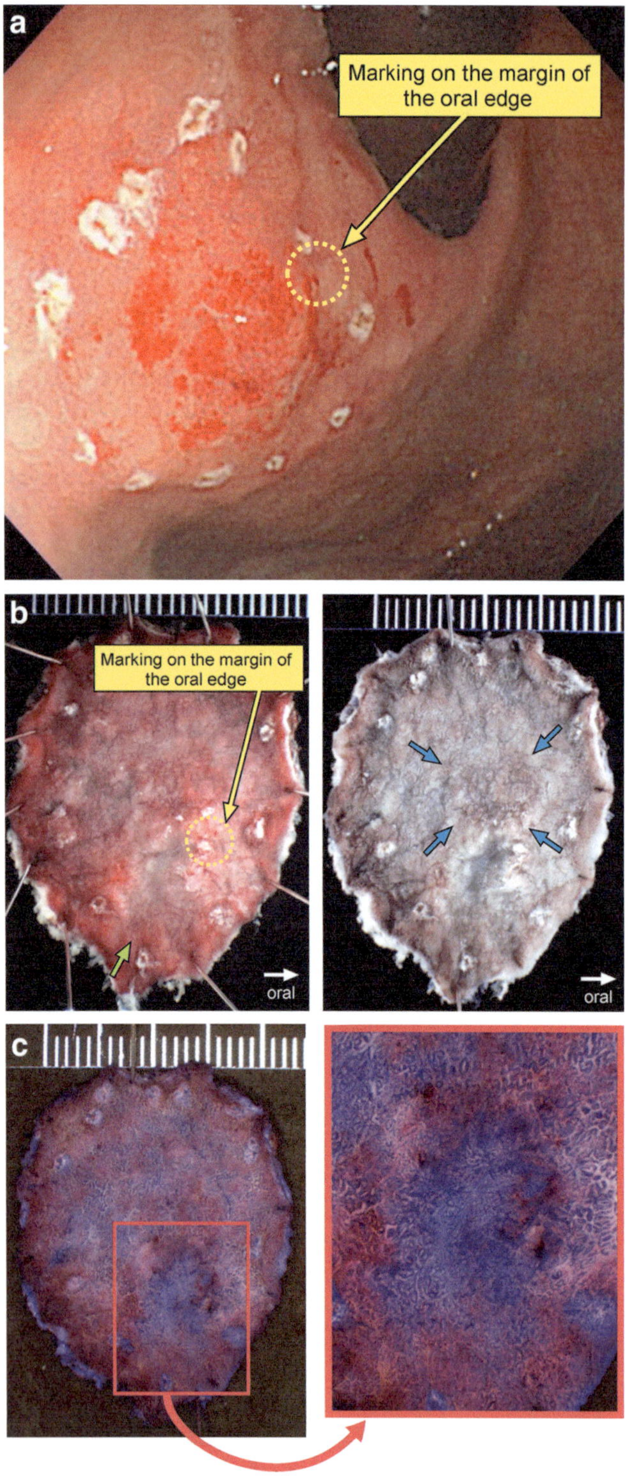

Fig. 29.4 (**a**) Magnified encoscopic image after marking by NBI (**b**) The freshly resected specimen taken by stereomicroscope, immediately after resection (*left*) The specimen after fixation with formalin (*right*) (**c**) The specimen after crystal violet staining (*left*) The magnifide view the lesion (*right*)

29.1.10 How About the Vascular Pattern?

- An irregular vascular pattern with partial network formations is seen just on the irregular surface demonstrated above, and a density of vessels is increased in this area. Though variable-sized vessels are seen, irregularity of vessels is not severe (Fig. 29.3f).
- According to the irregularity of vascular and surface pattern, the demarcation of this lesion is shown by the yellow dotted line.

29.2 Let's Compare Fixed Specimens with Resected Specimens

29.2.1 Let's Make Markings

- Using NBI magnified endoscopy, we made a marking just on the margin of the oral edge, and then we made markings in the surrounding mucosa outside of this lesion. But because of endoscopy contact during examination by NBI with magnification, not only this lesion but also surrounding mucosa became reddish and edematous.
- A marking just on the margin of the oral edge (this is to be placed in the yellow banner pointing to the yellow dotted circle) (Fig. 29.4a).
- These are images of the resected specimen taken by stereomicroscope, immediately after resection (Fig. 29.4b) and after fixation with formalin. In both figures, the right side is the oral side.

29.2.2 Let's Pay Attention to the Color Tone

- In the freshly resected specimen, although the relatively discolored mucosa is seen just on the depressed area, the demarcation on the anal and anterior side is unclear as marked by a green arrow. And the spreading of reddish mucosa is seen on the posterior side from the lesion (Fig. 29.4b).

29.2.3 Let's Pay Attention to the Surface Pattern

- In the fixed specimen, the surface pattern becomes clear, and the spreading of relatively nonstructured mucosa is seen just on the depressed area. There is no continuity between the lesion and the reddish mucosa seen in the fresh specimen (arrows), and the surface of this reddish mucosa is similar to the surrounding mucosa (Fig. 29.4b).

29.2.4 The Surface Pattern Becomes Even Clearer After Crystal Violet Staining

- These two images are the fixed resected specimen after crystal violet staining taken by stereomicroscope. And the right one is the magnified view of the lesion (Fig. 29.4c).
- Fine pitlike and irregular villi-like structures are seen in the depressed area.

This is a histological image of the center of the lesion (Figs. 29.5). Both irregularity of structure and cellular atypia are slightly severe, and cribriform is partially seen. Therefore, this lesion is diagnosed as MDA. Because there is no invasion to muscularis mucosa, the depth of the lesion is intramucosal.

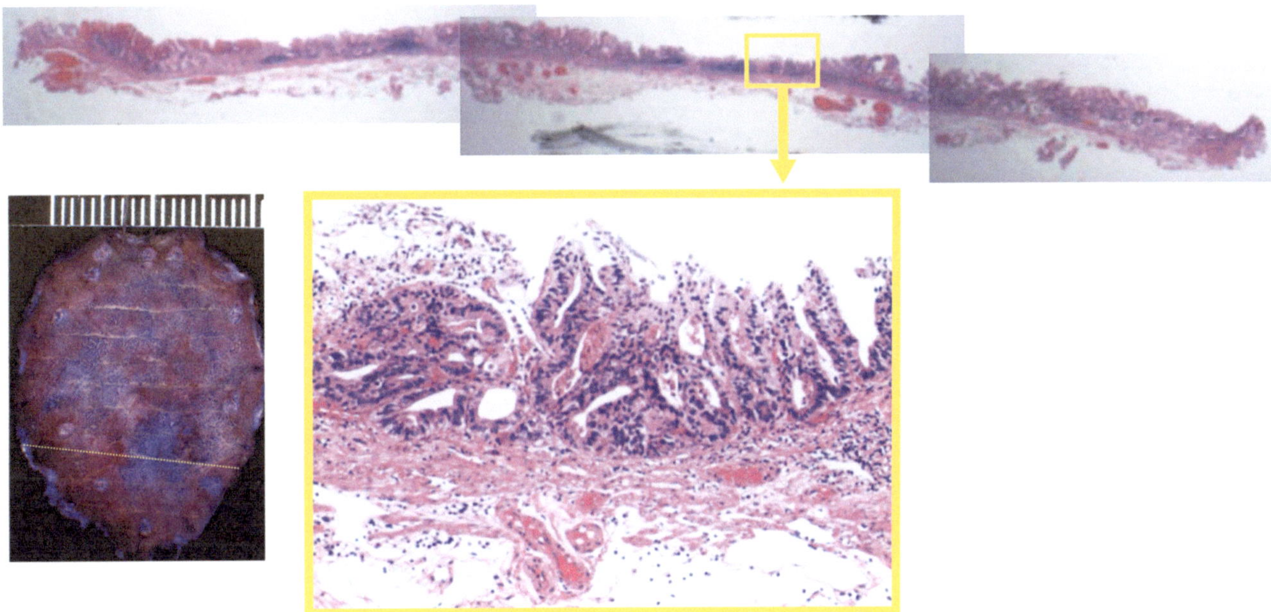

Fig. 29.5 Historogical image of the center of the lesion

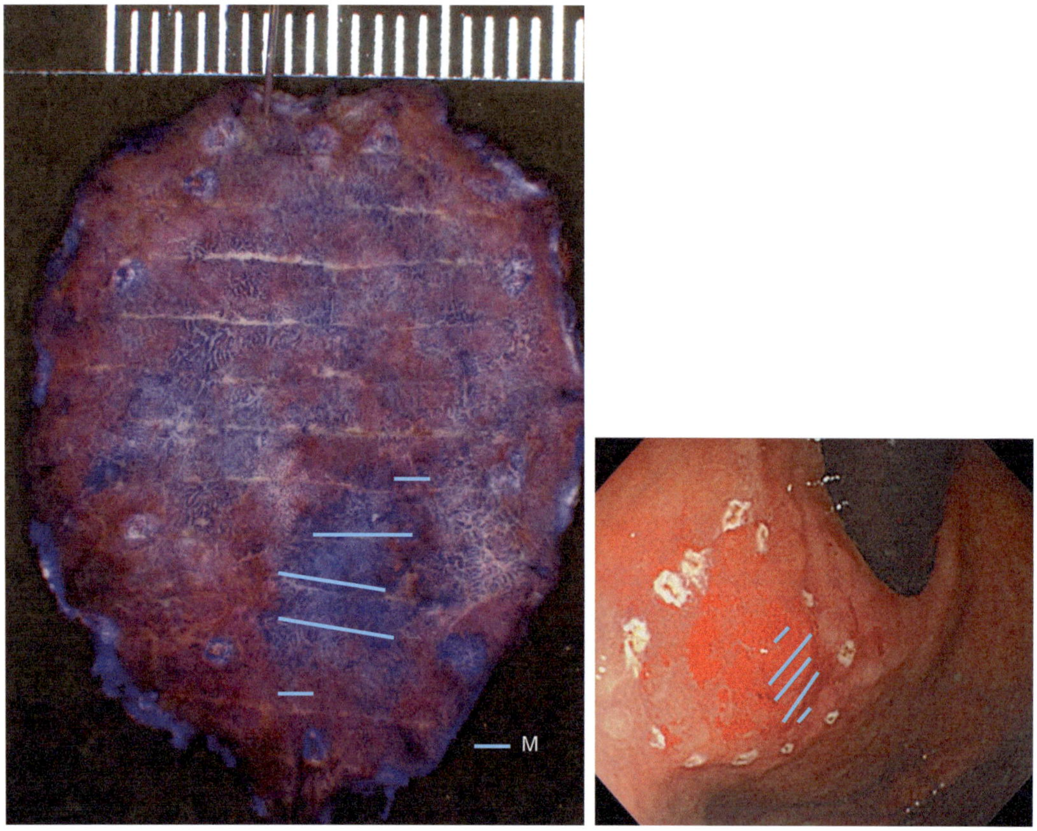

Fig. 29.6 Mapping of the cancer distribution on the specimen (*left*) and endoscopic image (*right*)

Conclusive Diagnosis (Fig. 29.6)
Gastric adenocarcinoma, tub2, T1(M), ly0, v0, LM (−), VM(−), pType 0-IIc, 11 × 6 mm, U, post.

Summary
In histological mapping, the lesion coincides with the depressed area seen endoscopically. Although this lesion is relatively well demarcated, the severe destruction in the surface pattern seen by magnified NBI as well as its scarcity of vascular networks suggests that histological differentiation is poor.

29.3 Answer

The correct demarcation of the lateral extension of this lesion is (1) white dotted line.

Question 16: Which Line Is the Lateral Margin of the Tumor?

30

Tokuma Tanuma

T. Tanuma (✉)
Department of Gastroenterology, Teine Keijinkai Hospital, 1-12-1-40
Maeda, Teine-ku, Sapporo, Hokkaido 006-0811, Japan
e-mail: tokuma@dk9.so-net.ne.jp

T. Oyama (ed.), *Endoscopic Diagnosis of Superficial Gastric Cancer for ESD*, DOI 10.1007/978-4-431-54469-2_30

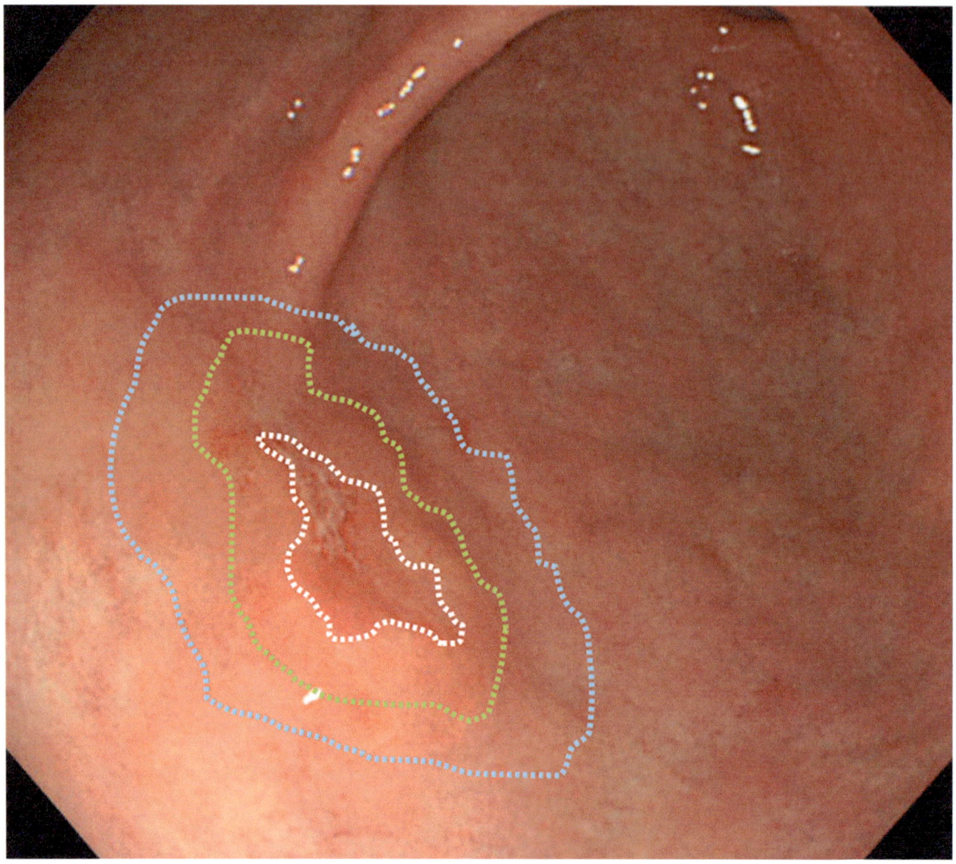

Fig. 30.1 Which line is the lateral margin of the tumor?

Which line is the lateral margin of the tumor? (Fig. 30.1)
Choose your answer from 1 to 3.

(1) White dotted line
(2) Green dotted line
(3) Blue dotted line

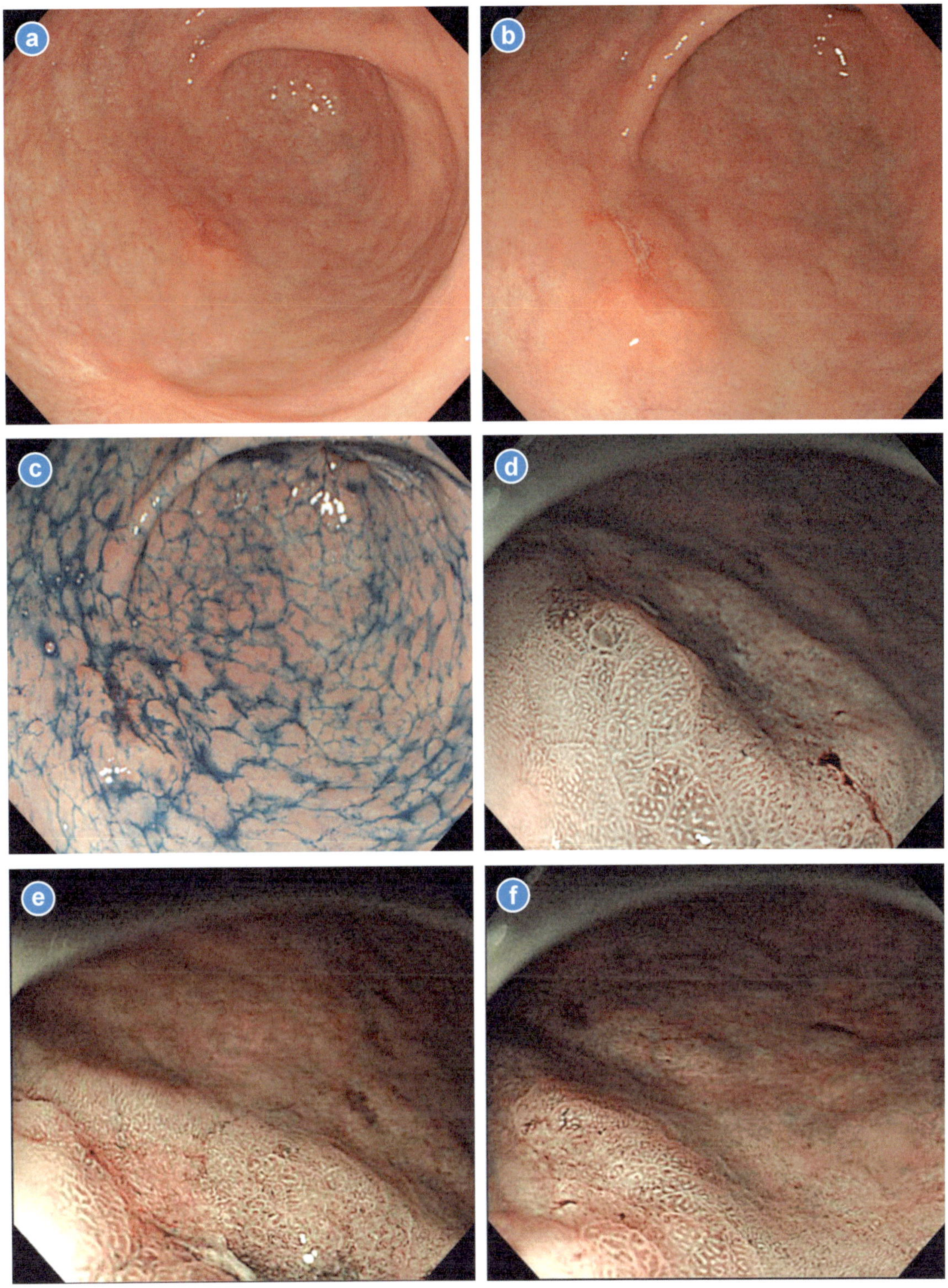

Fig. 30.2 Let's diagnose by observing these six images

30.1 Focus on These Points

30.1.1 Let's Pay Attention to the Reddish Area

- A slightly reddish depressed lesion is observed at the anterior wall in the gastric antrum (Fig. 30.3a).

30.1.2 Let's Pay Attention to Visibility of the Vessels in the Gastric Wall

- Vessels in the gastric wall are observed in the background mucosa, but few vessels are observed at the lesion (Fig. 30.3a).

30.1.3 How Do You Interpret These Findings?

- Because it is a singular lesion, it is more likely to be a neoplasm than inflammatory changes. Whether the extent of the lesion may be limited within the reddish depression or extending into the surrounding area with decreased vascular visibility must be evaluated in detail (Fig. 30.3a).

30.1.4 Let's Observe the Lesion Closely

- The margin of the depression is clear toward the greater curvature side but unclear toward the anterior wall side.
- The edge of the depressed lesion is slightly elevated, and the area of decreased vascular visibility extends further outside from there (Fig. 30.3b).

30.1.5 Let's Focus the Margin of the Depression and Its Surface Pattern

- After indigo carmine spraying, the edge of the depression is irregular, and the surface pattern is heterogeneous (Fig. 30.3c).
- The margin of the depression is clear on the greater curvature side but is unclear on the anterior wall side. There are some irregular pooling of indigo carmine in the surrounding area.
- The margin of the lesion is unclear. It is uncertain whether the extent of the lesion corresponds to the depression or includes the surrounding area.

30.1.6 What Shall We Do Next?

- We performed NBI magnified endoscopy with detailed examination (Fig. 30.3c).

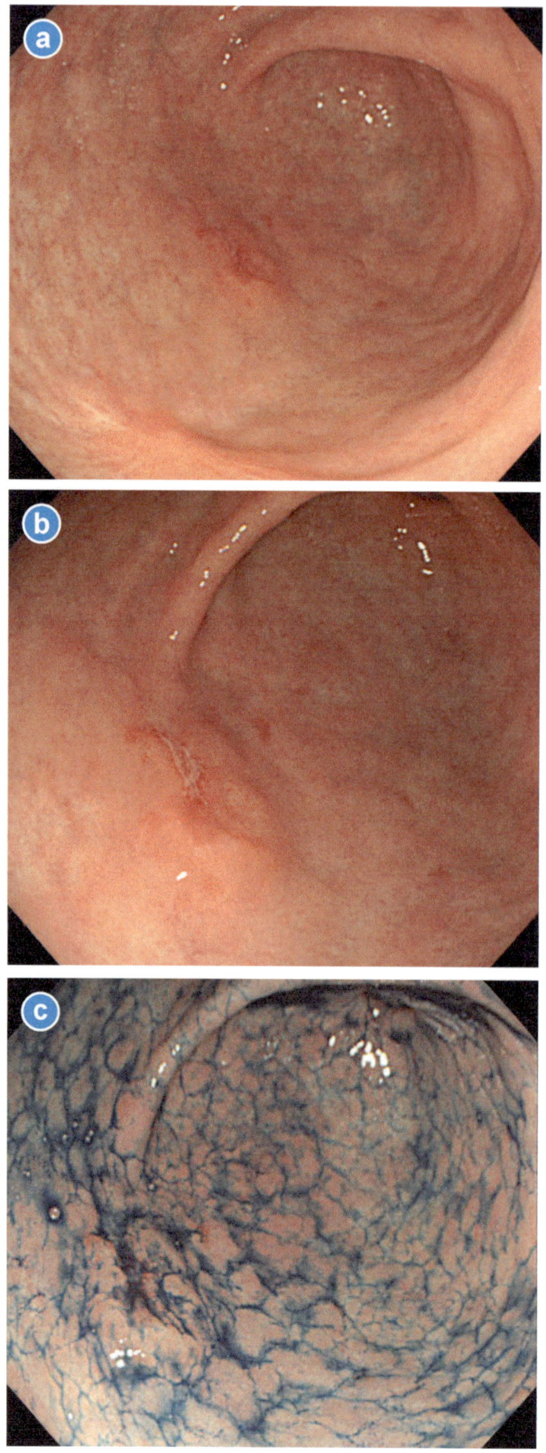

Fig. 30.3 Same images as Fig. 30.2

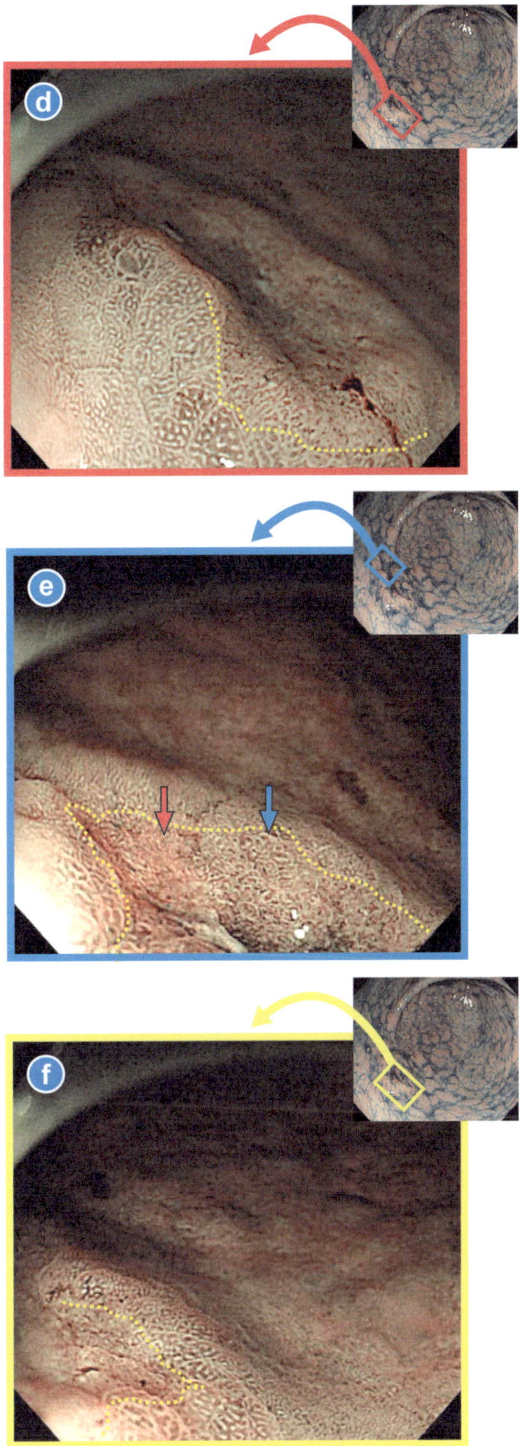

Fig. 30.3 (continued)

30.1.7 Let's Focus on the Surface Pattern in the Oral Side of the Lesion

- Regular pit pattern is observed in the oral side. But irregular villi of variable sizes are observed in the depression (Fig. 30.3d).
- The irregular pattern is noted to extend over to the elevated part surrounding the depression.
- The lateral extension of the lesion can be determined from the difference in surface patterns, so the margin of the lesion is recognized clearly as the yellow dotted line.

30.1.8 Let's Pay Attention to the Irregularities on the Surface Structure

- At the anterior part, the margin is unclear by conventional endoscopy (Fig. 30.3e).
- As marked with a blue arrow, irregular villi of variable sizes are observed suggesting a neoplasm.

30.1.9 Let's Pay Attention to Decreased Clearness of the Surface Structure

- As noted by a red arrow, the surface pattern is unclear, suggesting this area as PDA.
- In the background mucosa, regular pit pattern is observed, so we can determine the lateral margin of cancer as marked by yellow dotted line (Fig. 30.3e).

30.1.10 Let's Pay Attention to the Surface Pattern of the Grate Curvature Side

- This is an endoscopic image obtained by magnified NBI of the greater curvature side. The depressed part shows fine and irregular villi, but the surrounding elevated area shows a regular pit pattern. Therefore, the neoplasm is limited to the depressed area, and the surrounding area is diagnosed nonneoplastic.
- Based on above, the lateral extension of the tumor is thought of as being limited inside of the reddish depressed area. So the answer of the question is (1) the white dotted line.
- However, this cancer is potentially having a component of PDA, so we must consider the possibility of lateral invasion to the subepithelium (Fig. 30.3f).

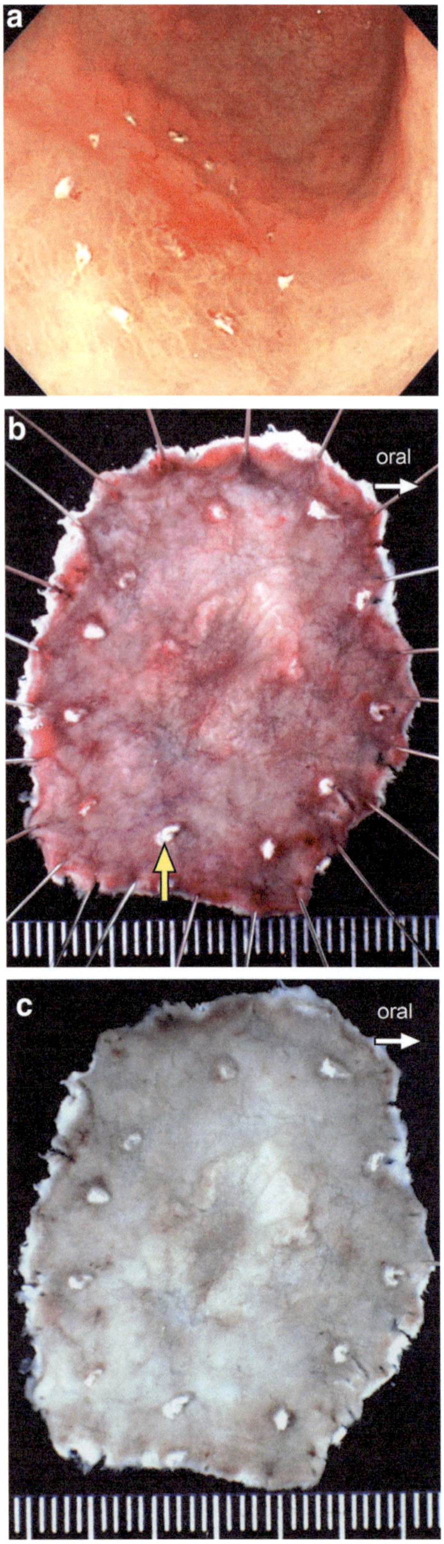

Fig. 30.4 (**a**) Encoscopic image after marking by NBI (**b**) The freshly resected specimen (**c**) The specimen after fixation with formalin

30.2 Let's Compare Fixed Specimens with Resected Specimens

30.2.1 Let's Place Markings

- We performed markings wider than usual before ESD because of a possibility of having a component of PDA (Fig. 30.4a).

30.2.2 Let's Pay Attention to Color Tone

- The right side of the picture is the oral side (Fig. 30.4b).
- A reddish depressed area and the surrounding white elevated area are observed at the center of the lesion.

30.2.3 Let's Pay Attention to "Bumps and Dents"

- At the oral side, the margin of cancer is clear, but at the anterior side and the anal side, it is unclear (Fig. 30.4b).
- At the anterior part, the depression seems to reach the marking spot as noted by a yellow arrow.

30.2.4 In the Fixed Specimen, the Surface Pattern of the Lesion Becomes Clearer

- The depressed area is noted inside of the marking. The surface pattern can be enhanced by lighting up the specimen so that the angle of the lighting becomes closer to the horizontal direction (Fig. 30.4c).

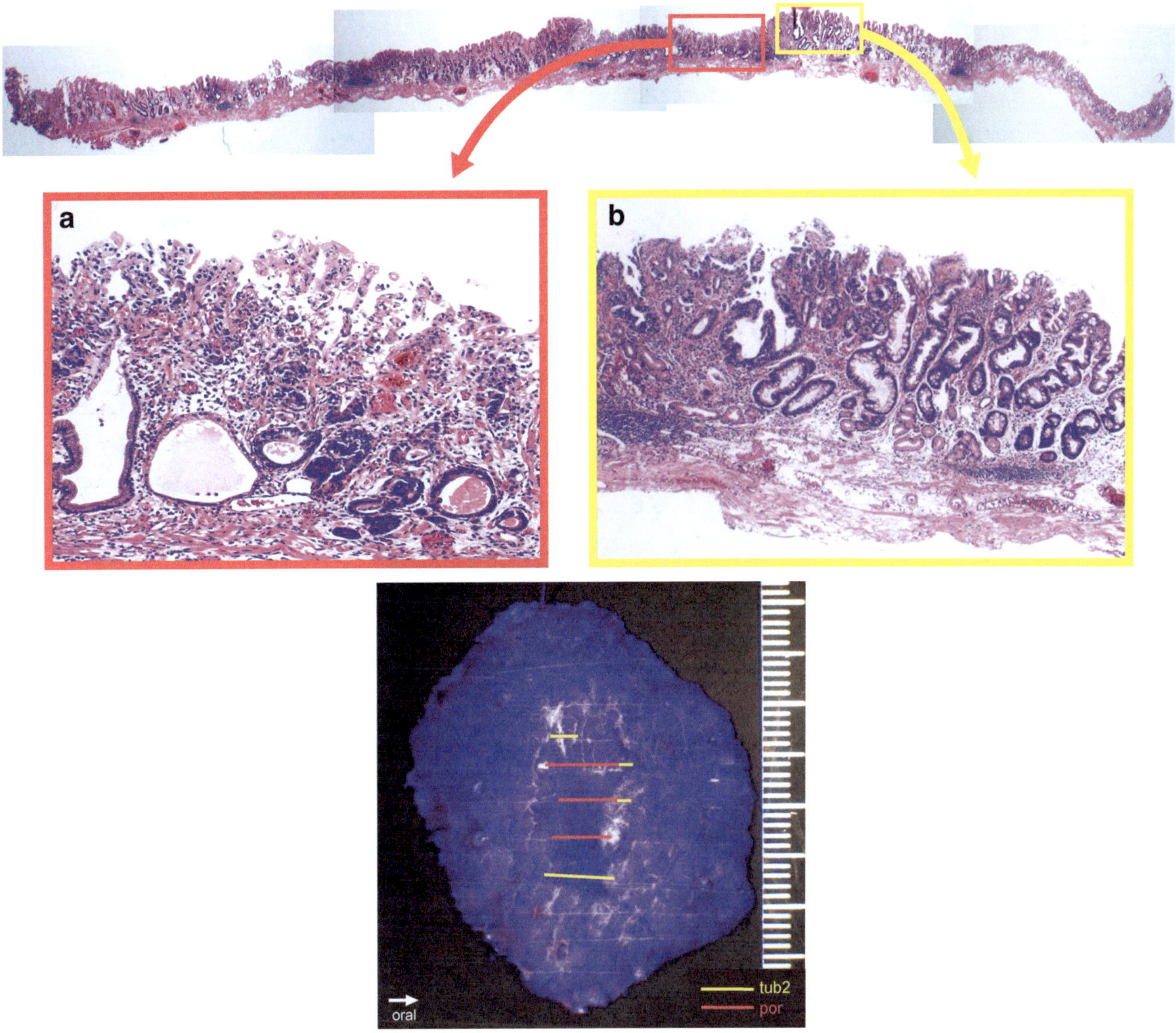

Fig. 30.5 (**a**) The histological image of the depressed part (**b**) The histological image of the elevated part (**c**) Mapping on the cancer distribution on the specimen

This is the histological image of the depressed part. No glands can be observed in the superficial layer, so it is diagnosed as PDA (Fig. 30.5a).

This is the histological image of the elevated part. Irregular small glands are observed, and this part is diagnosed as MDA (Fig. 30.5b).

Conclusive Diagnosis (Fig. 30.5c)

Gastric adenocarcinoma, por>tub2, T1(M), ly0, v0, LM(−), VM(−), pType 0-IIc, 15×10mm, L, Ant, Gre.

Summary
In this case, it is difficult to diagnose by conventional endoscopy, but the use of magnified NBI was helpful to appreciate a subtle difference in surface patterns between cancer and normal mucosa. The biopsy result was WDA, but we suspected that this cancer had possibility of having a component of PDA based on finding unclear surface pattern.

It is controversial whether to expand the criteria for ESD to include PDA. This case is not all PDA. It has MDA, but poorly differentiated component occupied more dominant portion.

30.3 Answer

The lateral expansion is (1) white dotted line.

31 Question 17: Where Is the Lateral Extension of This Lesion?

Tetsuro Yamazato

T. Yamazato (✉)
Department of Gastroenterology, Tokyo Metropolitan Cancer Detection Center, 2-9-2 Musashidai, Fuchu, Tokyo 183-0042, Japan
e-mail: yamazato5102086743@qa2.so-net.ne.jp

T. Oyama (ed.), *Endoscopic Diagnosis of Superficial Gastric Cancer for ESD*, DOI 10.1007/978-4-431-54469-2_31

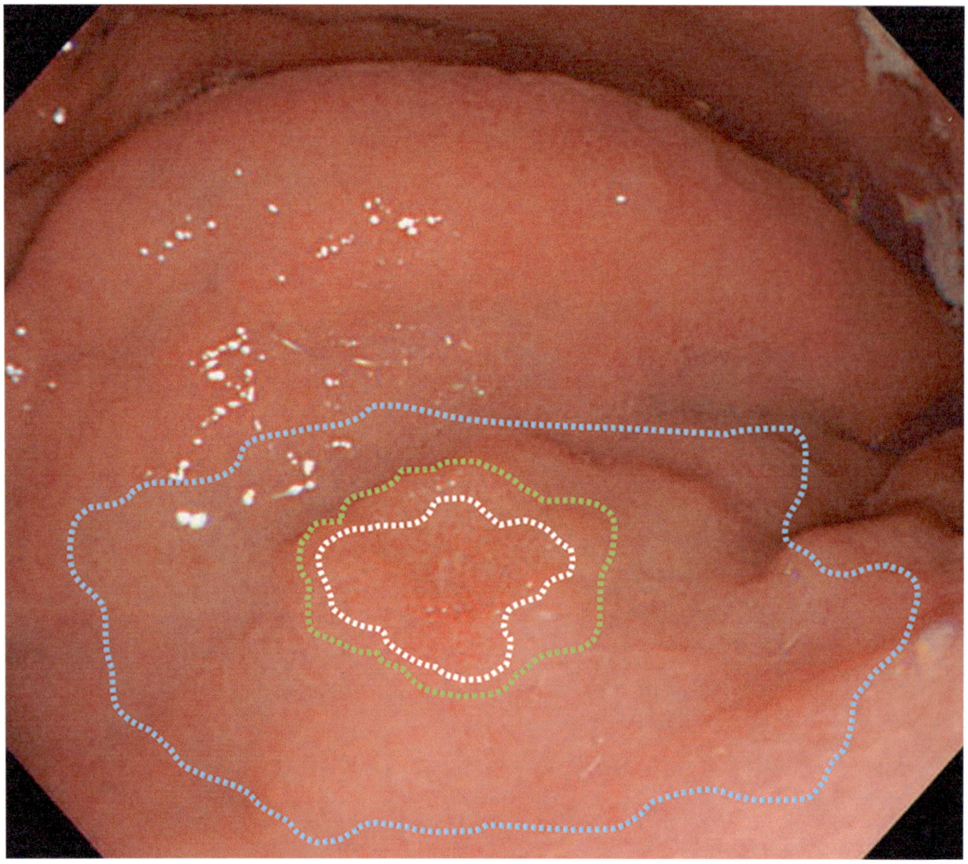

Fig. 31.1 Where is the lateral extension of this lesion?

Where is the lateral extension of this lesion? (Fig. 31.1)

Choose your answer from 1 to 3.

(1) White dotted line
(2) Green dotted line
(3) Blue dotted line

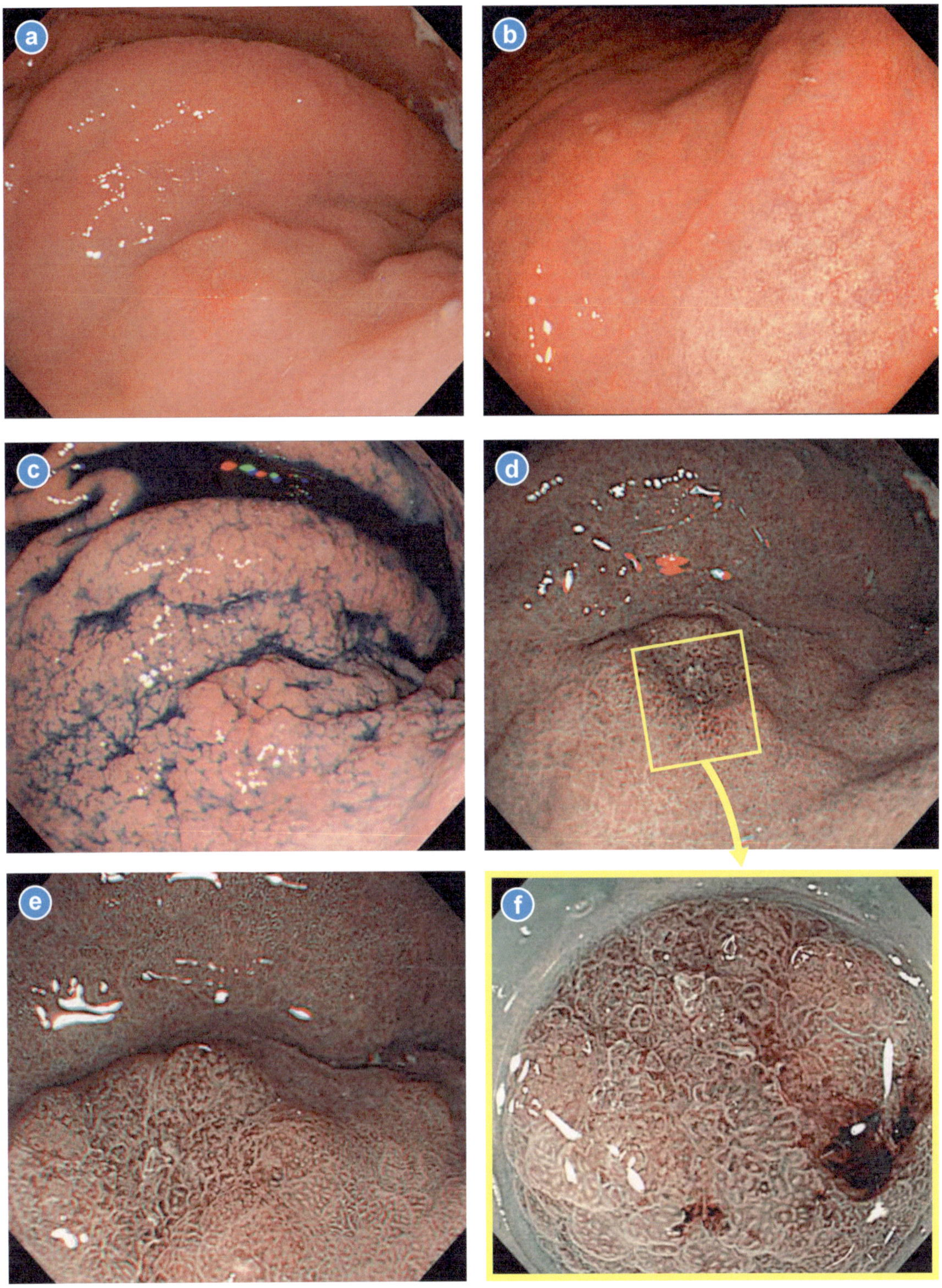

Fig. 31.2 Let's diagnose by observing these six images

31.1 Focus on These Points

31.1.1 Let's Observe the Red Color

- A slightly red and depressed lesion is shown in the posterior wall of the upper gastric body, and the background mucosa is of the fundic gland mucosa (Fig. 31.3a).
- The key to detection of such lesion is to notice slight color change of reddishness and depression. The lesion is more easily detectable when the air of the stomach deflated as seen in the first picture compared with the second one.

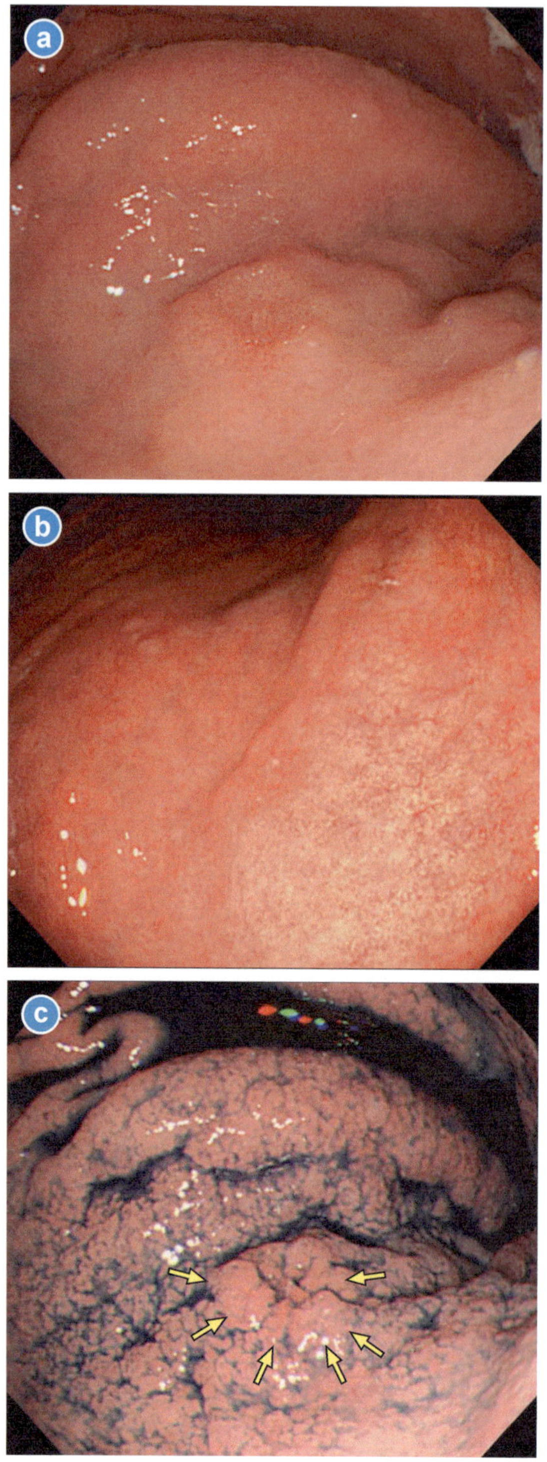

Fig. 31.3 (**a**-**c**) Same images as Fig. 31.2 a-c, (**d**, **e**) Same images as Fig. 31.2 e, f, (**f**) Endoscopic image after marking by NBI

31.1.2 Let's Observe the Surrounding Color

- A faded whitish area is observed surrounding the reddish and depressed lesion (Fig. 31.3a).
- The whitish area is matched to the marginal elevation.

31.1.3 How Shall We Interpret?

- The whitish area is spreading outside of the marginal elevation, but the margin is unclear (Fig. 31.3a).

31.1.4 Let's Observe the Red Color

- The second picture is obtained with full air insufflation of the stomach (Fig. 31.3b).
- Compared with the first picture, the unevenness of the lesion is unclear because the air has fully stretched the gastric wall, making mucosal elevations and depressions less prominent.

31.1.5 Let's Observe the Whitish Color

- The whitish area is seen on the oral side of the reddish area, but the margin is unclear (Fig. 31.3b).

31.1.6 Let's Pay Attention to the Surface "Bumps and Dents" (Unevenness)

- This is an image obtained after indigo carmine dye spraying from a distance (Fig. 31.3c).

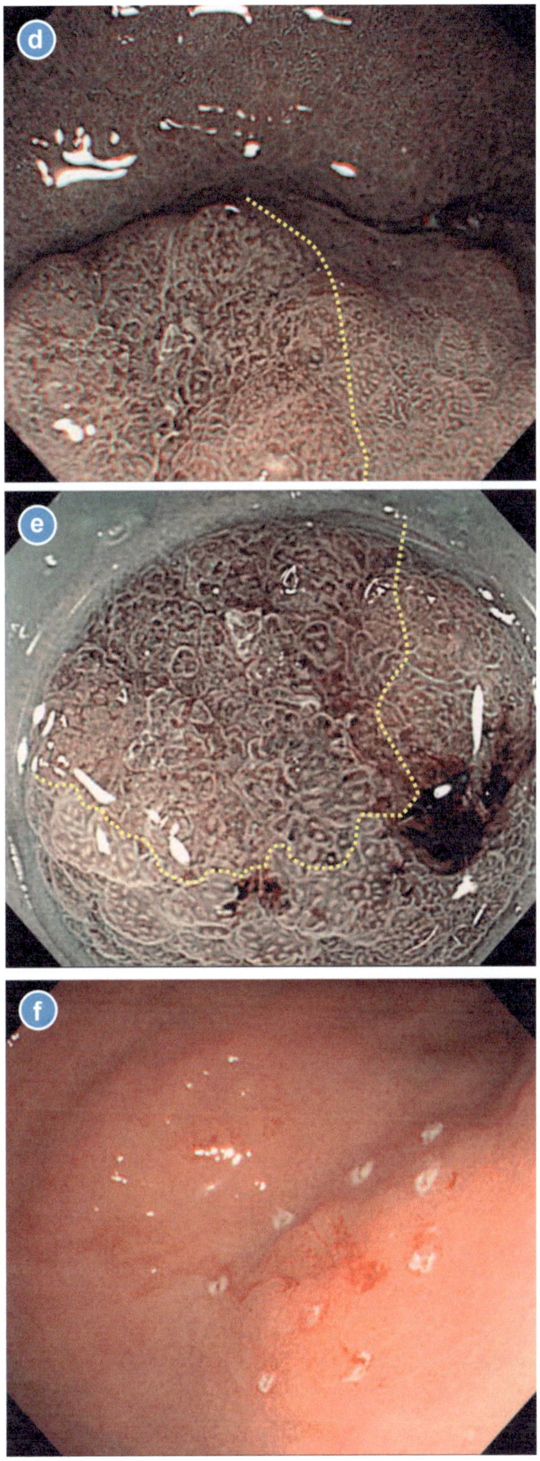

Fig. 31.3 (continued)

- Compared with areal patterns of the surrounding mucosa around the depressed area, coarse areal patterns are noted within the depression. The coarse areal patterns are extending beyond the depression up to the surrounding elevation as noted by yellow arrows. Coarse and larger areal patterns are seen at the marginal elevation, and the lesion may extend into the marginal elevation.

31.1.7 What Is the Next Step?

- NBI magnified endoscopy is performed to observe the details of the lesion (Fig. 31.3c).

31.1.8 Let's Observe the Surface Pattern

- The oral side of the lesion is shown with low-power NBI magnified endoscopy (Fig. 31.3d).
- The mixture of irregular villi and small pit patterns is found on the left side of the yellow dotted line, and regular pit patterns are found on the right side of the yellow dotted line.

31.1.9 Let's Observe the Shape and Size of the Villi

- The surface of the depressed area shows slightly large, variably sized, and irregular villi, part of which show fusion. Small pits of high density are found near the villi (Fig. 31.3d).
- A regular pit pattern is found on the right side of the yellow dotted line.
- Therefore, the lateral extension of the lesion could be diagnosed as starting from the marginal elevation to the lateral margin diagnosed at the yellow dotted line.

31.1.10 Let's Magnify More

- This image is obtained by medium-power NBI magnified endoscopy showing the oral side of the lesion (Fig. 31.3e).
- While the pit pattern is regular below the yellow dotted line, the surface pattern above the yellow dotted line shows larger, variably sized, and irregularly shaped villi.
- Therefore, the oral extension of the lesion can be diagnosed as the yellow dotted line.

- Markings are placed outside the area diagnosed as the lateral extension of the lesion by NBI magnified endoscopy (Fig. 31.3f).
- WL endoscopic image after the circumferential markings is placed.
- The area diagnosed by NBI magnified endoscopy (Fig. 31.3c) is corresponding to a large area after indigo carmine dying, and the answer to the question is (2) green dotted line.

31.2 Let's Compare Fixed Specimens with Resected Specimens

31.2.1 Let's Observe the Color Tone

- The right side of the figure is the oral side.
- The whitish area is found at the center of the specimen, and the margin is unclear (Fig. 31.4a).

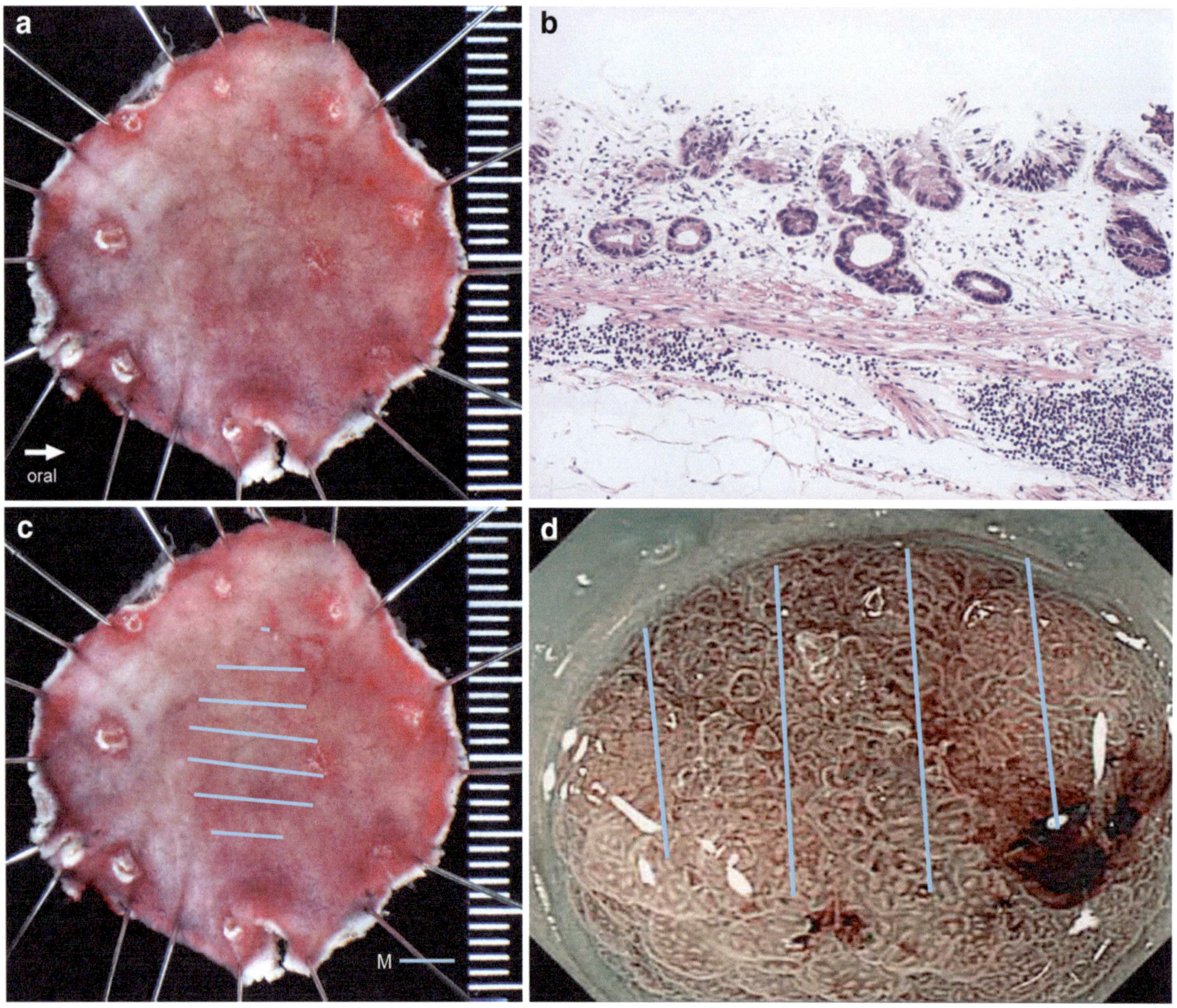

Fig. 31.4 (**a**) Freshly resected specimen marking by NBI (**b**) Histological image of the center of the specimen (**c**) Mapping of the cancer distribution projected on the freshly resected specimen (**d**) Mapping of the cancer distribution projected on the NBI endoscopic image

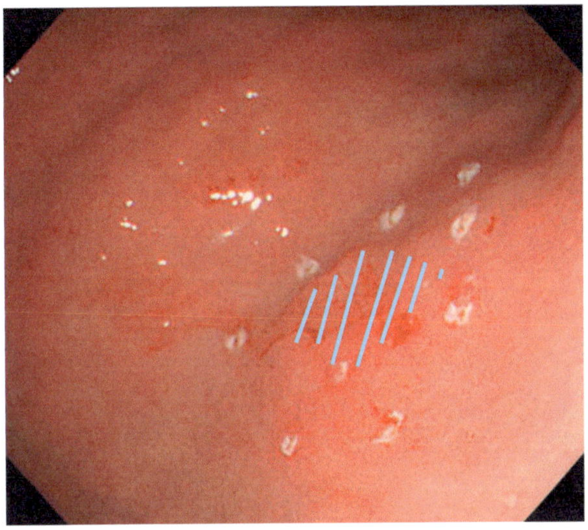
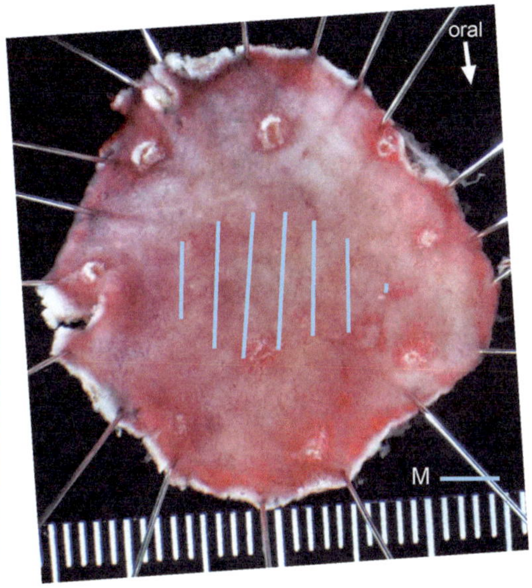

Fig. 31.5 Mapping of the cancer distribution on the WL image and resected specimen

31.2.2 Let's Observe the Surface Pattern

- A slightly depressed area is found at the center of the specimen (Fig. 31.4a).
- Villi patterns are found around the specimen, and a slightly large surface pattern is found at the center of the specimen, and the margin is unclear.

31.2.3 Let's Observe the Microscopic Findings

- Microscopic findings show WDA with structural irregularities at the center of the specimen (Fig. 31.4b).
- The freshly resected specimen is shown with superimposed mapping of the cancer area.
- The extension of the lesion is corresponding to the light blue lines, and its histological type is WDA with intramucosal depth of invasion (Fig. 31.4c).
- NBI magnified endoscopy with middle power magnification shows the oral side of the lesion with the superimposed mapping of the lesion.
- The lateral extension of the lesion corresponds to the area of the irregular villi pattern (Fig. 31.4d).

Conclusive Diagnosis (Fig. 31.5)
Gastric adenocarcinoma, tub1, T1(M), ly0, v0, LM (−), VM(−), pType 0-IIc, 14 × 10 mm, U, Post.

Summary
The image of the freshly resected specimen with superimposed mapping of the cancer area is rotated to align with the endoscopic image. The lateral extension of the lesion is shown with blue lines in the left endoscopic image. The lateral extension of the lesion is diagnosed only within the reddish depressed area by WL endoscopy. After indigo carmine spraying and NBI magnified endoscopy the lateral extension of the lesion is found to be extending to the marginal elevation in the lesser curvature side. The conclusive diagnosis of the lateral extension of the lesion is (2). If the lateral extension could not be diagnosed precisely, the lateral margin might have been positive for cancer even if an en bloc ESD is performed. It is important to observe lateral extensions carefully.

31.3 Answer

The lateral extension of the lesion is (2) green dotted line.

Question 18: Which Type of Gastric Carcinoma Do You Think This Is?

32

Tadashi Miike

T. Miike (✉)
Department of Gastroenterology and Hematology (Internal Medicine),
Faculty of Medicine of University of Miyazaki, 5200 Kiyotakecho,
Kihara, Miyazaki, Miyazaki 889-1692, Japan
e-mail: tadashi_miike@med.miyazaki-u.ac.jp

T. Oyama (ed.), *Endoscopic Diagnosis of Superficial Gastric Cancer for ESD*, DOI 10.1007/978-4-431-54469-2_32

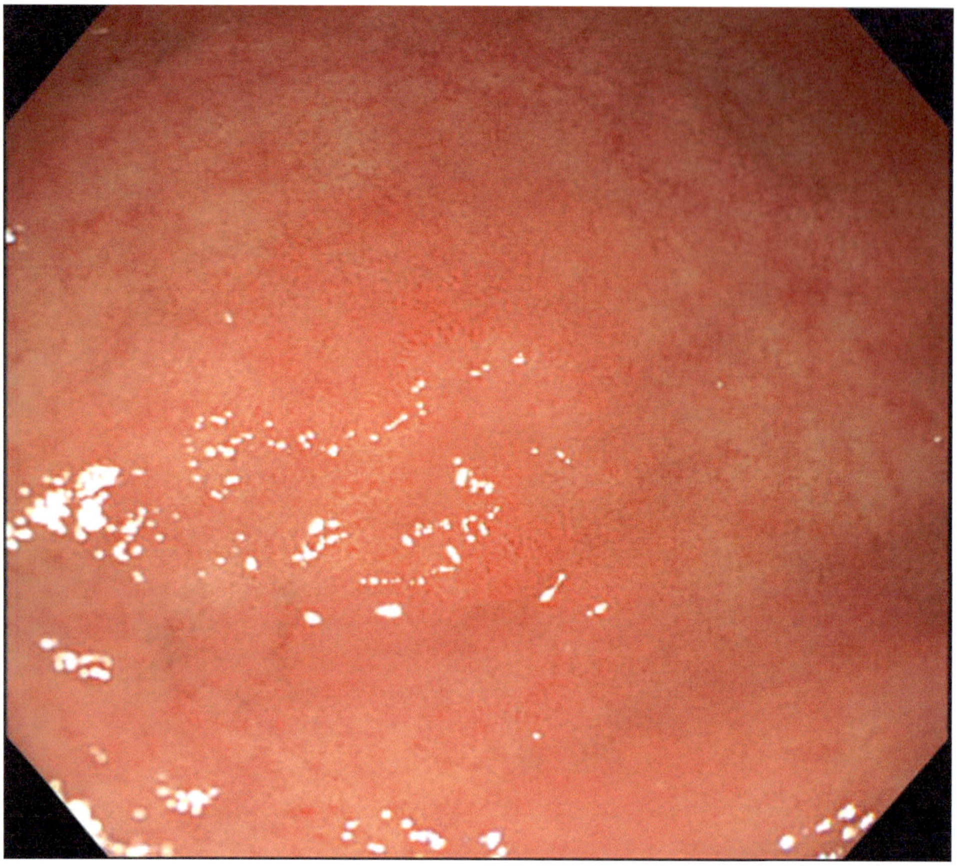

Fig. 32.1 Which type of gastric carcinoma do you think this is?

Which type of gastric carcinoma do you think this is? (Fig. 32.1)
Choose your answer from 1 to 3.

(1) WDA (tub1)
(2) MDA (tub2)
(3) PDA (por)

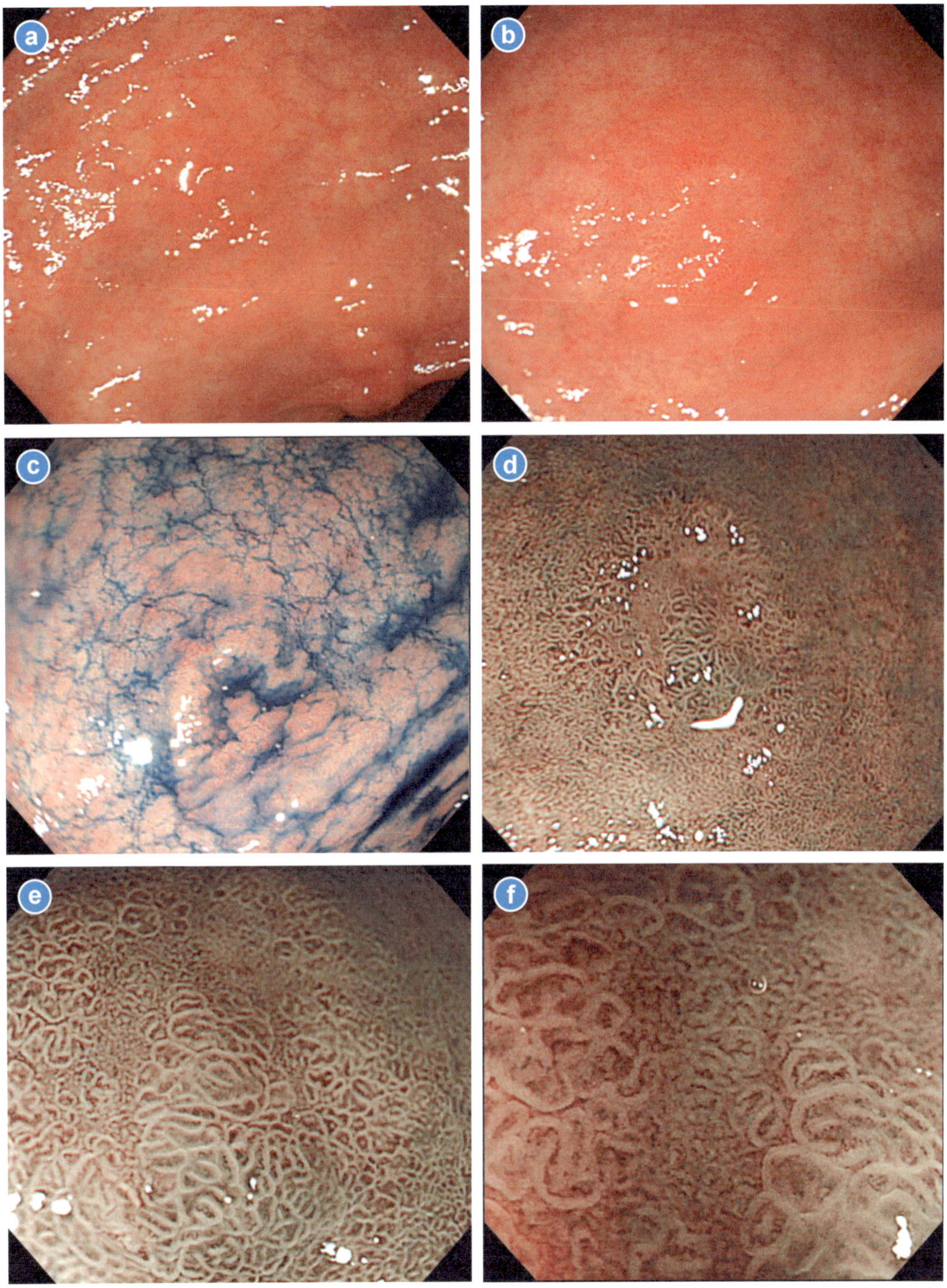

Fig. 32.2 Let's diagnose by observing these six images

32.1 Focus on These Points

32.1.1 Let's Watch an Area of Decreased Vascular Visibility

- The background mucosa is noted with an increase in vascular visibility and is diagnosed as atrophic gastritis.
- An area of decrease vascular visibility is noted in the antrum and the lesser curvature of stomach (Fig. 32.3a).

32.1.2 Let's Observe the Mucosa Closely

- With a very close observation, a pale depressed lesion is found in this area (Fig. 32.3b). The demarcation line as indicated by yellow arrows is partly distinct and irregular. The rest of the demarcation line is indistinct, and it is difficult to identify the entire shape of the lesion.

32.1.3 What Do You Make Out of This?

- The pale depressed lesion with a partly distinct demarcation line is isolated, and the edge is irregular, leading us to suspect a diagnosis of PDA (Fig. 32.3b).

32.1.4 Let's Spray the Lesion with Indigo Carmine

- After spraying the lesion with indigo carmine, a depressed lesion with a surrounding elevation has become evident.
- But the demarcation of the pale depressed area has become indistinct by indigo carmine (Fig. 32.3c).

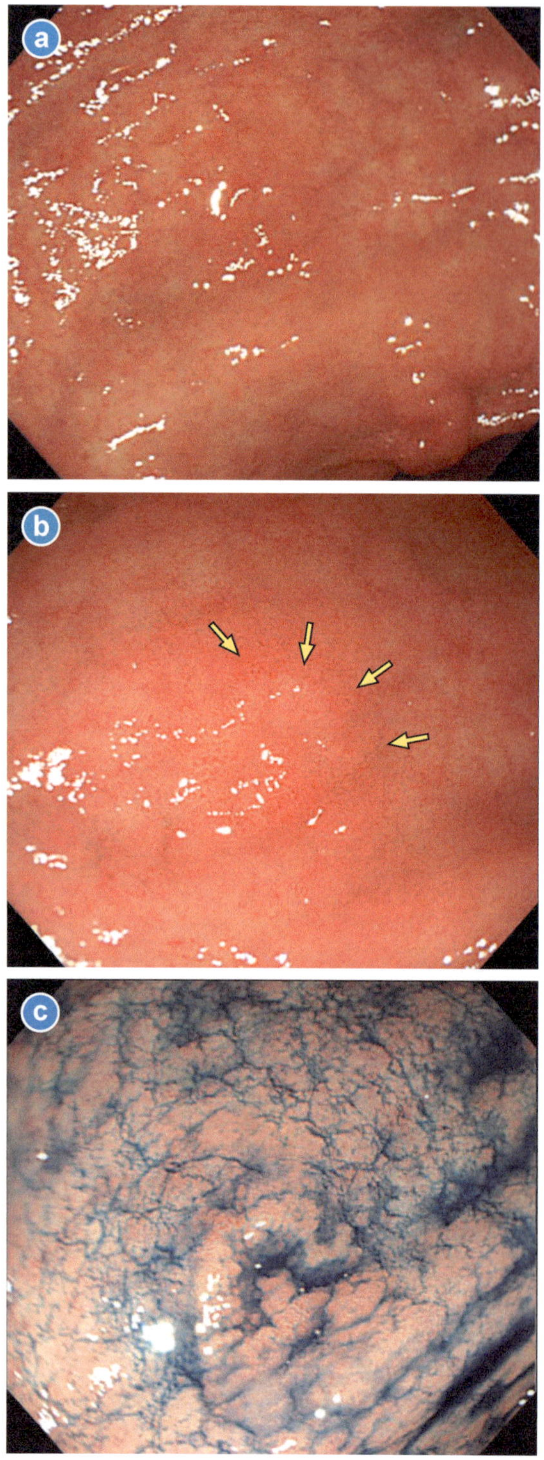

Fig. 32.3 Same images as Fig. 32.2

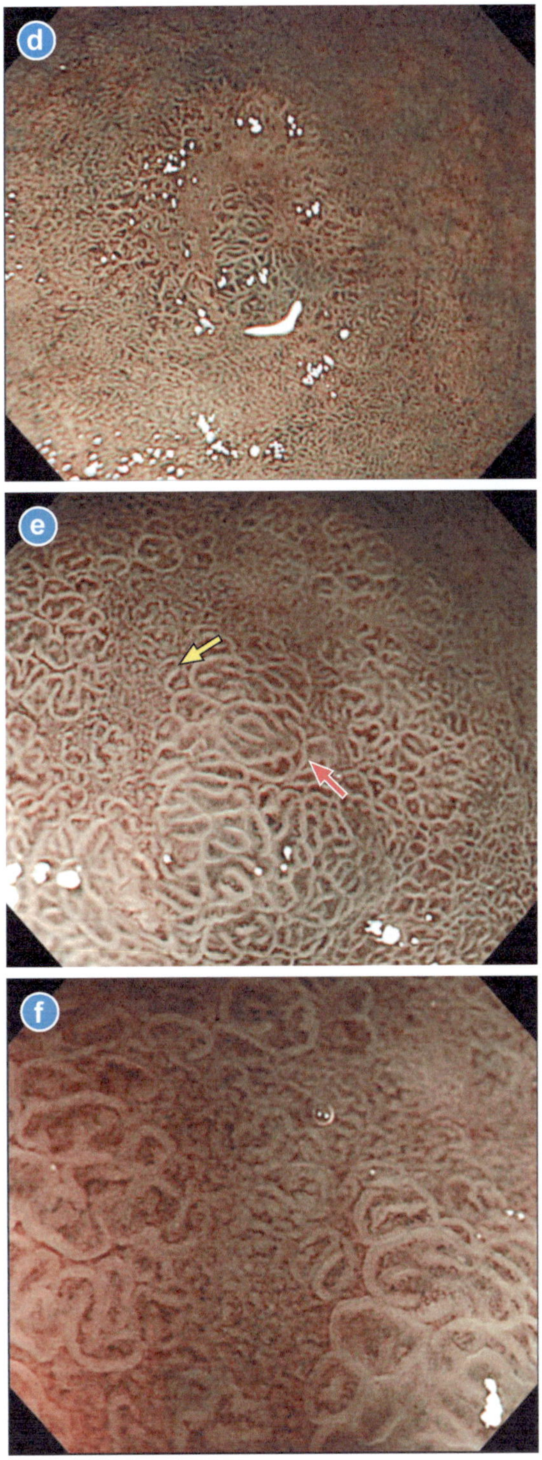

Fig. 32.3 (continued)

32.1.5 Let's Observe with Magnified NBI

- The depressed lesion with a prominent border can be appreciated by NBI without magnification.
- The demarcation of the depressed area and the prominent border is distinct, but the demarcation of the prominent border and the background mucosa is indistinct (Fig. 32.3d).

32.1.6 Let's Observe with Moderate-Power Magnified NBI

- The surface pattern is observed distinctly with moderate-power NBI (Fig. 32.3e).
- A prominent elevation surrounding the depressed area indicated by a red arrow shows enlarged villi pattern and partly pitlike pattern. Both of these surface patterns are regular, and neither is found nonneoplastic (Fig. 32.3d).
- The depressed area indicated by a yellow arrow is found with a mixture irregular of dense pit and villi pattern (Fig. 32.3e). So we diagnose the lesion as neoplastic.

32.1.7 Let's Magnify the Lesion by High-Power Magnified NBI

- With high-power magnified NBI, vascular patterns of the lesion are observed as well.
- Since vascular patterns appear regular, the lesion is diagnosed as WDA (Fig. 32.3f).

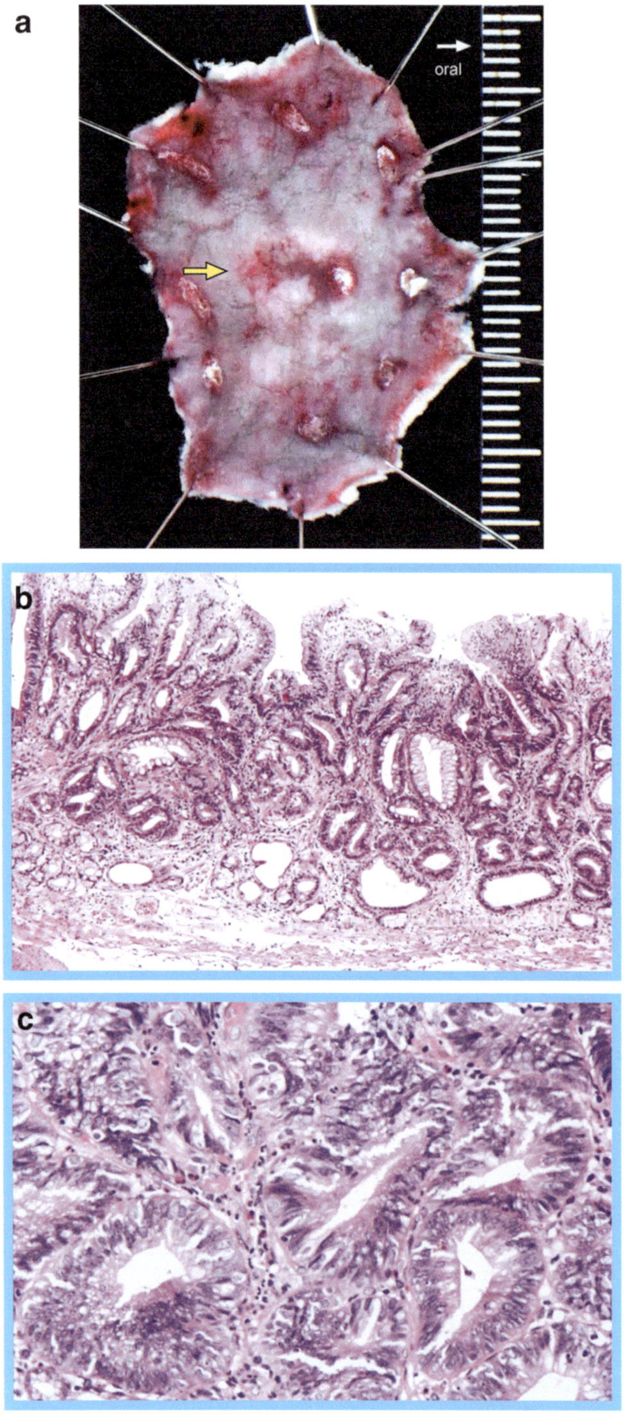

Fig. 32.4 (**a**) The resected specimen marking by NBI (**b**) The histological image of the center part of the lesion (**c**) The magnified image of the lesion

32.2 Let's Compare Fixed Specimens with Resected Specimens

32.2.1 Let's Observe the Freshly Resected Specimen

- The right side of the figure is the oral side (Fig. 32.4a).
- An irregularly shaped reddish depressed lesion is noted in the central region.
- The demarcation of the lesion can be noted mostly by the difference of color tone, but the anal border as indicated by a yellow arrow is indistinct.

32.2.2 Let's Observe the Pathological Specimen

- The pathological specimen of the central part of the lesion (hematoxylin-eosin stained) (Fig. 32.4b).
- We could watch the irregular proliferation of tubular gland with structural atypia.
- The surface layer of neoplastic region and the deep layer of nonneoplastic region form a two-layer structure.

32.2.3 Let's Observe with High-Power Magnification

- The proliferation of neoplastic cells with irregular nuclei is noted (Fig. 32.4c).
- An increased N/C ratio and disorderly nuclei with loss of polarity are observed leading to the diagnosis of WDA (tub1).

32.2.4 Let's Compare the Freshly Resected Specimen with the Endoscopic Image

- The image of the resected specimen is rotated to align the oral mark indicated by a yellow arrow (Fig. 32.5a) on WL endoscopy with the oral mark indicated by a yellow arrow (Fig. 32.5b) of the freshly resected specimen (Fig. 32.5c).

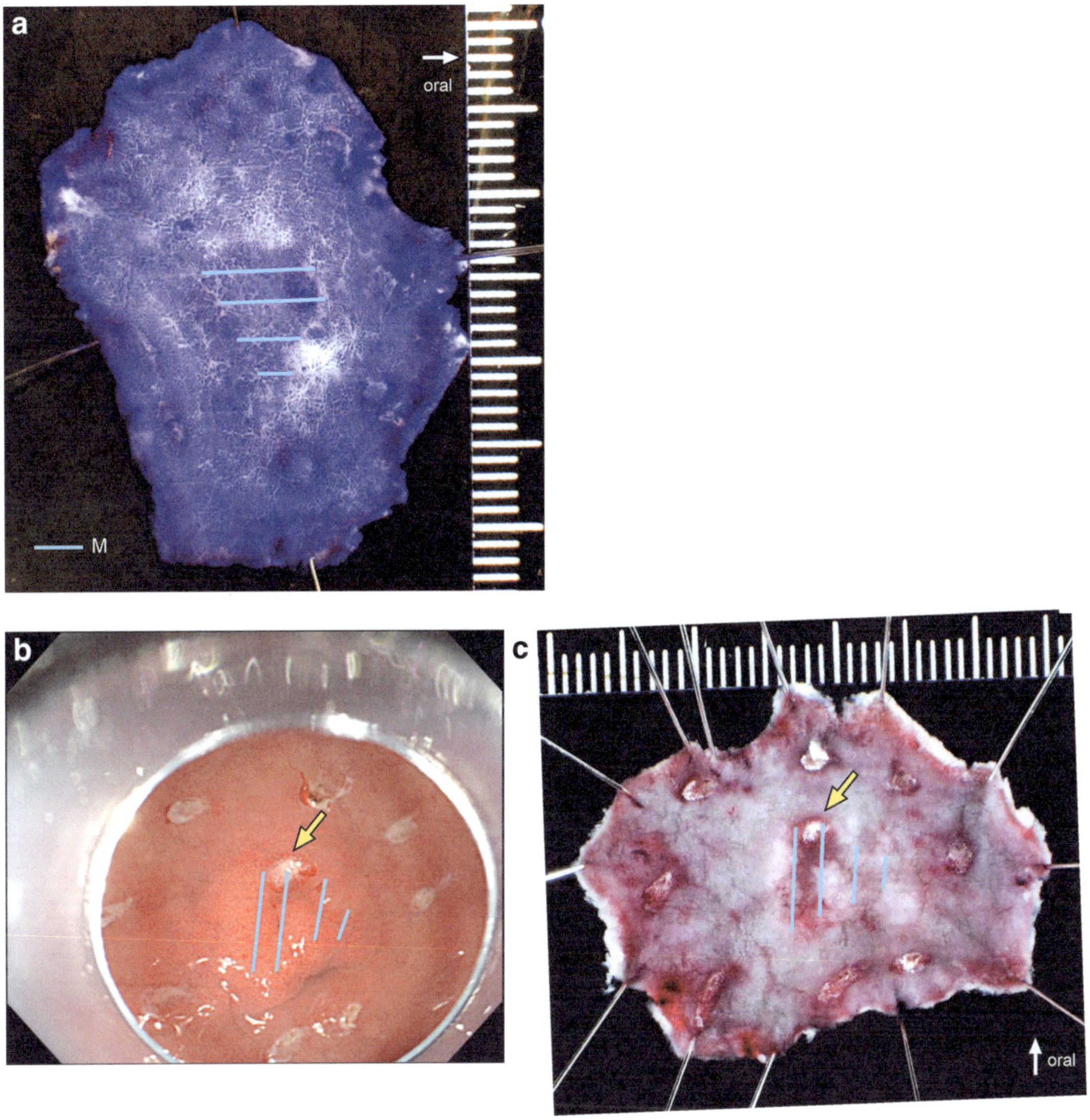

Fig. 32.5 Comparison between the endscopic image with the resected specimen. The mapping of the cancer distribution projected on the lesion

Conclusive Diagnosis
Gastric adenocarcinoma, tub1, T1(M), ly0, v0, LM (−), VM(−), pType 0-IIc, 8 × 6 mm, L, Less.

Summary
A pale and poorly demarcated depressed lesion is noted at the antrum and the lesser curvature of the stomach and is suspected of PDA by WL. Indigo carmine spraying is applied, but the lesion has turned indistinct. With high-power magnified NBI, mixed irregular pitlike and villi-like patterns are noted in the depressed area. Irregular vascular pattern, but with regular distribution, is noted, consistent with the diagnosis of WDA (tub1). Initially, the lesion thought of as PDA by WL later was diagnosed as WDA (tub1) by high-power magnified NBI. This case demonstrates the usefulness of NBI magnified endoscopy for diagnosing neoplastic lesions.

32.3 Answer

The pathological tissue type is (1) WDA (tub1).

Question 19: Where Is the Lateral Extension?

33

Kou Yoshida

K. Yoshida (✉)
Department of Internal Medicine, Obihiro Kosei General Hospital, 8-1, Nishi, 6jominami, Obihiro, Hokkaido 080-0016, Japan
e-mail: kospider2324@yahoo.co.jp

T. Oyama (ed.), *Endoscopic Diagnosis of Superficial Gastric Cancer for ESD*, DOI 10.1007/978-4-431-54469-2_33

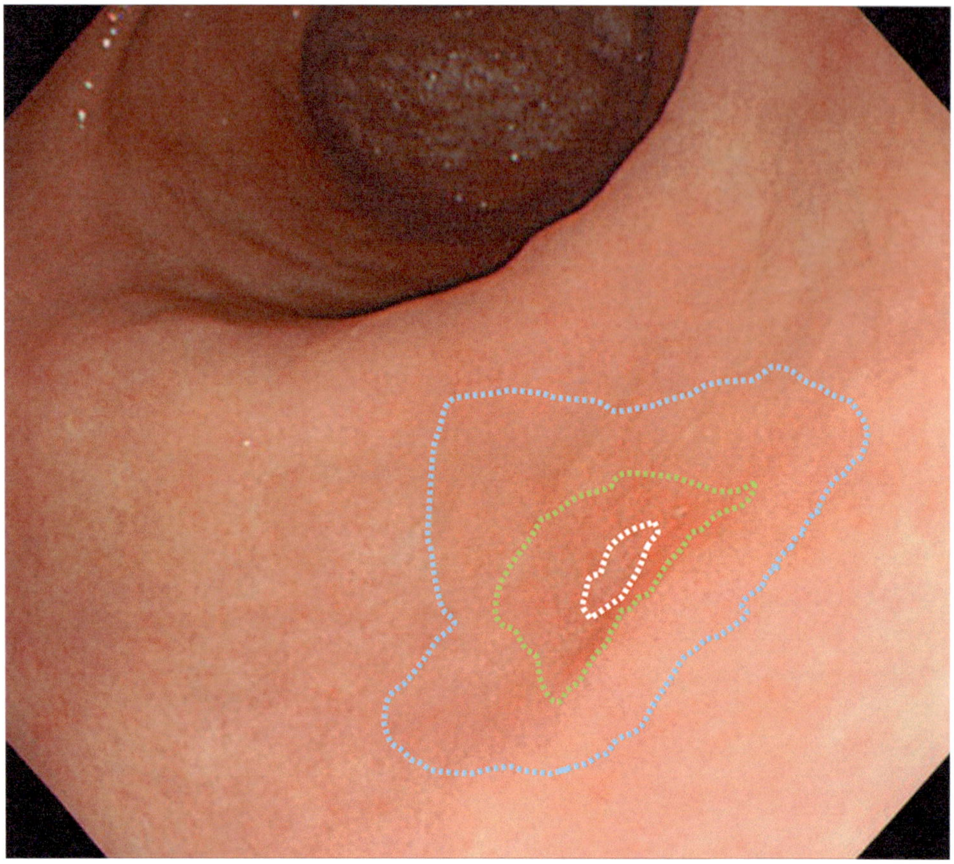

Fig. 33.1 Where is the lateral extension?

Where is the lateral extension? (Fig. 33.1)
Choose your answer from 1 to 3.

(1) White dotted line
(2) Green dotted line
(3) Blue dotted line.

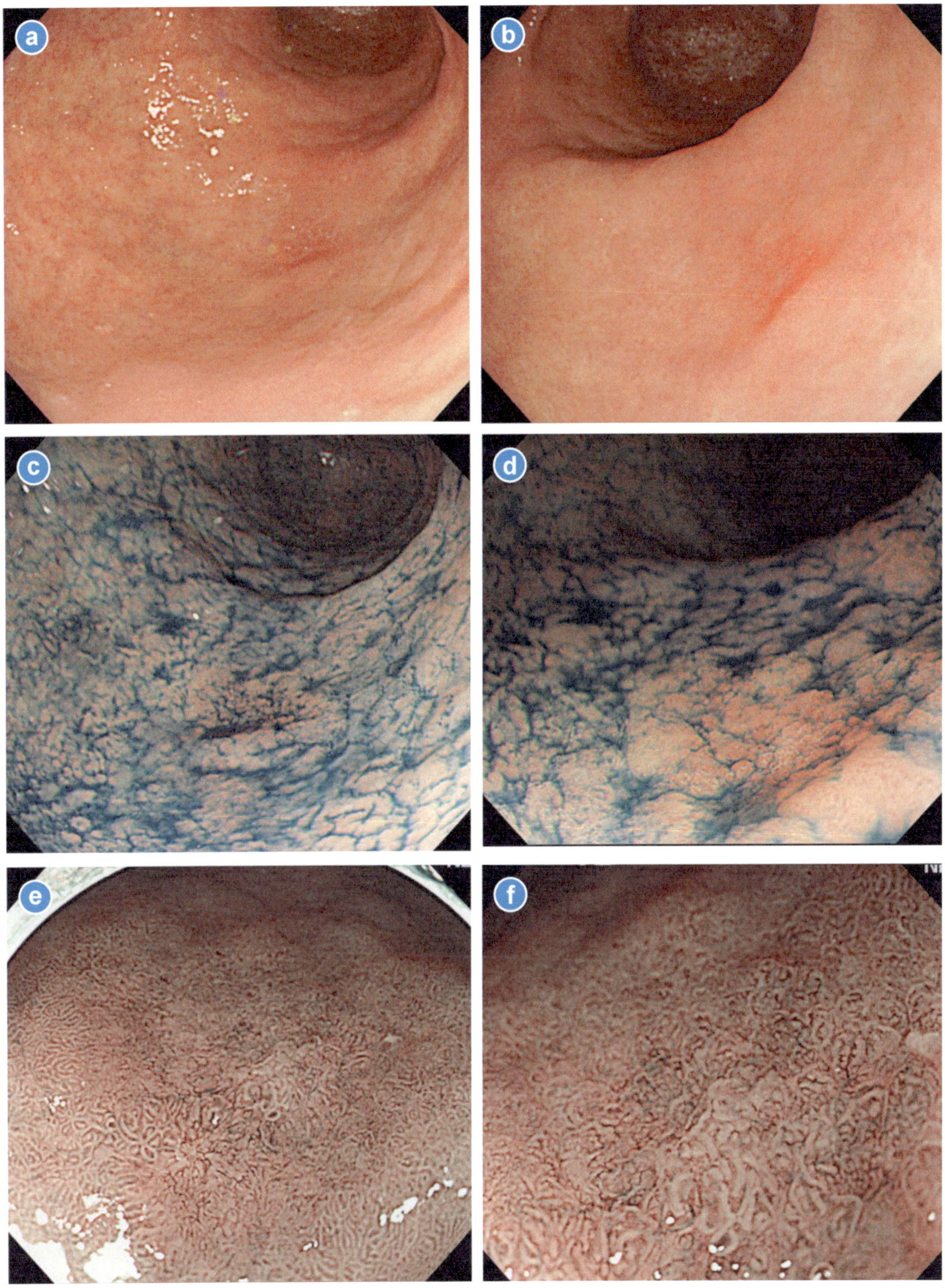

Fig. 33.2 Let's diagnose by observing these six images

33.1 Focus on These Points

33.1.1 Let's Observe with WL Endoscopy

- The background mucosa shows an increased vascular visibility in whitish mucosa with patchy redness, consistent with atrophic gastritis (Fig. 33.3a).
- A reddish depressed lesion is noted in the greater curvature of the antrum. Its border anally is somewhat obscure, but its oral border appears distinct by color tone differences as marked by green arrows, and an epithelial tumor is suspected.

33.1.2 Let's Observe Closely

- On close observation, no clear border can be found (Fig. 33.3b).
- The area is slightly depressed with slight elevation laterally without clear border of the elevation.
- No remarkable bumps or dents are noted in the depressed area.

33.1.3 Let's Observe After Indigo Carmine Spray

- With indigo carmine spray, a pooling of the dye is noted inside the depression (Fig. 33.3c).
- There is a slight elevation surrounding the depressed area, but no clear demarcation is noted of the elevation.
- On the other hand, there are fine surface patterns in the depressed area, making the difference in surface patterns distinct.

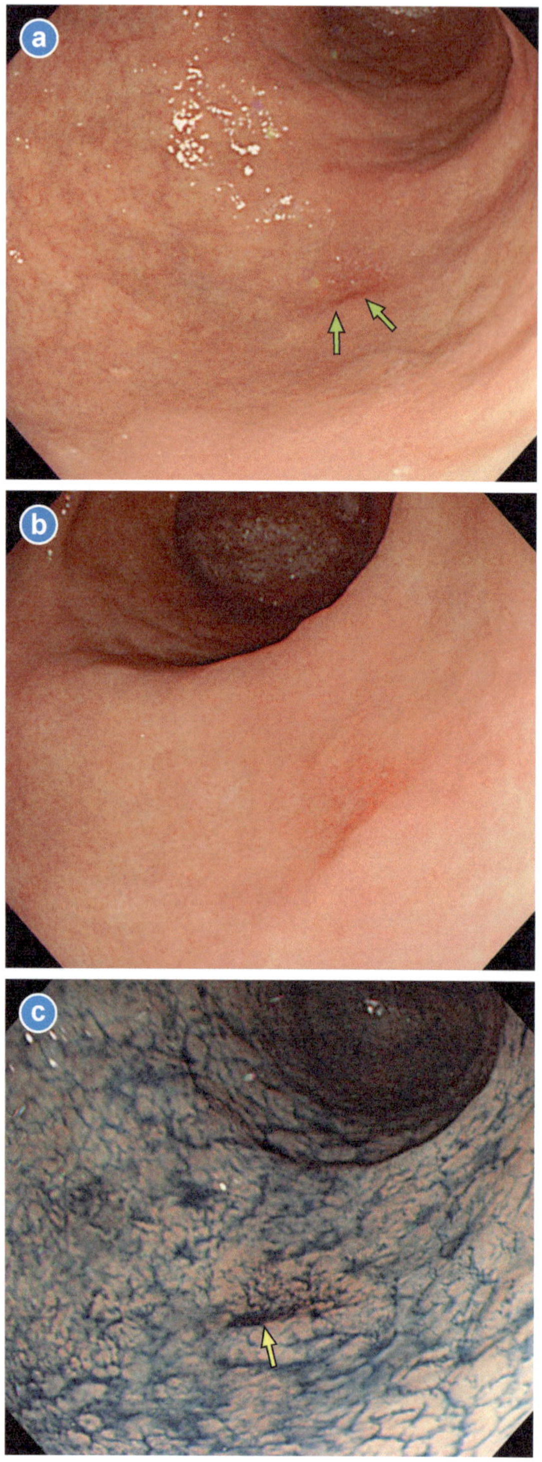

Fig. 33.3 Same images as Fig. 33.2

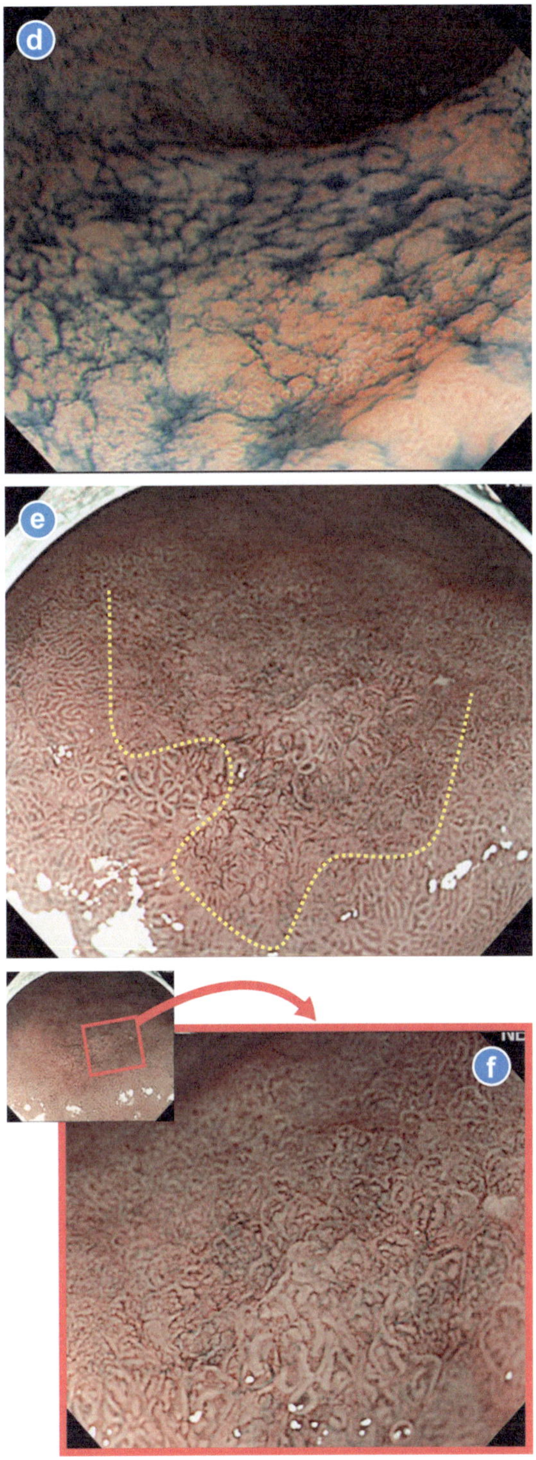

Fig. 33.3 (continued)

33.1.4 Let's Observe Closely

- On closer observation, variably sized irregular surface patterns are noted in the depressed area compared with regularly appearing surrounding surface patterns. But no distinct border is noted (Fig. 33.3d).
- Based on partly clear border on WL observation and irregular surface patterns within the depressed area by indigo carmine spray, an epithelial neoplasm and 0IIc WDA may be included in differential diagnosis.
- To further evaluate in detail, NBI magnified endoscopy is performed.

33.1.5 Let's Observe with NBI Magnified Endoscopy

- The observation with NBI magnified endoscopy shows a regular villi pattern of the surrounding mucosa but highly dense and finely irregular villi within the lesion. The border can be traced by the difference in surface structures and villous densities as marked by the yellow dotted line (Fig. 33.3e).
- The observation with NBI magnified endoscopy shows irregular villi with a clear demarcation, consistent with the diagnosis of WDA.
- Higher-power magnification is used to observe the internal structures in detail.

33.1.6 Let's Magnify Further

- On magnifying the lesion further, the basic structure is found to be a pit pattern (Fig. 33.3f).
- Pits are variably sized and irregular, irregular microvessels form networks, and the lesion is diagnosed as WDA.
- Based on the observations by WL endoscopy, indigo carmine chromoendoscopy, and NBI magnified endoscopy, the lesion is diagnosed as 0-IIc, WDA, with the intramucosal invasion depth.

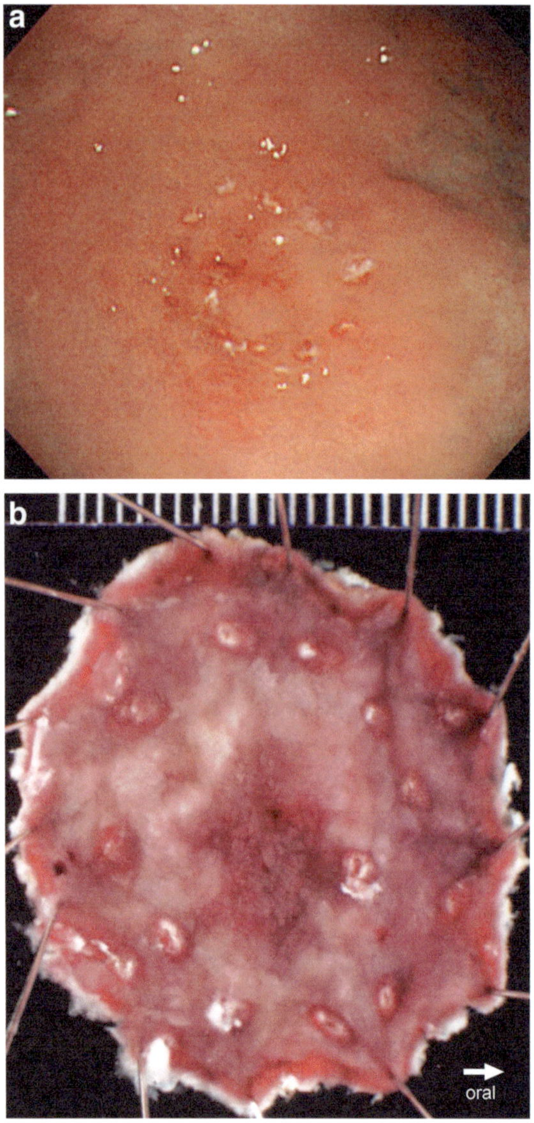

Fig. 33.4 (**a**) WL endoscopic image after marking (**b**) Freshly resected specimen

33.2 Let's Compare Fixed Specimens with Resected Specimens

33.2.1 Let's Place Markings

- The lateral extension of the lesion is identified using magnified NBI, and markings are placed outside the lesion as shown in the figure (Fig. 33.4a).
- Under magnified NBI, the extent of the lesion corresponds to the area with a different surface texture after indigo carmine staining.
- ESD for en bloc resection was performed.

33.2.2 Let's Observe the Freshly Resected Specimen

- The right side of the figure is the oral side (Fig. 33.4b).
- An erythematous lesion with an irregular depression and an elevated margin is seen in the central part of the specimen.
- Due to differences in color tone and surface texture, the margin of the lesion is clearly seen.
- The surrounding elevation is not different in color from the surrounding mucosa and hence is considered benign.

This is a histological image of a depressed region. Atypical ductal structures lined with cells having enlarged nuclei are seen. A WDA is diagnosed (tub1) (Fig. 33.5).

The blue lines mapped on the crystal violet-stained fixed specimen correspond with the WDA (tub1). The mapping is superimposed on an endoscopic image. The lateral extension of the lesion is (2).

The villous structures observed using magnified NBI correspond to the erythematous area under normal observation and the area of structural irregularity observed after indigo carmine staining (Fig. 33.6).

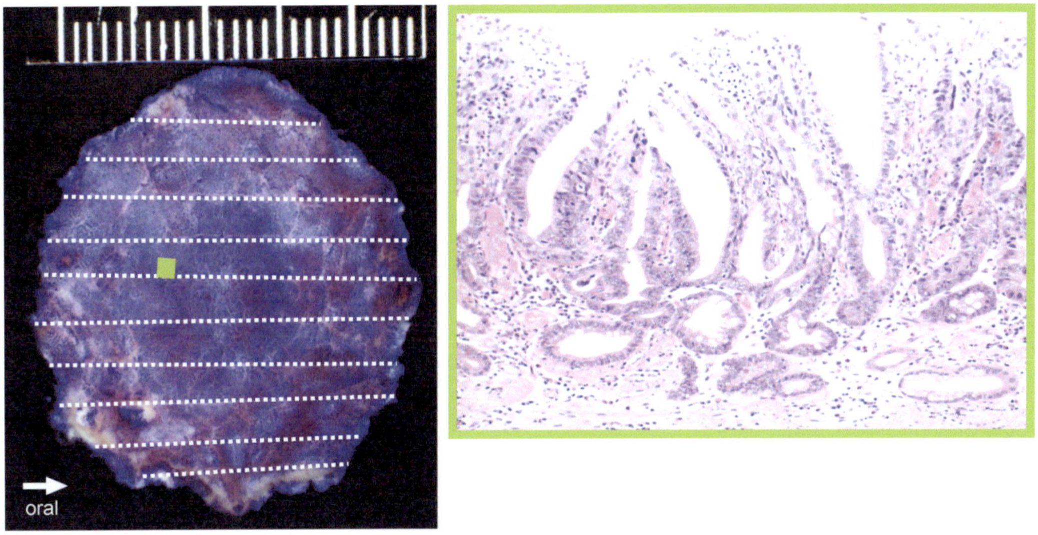

Fig. 33.5 Marking on the resected spacimen and histology image of the lesion

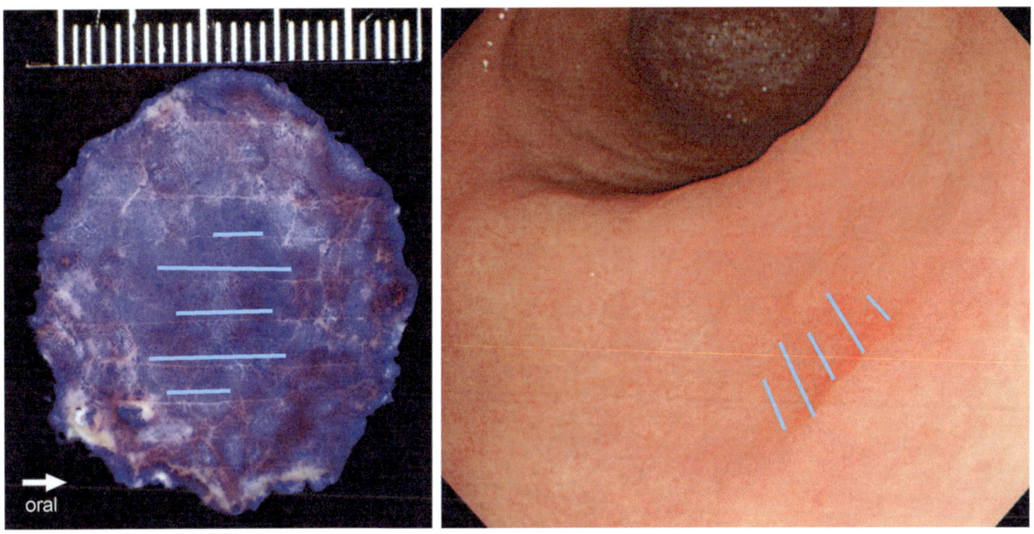

Fig. 33.6 Mapping of the cancer distribution projected on the resected spacimen and on the endoscopic image of the lesion

Conclusive Diagnosis

Gastric adenocarcinoma, tub1, T1 (M), ly0, v0, UL(−), LM(−), VM(−), pType 0–IIc, 12 × 9 mm, L, Gre.

Summary

The margin of the lesion is unclear under WL observation and indigo carmine staining. However, the extent of the lesion can be judged by observing the details of the surface texture.

33.3 Answer

The lateral extension of the lesion is (2) green dotted line.

Question 20: What Is the Depth of Invasion for This Cancer?

34

Tokuma Tanuma

T. Tanuma (✉)
Department of Gastroenterology, Teine Keijinkai Hospital, 1-12-1-40
Maeda, Teine-ku, Sapporo, Hokkaido 006-0811, Japan
e-mail: tokuma@dk9.so-net.ne.jp

T. Oyama (ed.), *Endoscopic Diagnosis of Superficial Gastric Cancer for ESD*, DOI 10.1007/978-4-431-54469-2_34

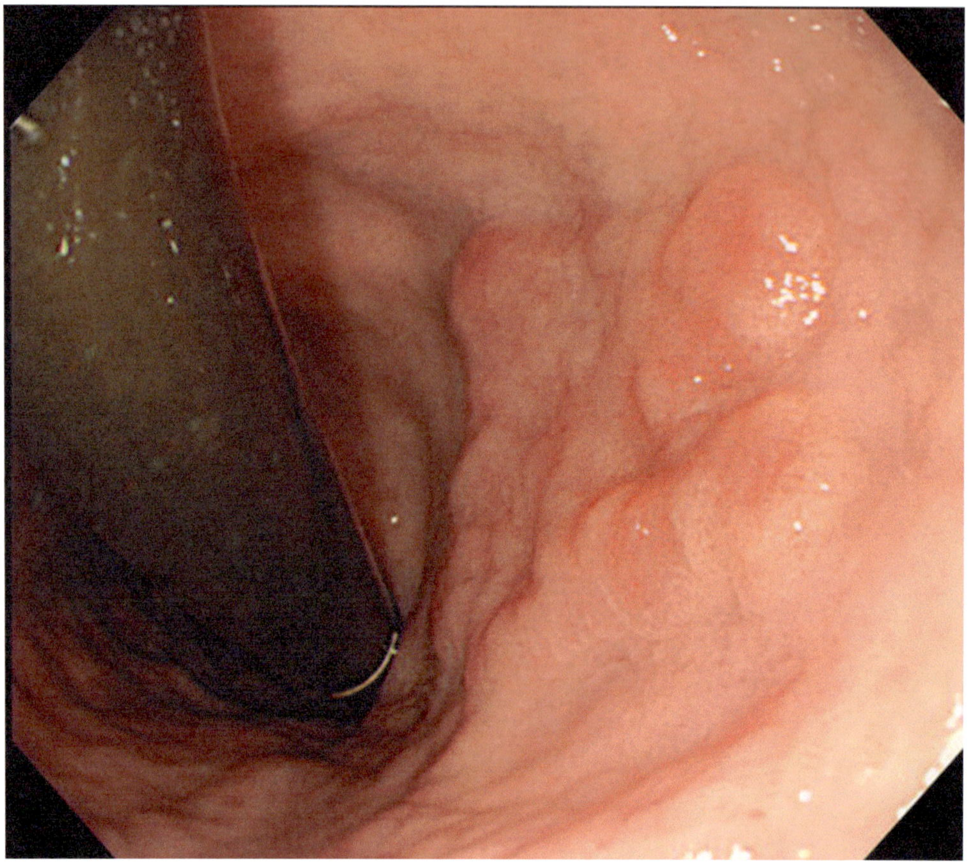

Fig. 34.1 What is the depth of invasion for this cancer?

What is the depth of invasion for this cancer? (Fig. 34.1)

Choose your answer from 1 to 3.

(1) M (mucosal)
(2) SM1 (submucosal level 1)
(3) SM2 (submucosal level 2)

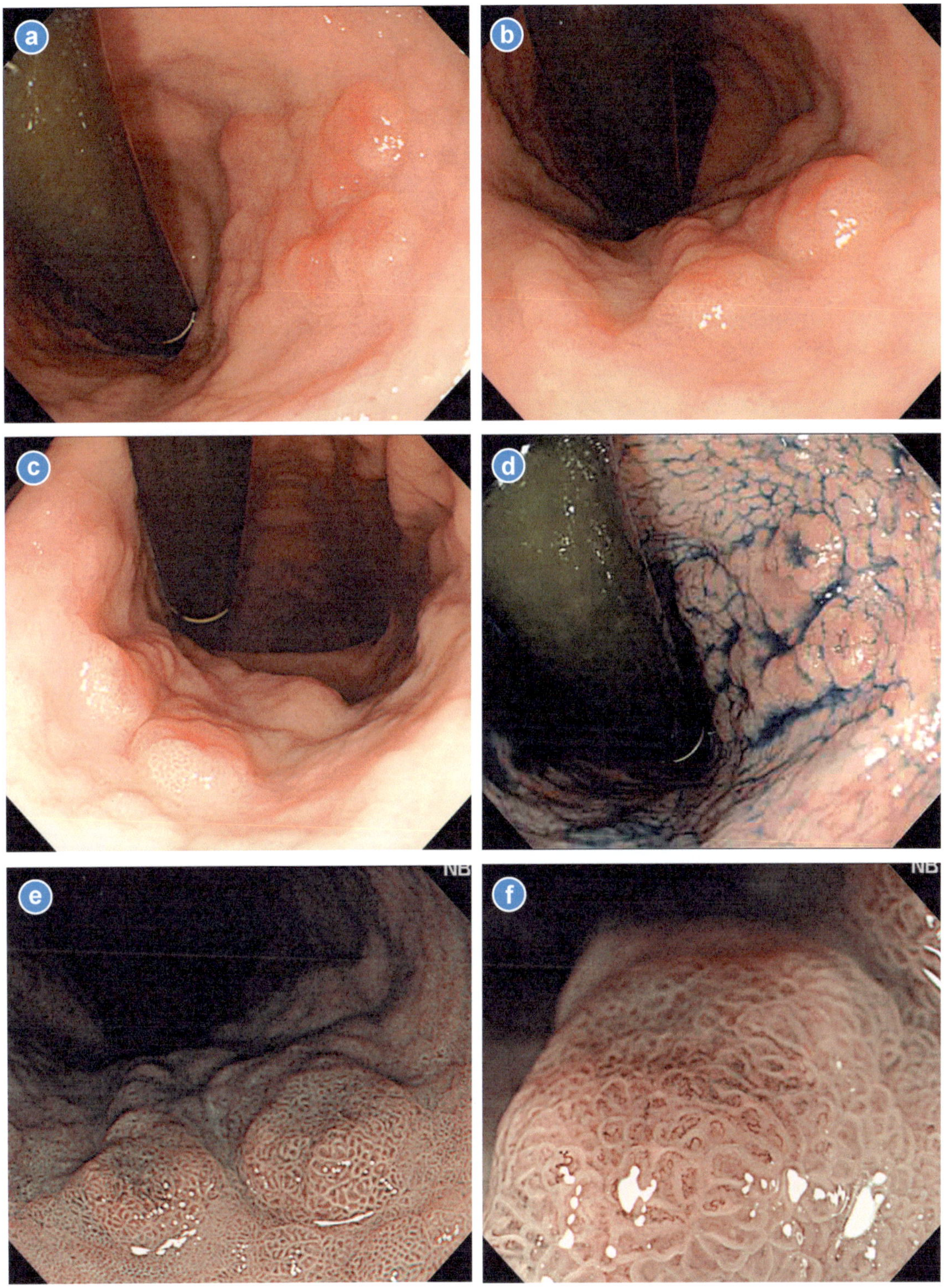

Fig. 34.2 Let's diagnose by observing these six images

34.1 Focus on These Points

34.1.1 Let's Pay Attention to the Elevation

- A reddish, elevated lesion is seen at the lesser curvature in the gastric upper body. It looks like a cluster of large and small nodules. It is a big lesion of over 3 cm compared with the scope width (Fig. 34.3a).

34.1.2 Let's Pay Attention to the Extensibility of the Lesion

- By filling air to the stomach, the lesion is extended well (Fig. 34.3a).

34.1.3 How Do You Interpret These Findings?

- It is highly suspicious of a WDA, because it is reddish in color with an irregularly elevated lesion with a clear margin (Fig. 34.3a).
- This cancer appears rather shallow not invading the submucosal layer because of good extensibility with air inflation.

34.1.4 Let's Observe from the Tangential Angle

- The thickness of the lesion can be better appreciated by observing from the tangential angle (Fig. 34.3b).
- The lesion is a few millimeter in height, does not have much thickness submucosally, and does not show any deformity of the gastric wall line.

34.1.5 Let's Observe Carefully by Adjusting Air Volume

- The shape of the lesion is easily changed by the amount of air, suggesting this lesion is soft (Fig. 34.3c).

34.1.6 How Do You Interpret These Findings?

- The lesion is suspected to an intramucosal lesion, because the lesion is soft and the gastric wall line is smooth (Fig. 34.3c).
- The answer to the question is number (1) the invasion depth of M (mucosal).

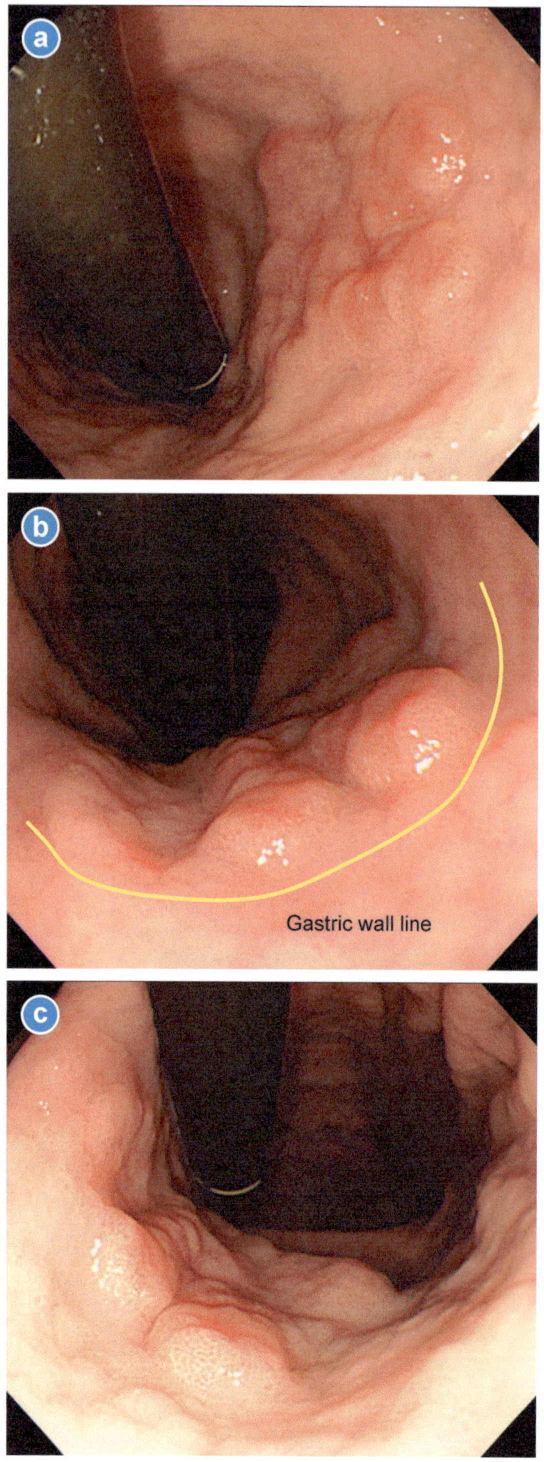

Fig. 34.3 Same images as Fig. 34.2

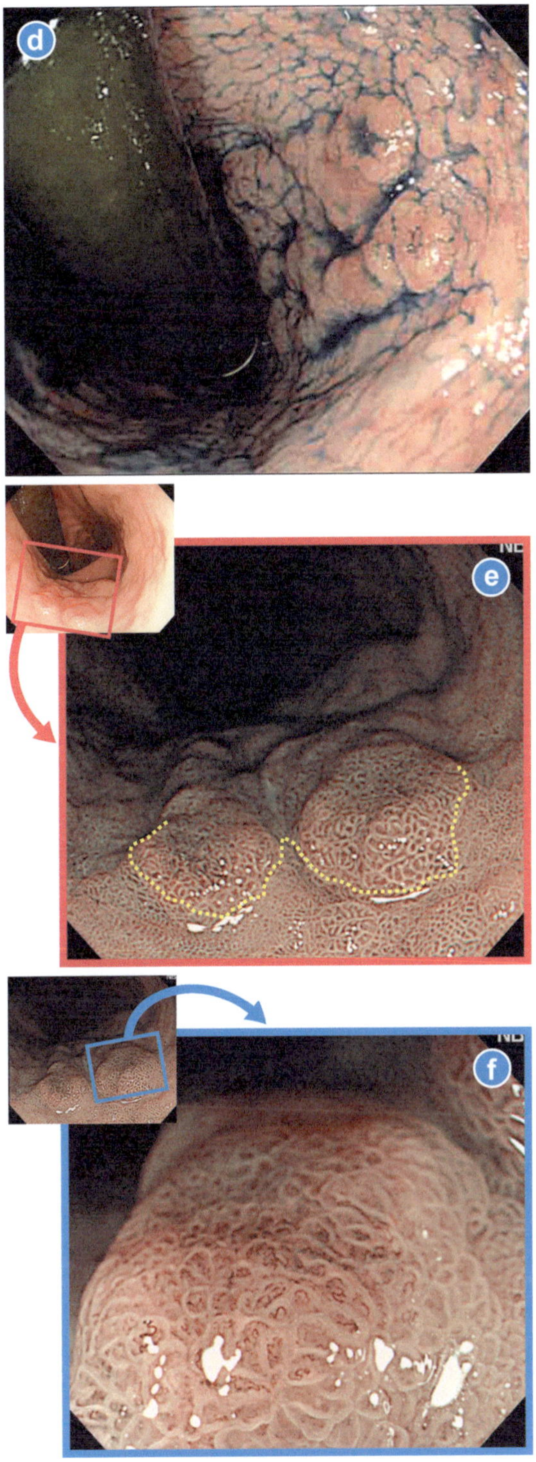

Fig. 34.3 (continued)

34.1.7 Let's Focus on the Margin of the Lesion and Its Surface Pattern

- After indigo carmine spraying, the demarcation line of the elevated lesion becomes clearer (Fig. 34.3d).
- And an irregular surface pooling of indigo carmine dye appears which is different from the areas of the surrounding mucosa.
- These findings are consistent with that this lesion is WDA.

34.1.8 Let's Focus on the Surface Pattern

- NBI magnified endoscopy is used to observe the anal side of the lesion. Intermediate-power magnified NBI shows regular villous patterns in the background mucosa, but an irregular villous pattern is observed at the elevated lesion (Fig. 34.3e).
- The lateral margin of the tumor is the same as the margin of the elevated lesion as noted by yellow dotted line.

34.1.9 Let's Focus on Microvascular Patterns in the Villi

- High-power view of NBI magnified endoscopy allows observation of microvessels in the villi (Fig. 34.3f).
- The lesion has mildly size-variable microvessels and irregularly running microvessels regardless of having a slight change of shape.
- In conclusion, this lesion is diagnosed as WDA, 0-IIa, with the invasion depth of M, and greater than 2 cm in diameter. This meets expanded criteria for an indication of ESD.

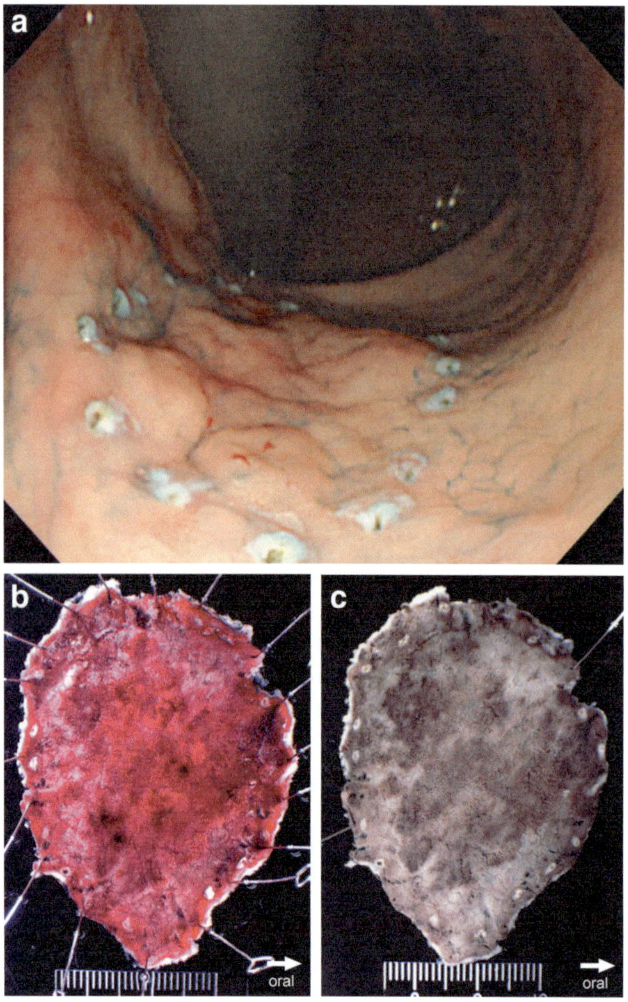

Fig. 34.4 (**a**) WL endoscopic image after marking (**b**) Freshly resected specimen (**c**) Fixed resected specimen

34.2 Let's Compare Fixed Specimens With Resected Specimens

34.2.1 Markings Are Placed Around the Elevated Lesion

- The lesion ranges widely, extending from the upper to the middle gastric body (Fig. 34.4a).

34.2.2 Let's Note the Color Tone

- The elevated lesion is reddish as a whole (Fig. 34.4b).

34.2.3 Let's Note the Surface Elevations and Depressions

- The lesion is noted with irregular elevations and depressions, as well as variably sized granular structures (Fig. 34.4b).

34.2.4 Formalin Fixation of the Resected Specimen Makes the Surface Pattern of the Lesion Clearer

- In the fixed specimen, the reddish area has turned brownish (Fig. 34.4c).
- The lighting on the specimen should be directed so that the angle of lighting becomes nearly horizontal to enhance the surface elevations and depressions.

This is a histological image of the elevated lesion. The cancer grows leaving the glandular structures intact, and the lesion is diagnosed as WDA (Fig. 34.5a).

The margin of the elevation coincided with the margin of the tumor (Fig. 34.5b).

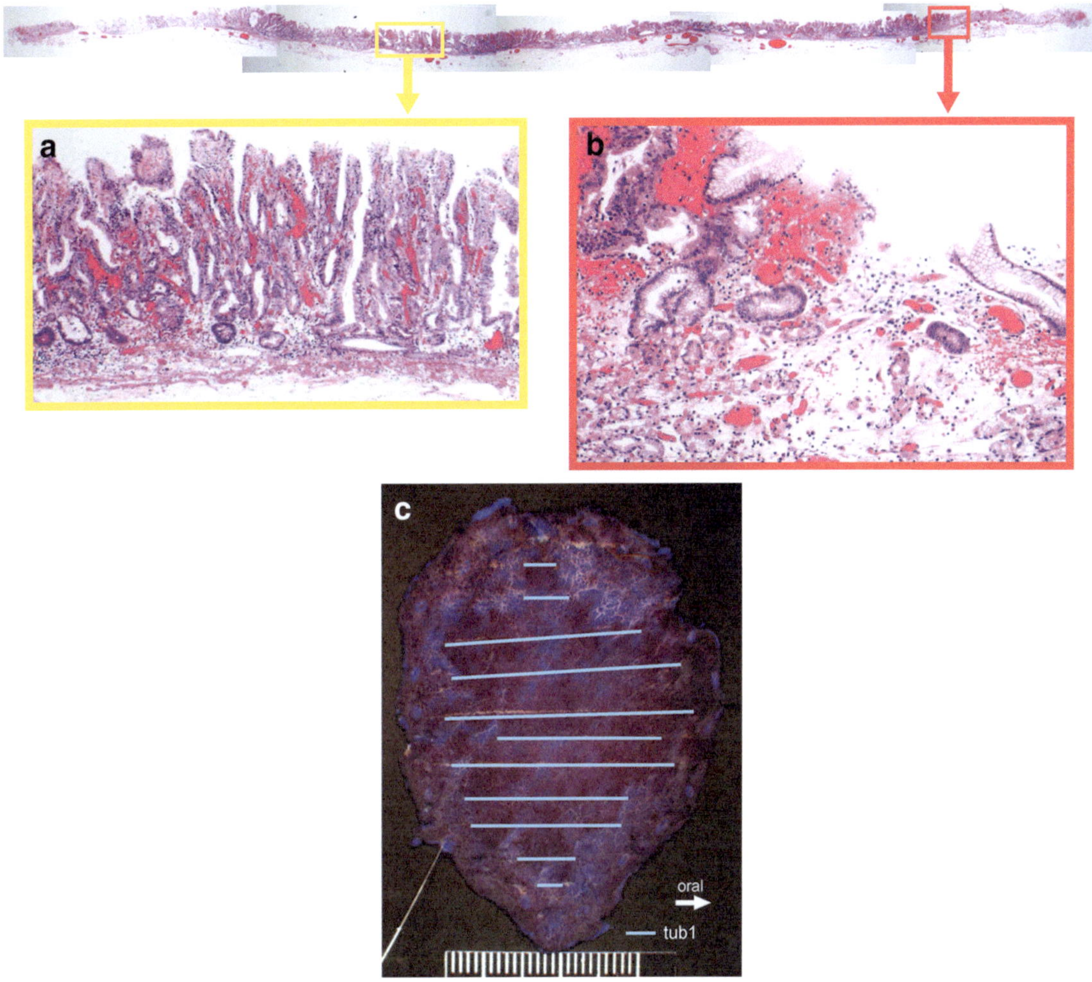

Fig. 34.5 (**a**) Histological image of the elevated lesion (**b**) Histological image of the margin of the elevation (**c**) Mapping of the cancer distribution projected on the resected specimen

Conclusive Diagnosis
Gastric adenocarcinoma, tub1, T1(M), ly0, v0, LM (−), VM(−), pType 0-IIa, 38 × 30 mm, M, Less.

Summary
This is a large tumor, but it doesn't invade the submucosal layer. For diagnosis of the depth of invasion like this case, it is important to observe from the tangential angle and check extensibility of the lesion by adjusting air volume. If the lesion has good extensibility and doesn't have elevation like a SMT, it can be diagnosed as an intramucosal lesion. It is possible therefore to perform ESD to this lesion.

34.3 Answer

The depth of invasion for this lesion is (1) M (mucosal).

MIX
Papier aus verantwortungsvollen Quellen
Paper from responsible sources
FSC® C105338

If you have any concerns about our products,
you can contact us on
ProductSafety@springernature.com

In case Publisher is established outside the EU,
the EU authorized representative is:
Springer Nature Customer Service Center GmbH
Europaplatz 3, 69115 Heidelberg, Germany

Printed by Libri Plureos GmbH
in Hamburg, Germany